Health Is Simple
Disease Is Complicated

Health Is Simple
Disease Is Complicated

A Systems Approach
to Vibrant Health

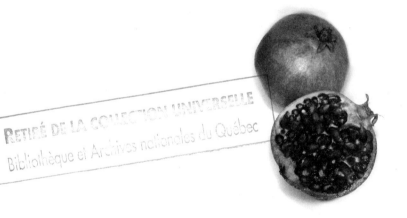

JAMES FORLEO, DC

North Atlantic Books
Berkeley, California

Published by North Atlantic Books
P.O. Box 12327
Berkeley, California 94712

Cover photograph by Ricardo Sousa
Illustrations by Carly DeLong
Cover and book design by Brad Greene
Printed in the United States of America

Health Is Simple, Disease Is Complicated: A Systems Approach to Vibrant Health is sponsored by the Society for the Study of Native Arts and Sciences, a nonprofit educational corporation whose goals are to develop an educational and cross-cultural perspective linking various scientific, social, and artistic fields; to nurture a holistic view of arts, sciences, humanities, and healing; and to publish and distribute literature on the relationship of mind, body, and nature.

North Atlantic Books' publications are available through most bookstores. For further information, call 800-733-3000 or visit our website at www.northatlanticbooks.com.

MEDICAL DISCLAIMER: The following information is intended for general information purposes only. Individuals should always see their health care provider before administering any suggestions made in this book. Any application of the material set forth in the following pages is at the reader's discretion and is his or her sole responsibility.

Library of Congress Cataloging-in-Publication Data

Forleo, James, 1948–
Health is simple, disease is complicated : a systems approach to vibrant health / James Forleo.
    p. cm.
  ISBN-13: 978-1-55643-718-2
  ISBN-10: 1-55643-718-8
  1. Holistic health. 2. Self-care, Health. 3. Human physiology—Popular works. 4. Health. I. Title.
  R733.F7253 2008
  613—dc22

2008011660
CIP

1 2 3 4 5 6 7 8 9 VERSA 14 13 12 11 10 09 08

This book is dedicated to my first patients, my parents Joseph and Mae Forleo, for their trust and for their willingness to change their ways; to my wife Julianne for putting up with me during the never-ending process of writing this book; and to my friend and mentor Bill Bahan, DC, for providing me with a lifetime of inspiration.

Acknowledgments

I would like to acknowledge the influence that Dr. William Bahan, Dr. Joe Houlton and June Houlton, Dr. Randolf Stone, Dr. Bernard Jensen, Mark Anderson, Dr. George Goodheart, Dr. John Bandy, Dr. Wally Schmitt, and Dr. Burl Pettibon have had on my life and on my book. I also wish to thank my writing coach, Michael Thunder, my editor Caroline Pincus for her guidance and encouragement, and Dr. John Travis, Dr. Bernie Siegel, and Dr. Andrew Weil for their trust and support.

Contents

Chapter 6: **The Endocrine System** . . . 147

Chapter 7: Insightful Nutrition . . . 187

Chapter 8: **Digestion and Elimination** . . . 219

Chapter 9: **The Immune System** . . . 263

Chapter 10: Respiration and Circulation . . . 303

Illustrations, Photos, and Charts

Introduction

MOST OF US only go to a doctor or other health care provider when we're feeling pretty miserable. We seek out health care to deal with troubling symptoms or severe pain. We even approach "alternative" health care with a focus on alleviating our latest variety of symptoms. But is that what health is all about, an *absence* of disease or pain? Or is it possible that health is an active *presence,* a power, a grand feeling of being alive and in tune with yourself and the world around you? And if that's the case, why aren't we focusing our efforts on building that power in order to create vibrant health?

If you think I'm just splitting hairs, I ask you to reconsider. As far as our health is concerned, we have all been settling for far less than we should be. We have become reasonably satisfied with being free of our obvious ailments, without considering what these ailments really signify. I have been providing health care to patients for nearly thirty years, and I can tell you that health is far more than the mere absence of disease or pain. Health is a positive and powerful *presence.* Symptoms and disease are the result of the absence of that presence.

Rather than looking so intently at what has gone wrong with us, we should be looking at the causes of health within ourselves. What I am proposing is that the human body isn't just a machine that breaks down and needs its parts replaced, like an automobile; it is a magnificently intelligent, self-healing organism that is capable of creating vibrant health and well-being—not only for our physical bodies but for all levels of human experience. To have this experience we must understand our amazing human bodies and learn how best to care for them.

As you read this book you will discover how you can have an ongoing experience of health that goes far beyond the absence of symptoms, disease, or pain. To begin the process, I will help you understand how your body works, and how you can work along with it, not only to alleviate your symptoms but also to correct the underlying causes that create the experience of symptoms and disease in the first place.

I will help you decode the signs and symptoms of dis-ease that might be present in your experience and guide you toward correcting their underlying cause. I will show you how each of the major systems within the body works, including the often-overlooked neuromusculoskeletal system, and how you can bring each system into balance by working with the awesome healing presence that is within you and everywhere around you. I will introduce you to a series of simple, powerful practices to get you in touch with that healing presence. In short, I will help you become actively engaged in the process of *creating* your own health.

These practices will not only help you to break through to a more vibrant level of health, but they will significantly lighten your financial burden as well. If you are like most of us, you have been paying through the nose for disease care, so much so that you don't really do much about your health until it is too late and you need the expensive heroics of modern medicine. I am going to show you another way— the way of building health, the way of listening to your body's needs and making the appropriate changes before you become another diagnostic statistic.

★ ★ ★

Creating health begins with a shift to the perspective that the whole (body) really is something much greater than the sum of its parts. A shift that recognizes that health is our birthright and represents the natural state of affairs for human beings on planet Earth.

I remember the first time this shift in perspective began to occur for me. I was starting chiropractic school and beginning my journey toward understanding how the body works. I attempted to piece together everything I was learning in the basic sciences into a working model, which was quite a chore. There was so much I didn't know and so many relationships in the body I didn't understand.

I began to realize that health was really the normal state and that the experience of disease was totally abnormal. This realization startled me because everyone else I knew in the health field was focused on disease and on what was wrong with us. From that moment on, I began to focus on building health. The half-empty glass forevermore became half full.

This seems so obvious to me now, and perhaps to you as well, but the moment I focused on health instead of disease, my perspective about everything totally changed. Even the word "disease" became a reflection of the true state of affairs. Dis-ease, in medical terminology, means being away from ease, or away from health. Because of this change in my *perspective,* I soon began to see my whole world differently. And as my *perception* shifted, so, ultimately, did my (and my patients') *experience.*

This formula has become key for me in translating the inner experience of body, mind, heart, and spirit into the outer experience of health and vitality. A change in your perspective → changes your perception → which changes your experience.

Until now, our perspective has been one of separation—a separation that not only pertains to the condition of different parts of the body but includes the internal separation between our own body, mind, heart, and spirit. This perspective of separation has given us the idea that we need to consult a specialist to treat each separate part of our body, as well as specialists for our mind, emotions, and spirit. We have divided ourselves into such small pieces that there seems no one left who has the ability to put us back together again, back to the whole person who started this life journey. But there is one person who can bring you back to health and wholeness, and that person is you.

Hundreds of my patients have set a new course to reclaim their health and well-being. When they initially arrived at my office, patients perceived themselves as a combination of ailments and conditions with little or no whole person in sight. As this new perspective started to take hold, as they started to own it for themselves, people began to perceive that they weren't their ailments or conditions anymore. They began to perceive their conditions as direct feedback from the Intelligence of their bodies about their diet and lifestyle, the alignment of their spinal and structural system, and the state of their mental, emotional, and spiritual selves. They began to see through the layers of their past experiences, which had dimmed their perceptions and made separation and dis-ease seem normal.

Their conditions covered the entire gamut of human experience, from headaches, depression, mental confusion, and developmental disabilities to a host of female imbalances, male impotence, exhaustion, autoimmune disorders, childhood immune system problems, allergies and respiratory disorders, to the multitude of structural and spinal problems that chiropractors have been resolving for over a hundred years. When the underlying cause of the problem was corrected, the resulting condition was completely resolved in an overwhelming majority of these cases.

When imbalances in the body are small, the course back to health is a relatively easy one. When we treat our symptoms and dis-ease for years and allow these conditions to degenerate, our problems become compounded, and we need more and more time, effort, and money to keep them at bay. Unfortunately, with a disease-care approach to health, we never really correct the underlying cause of our problems, and we never make the important correlation between the effects that we experience and the underlying cause within ourselves. Instead, we simply settle for being more comfortable in our state of dis-ease. As one of my patients (and teachers) proclaims, "It makes a difference how soon you start to take care of yourself—the earlier the better." He is ninety-two years old and still going strong.

The truth is that we have become separated from ourselves, from other human beings, and from the powerful force of nature that exists both inside and outside of us. This perspective of separation has adversely effected our perception of what is possible and, ultimately, our experience of life and health.

From the perspective of wholeness, which includes the multidimensional nature of life, everything looks different. Physically, we see that nature follows certain laws and principles, and in order for us to experience physical health we need to understand and live by these natural laws. Mentally, we can see that it is our system of beliefs about the nature of the world in which we live that determines our experience of it. Emotionally, we see that it is the internal power of our feelings and emotions that help to create our external circumstances. Spiritually, we find that it is our own unique connection with Spirit that creates a world centered in wholeness, with us in the middle.

This shift in perspective calls upon us to embrace a new way of listening, seeing, understanding, and feeling—with everything and everyone in our world; it awakens in us a whole new way of *perceiving* what our bodies have been trying to tell us all this time.

In over thirty years of observation and study, I have repeatedly been a witness to the magnificent Intelligence of the human body. This internal Intelligence is trying to tell us exactly what is going on inside our bodies, and what it wants and doesn't want from us. This healing *presence* can guide us toward a state of true multidimensional health, far beyond anything we have ever experienced before. But first we must understand its language.

And that's what this book is all about—helping you tap into the magnificent Intelligence of your own body and understand its profound language. If I have done my job well, by the end of the book you will have all the tools you need—both the insights and practices—to support a self-styled program for creating vibrant health and well-being. Each of us has the capacity to experience much higher states of health, but these states must first be awakened and unleashed. Come, join me on a journey to vibrant health.

Chapter 1

The Whole Enchilada

LIFE ON PLANET EARTH is guided and directed by the laws and principles of nature. These universal laws govern the movement of the planets, the stars, and the galaxies that compose the living system of our universe, and, whether we realize it or not, the life experience of human beings on planet Earth is governed by the same laws and principles.

Consider this: We live on a giant rock called Earth that is nine thousand miles in diameter and sits in the middle of nothingness. This never-ending nothingness is so huge that scientifically it could be described as infinite.

We estimate this giant rock to be some 4.5 billion years old and to weigh some 6 sextillion tons, but we are not entirely certain about any of this information. The earth is composed of many different kinds of rocks, gases, metals, and crystals, and has a liquid center of molten lava that is estimated at 9,000 degrees.

This giant rock is traveling through endless space at over 66,000 miles an hour on its yearly 600-million-mile journey to encircle the sun, only to return and begin the journey again. While it is traveling at this enormous speed, it is also rotating around an invisible axis, which creates periods of darkness and light on the surface of the earth. In addition to these movements, the earth and sun travel as part of the Milky Way galaxy at a whopping 43,000 miles an hour.

By some miracle, we are able to stand still on this planet as it travels at these enormous speeds. Somehow we are able to breathe, move, and live on this beautiful planet at the most comfortable of temperatures. Our scientific theories make it sound like we know exactly how all of this is possible, but in reality, this whole experience is still a mystery that is light years ahead of our comprehension.

This is the incredible underlying context that is present at the core of our life experience. We can only attribute this amazing miracle to the powerful invisible force of nature, which is intimately connected to human beings.

We do know that 75 percent of the surface of our earth is water, which is also the same amount of water contained in our human bodies. We know that the earth is a living organism and that the living organism of the human body is composed of the same earth elements. We know that we live in a symbiotic relationship with the earth, and we innately feel that somehow the earth is our mother. We know that the ecosystems of the universe provide the same life-giving environment provided by the internal systems that comprise the human body. We need to know how else this important connection impacts us. Somehow our perspective of the world needs to include our conscious relationship with the power of the natural world.

When we as human beings consciously reconnect ourselves and our lives with the force of nature, we will realize that we are an integral part of the natural world and everything that resides within it. This implies that not only does nature have a direct influence on human beings, but because we are so intimately connected, the experience of human beings also has an influence on the cycles of nature.

Experiencing vibrant health on the levels of body, mind, heart, and spirit means consciously reconnecting with the external force of nature and its internal counterpart—our innate body wisdom. It also means realigning ourselves as best we can with the expanded perspective that goes along with it. This shift in perspective provides us with the total body awareness to create vibrant health on every level of our experience and to understand the reasons why this is possible. In order to continue to create health and happiness on a daily basis, we need to know its source.

Our Inner and Outer Worlds of Experience

Along with the macrocosmic view of the earth in relation to the cosmos, human beings must also appreciate the perspective of an interconnected microcosm. This microcosm includes the world of atoms, electrons, neutrons, quarks, waves, particles, and microorganisms that are also governed by the laws and principles of nature. The laws and principles of nature govern the world of the very small, both inside and outside the skin of human beings. The inner world of the body and the outer world of nature are not only interconnected; in reality, they are two ends of the same stick. The external reality of nature is coupled with an internal reality of equal proportions. In other words, the inner world of our bodies, minds, hearts, and spirits mirrors the external world of the planets and stars. The ecosystems outside the human body are directly connected to the ecosystems within it.

This systems view of the universe and the systems view of the human body, mind, heart, and spirit are both interconnected and interdependent. This is the perspective presented throughout this text. This perspective not only provides an understanding of how our magnificent body works, it also provides an understanding of how we can create our own health and well-being as a result.

It is a little known fact in the reality of human beings that whatever is contained in the inner world of our mind, heart, and spirit is ultimately re-created in our body and in our outer world experiences. Perhaps it was Henry David Thoreau who said it best: "In due course, the inner becomes the outer." Our internal experience will soon manifest in our external circumstances. The awareness of this principle puts us in the rightful place of being the authors of our experience. This simple act of awareness places the responsibility for our health squarely upon our own shoulders.

When we shift our perspective and become attuned to the rhythms and frequencies of nature and the inner world of our highly intelligent body, we become consciously aware that we *are* the connecting link between the inner world of our body, mind, heart, and spirit and the outer world of our experience.

Attunement with Nature

One way of experiencing attunement with the external world is by direct contact with nature. Many of us have had this experience of attuning ourselves to the frequency patterns of nature when we go camping, hiking, fishing, or even hunting. This attunement occurs naturally when we spend enough time outside in the world of nature, away from the city lights and the world that human beings have created. Attunement happens, for example, when we return to the natural cycles of life and are awakened by the sun and ushered to sleep by the darkness of night.

Unfortunately for most of us, it is impossible to permanently live outside in nature, so we have to look for other ways of tuning our body, mind, heart, and spirit to these natural frequencies. As a messenger, I will introduce several of these "ways" throughout the book, ways for our whole selves to attune to a higher frequency, much as a tuning fork does for a musical instrument.

When we become more internally directed by the natural rhythms and cycles of life, rather than by the self-directed rhythms, stresses, and demands of our external world, attunement naturally and regularly occurs. After all, our own internal Intelligence is already in tune with nature. In fact, the two have an inherent resonant frequency, and, depending on the state of our own attunement, our health and well-being are a naturally occurring result.

Resonance is perhaps most clearly illustrated through music. If we were to put two grand pianos side by side in the same room and strike middle C on one of them, middle C on the other would resonate as if it, too, were being played. (If you try this, hold down the right pedal.) This is a resonant system. If the pianos were tuned correctly, these two strings would resonate together at the same frequency, as if they were one string.

In the same way, we can attune ourselves to the external rhythms and frequency of nature and to the internal wisdom of our body. Both ends of this continuum, so to speak, provide the same opportunity for attunement.

Even our original piano has a tuner, who returns the piano to the established sound frequencies. In fact, some tuners do this with a tuning fork, or use a scientific instrument to determine the tones, but the really great piano tuners use their own inner middle C to tune the piano. They tune by ear. Tuning by ear is nothing more than the art of tuning the notes of a piano to the tones that resonate within the piano tuner. These tones within the piano tuner are the tones of our Inner Intelligence.

Bringing this back to our discussion of health, our present level of health is a reflection of our current attunement with life. This experience of attunement gradually replaces our experience of separation from nature, from other parts of ourselves, and from other human beings. In the process of tuning ourselves back to middle C, we release the perspective of separation and begin to live from the integrated perspective of wholeness.

The Resonant System of the Body

As we become more and more responsive to the frequency of the natural world, we soon find that everything in our life begins to change. Scientifically speaking, this frequency has an actual numerical value.

When I began studying this frequency some thirty years ago, the numerical value was approximately seven cycles per second, or 7 hertz. This was the vibrational frequency of sound waves emitting from the earth (similar to radio waves) that vibrated at a rate of seven times per second. Today, that frequency has increased to 10 hertz (and you thought that only your world had speeded up). This frequency, which has also been called Schumann Resonance (SR), is the means by which human beings can become connected to the electromagnetic fields of the earth. This is the way used by planet Earth to tune human beings to the frequency of health.

If we focus our attention on the chaos of the world, we will entrain ourselves to that frequency, which will attune us to chaos and dis-ease. If we focus our attention in the direction of these SR waves, we can entrain ourselves to this healthy frequency, which is what we do when we are outside in nature.

There is an actual physical apparatus within the human body that enables this entrainment to occur. A resonant system is present in our cardiovascular system and is activated by sound waves from the heart and the aorta, the huge artery that is attached to the left ventricle of the heart. When blood is ejected from the left side of the heart it goes through the aorta, down the trunk of the body, and out to our legs and feet.

Our heartbeat sends sound waves down this huge artery, which bounce off the lower end of our aorta, setting up a resonant system within the body. This sound frequency wave extends out to the lungs and diaphragm in order to regulate the resonant system. As the sound waves expand outwards, it takes very little effort for the entire body to entrain to a new vibrational frequency.

This is how the body attunes to the frequency patterns of its user. Whatever tonal frequency we express ultimately manifests throughout the entire body. Every cell, tissue, organ, and system reflects the vibrational tone to which we pay attention. If we embrace fear, every cell knows about it; if we embrace love, our body is bathed in it.

These tonal frequency patterns are also reflected in our patterns of movement and, ultimately, in our patterns of behavior. Our movement and behavior patterns are a direct extension of the way we think, act, and feel—and of the spirit and tone that we embrace. Think about that the next time you're about to lose your temper.

Our View of the World

Human beings have had a collective view of the world that has been appropriate for hundreds of years. Scientifically speaking, we began to assume a reductionist view of the world in the beginning of the seventeenth century. We suddenly became interested in the purely physical and scientific. By analyzing the sum of the parts, it was assumed that a scientist would be able to determine the state and condition of the whole. Scientists and philosophers felt that the whole of the universe could be totally explained, and even its future predicted.

The mechanistic model succeeded in separating man from nature. It even pitted us against her in a struggle for control and dominance. This model of the world also completed the separation in ourselves by separating our mind, heart, and spirit from our physicality, and it succeeded in separating us as human beings, one from another.

René Descartes, the father of the mechanistic view, believed that man, through his mind and through the collective mind of science, could become an independent observer and determine the ultimate truth. His famous phrase, "I think, therefore I am," made us out to be the original cause of our human experience, successfully extracting us from the wholeness and Intelligence of life.

But major scientific breakthroughs in the past half century have changed the perception of the world in which we live. Beginning in the 1930s our scientific viewpoint began to change from a reductionist, mechanistic view of the world to a more inclusive, holistic one. While most human beings still live their lives from the old and outdated perspective, science changed its view of the world long ago.

This change is similar to what happened when Columbus sailed the seas to America. Most of the world at the time thought that they would never see Columbus again. They thought he would sail right off the edge of what was then considered a very flat world. Well, we all know what happened to Columbus.

After his success, people's view of the world changed, and consequently their experience of the world changed right along with it. In a relatively short time, no one was afraid of sailing off the edge of the earth anymore. In any new exploration, the unknown eventually becomes known. Changes in our perspective of the world change our perception and create a different world of experience.

For over two centuries all of science and most other areas of human endeavor followed the lead of the mechanistic scientists. This included the field of medicine, which, for the most part, still subscribes to the ideas of separation and independence presented in the mechanistic model.

Our current medical model still views the human body as a machine whose parts can be studied to determine what makes it tick. If something breaks, we simply replace the part, and on we go, as if nothing ever happened. In a context of health, treating symptoms and disease with drugs, as if they were the real cause, is somewhat similar to the fear of sailing off the end of a flat world.

The Experience of Wholeness

In terms of the human body, wholeness relates to every level of human experience. The cell is a complete whole that is composed of parts that are also wholes. Our cells compose tissues that are wholes, and are also parts of organs that are wholes. These organs are parts of whole systems, which in turn are integral parts of the workings of the whole body. The body, mind, heart and spirit are wholes that are simply parts of a whole person. A whole person is a part of the wholeness of the body of mankind, which in turn is only a part of the wholeness of Being.

This may sound silly, but a perspective of wholeness is fundamental to the experience of vibrant health. The wondrous fact is that human beings are already hardwired for the experience of wholeness, which manifests itself as multidimensional health and well-being.

Wholeness naturally contains a worldview that includes the organizing principle of the universe and the belief that ultimately the world is a healthy, safe, and wonderful place in which to live—a place where all human beings are interconnected and interrelated. This is not the experience of most human beings on planet Earth. It is, however, an experience that is currently available to anyone with the perspective of wholeness.

In relation to health, wholeness is the most important principle to have in place. If we can trust that the inherent wholeness within our body is the same perfection contained in our vast universe, we will soon learn that we can always trust our body to create health.

On the surface, many of us accept that the whole is greater than the sum of the parts, but as we investigate this further, we may get confused by questions like "How can this be so? How can something be created out of nothing? Where does this something extra come from, and what is it?"

This extra something comes from the world of Spirit. It is invisible and cannot be detected or measured; nevertheless, it is the wellspring of our life and health. In order to be vibrantly healthy, the essence of Spirit must move through our hearts, into our minds, through our bodies, and out into the world of our experience. Without this invisible cause of health, we as human beings are reduced to mere machines.

Human beings currently do not have a coherent or interconnected worldview. We function as if everything is separate, especially ourselves. Our actions indicate that we are not even connected to each other as people and as a human race, and neither do they indicate that we are consciously connected to nature.

But when we look at the world from the vantage point of wholeness, we discover that everything is interdependent and interconnected to everything and everyone else. This expanded perspective provides the understanding that we are forever connected to the wholeness of life, and this wholeness provides a view of the world that can actually guide us on our life journey. This change in perspective alone makes a world of difference and truly makes for a different world of experience. Now is the time to put our whole selves back together again.

Co-creation

The more we explore the cosmos, the more we become aware of a new view of reality that demonstrates the presence of a self-organizing Intelligence. The more we look at the macrocosm, the more we see wholeness. The more closely we look, the more wholeness appears to be the most integral part of life.

We suddenly find a universe that at its core is composed of interchangeable waves and particles of matter. This idea expands to include the theory that the matrix of the universe is always in a wave form until we interact with it. And, at the point of interaction, the wave form becomes form itself. I feel that this is perhaps the most profound explanation of how we co-create with the Intelligence of life. As we interact, so is our experience.

The physicist Nick Herbert says, *"Everything we touch turns to matter."* Perhaps waves are the matrix of our entire world, the underlying reality of everything. Waves, after all, are everywhere. There are ocean waves, heat waves, sound waves, radio waves, electromagnetic waves, and even brain waves. Whenever we interact with these waves, we create something that is somehow encoded with the frequency of our intent. Somehow who we are and what we intend appear in the final creation.

In essence, we live in an interactive universe. Whenever we interact with the blank slate of the universe, which is in waveform, a particle of matter comes into being. And, as our interaction becomes more conscious and specific, we are capable of creating forms that reflect our level of consciousness and intention. In this way, the world of our experience can change into a place of love, health, abundance, and beauty. We as human beings have the choice to go from the world of "I think, therefore I am" to the world of "I am, therefore I think."

Chapter 2

Health and Disease

The Wisdom of Our Inner Intelligence

IN THE WORLD of natural health and healing, we know that all life is organized and intelligent. This organized and intelligent life force is not only responsible for creating all life on planet Earth, but functions to maintain human beings in a state of health and harmony.

Everything in the universe is permeated by this life force, which resides outside of us as nature and inside of us as our Internal Intelligence. I like to refer to the internal aspect of our life force as our Innate Body Wisdom.

What is this invisible force that is responsible for directing our hearts to beat and our digestive system to process our last meal while we simultaneously read these simple lines? How is it that this Intelligence not only gives us the breath of life, but constantly works to maintain us in an optimal state of health? This force is truly magical, and in this magnificent multidimensional life of ours we often take such things for granted. As a matter of fact, we often act as if we feel thoroughly entitled to the host of incredible things that happen to us all the time. What I am suggesting is that to be in a state of vibrant health, we need to consciously align ourselves with this awesome power. When we align ourselves with our Innate Body Wisdom, we receive instructions to heal all of our multidimensional ills. My goal throughout this book is to teach you how to access this power.

As you become aware of your relationship to this healing Presence, you will discover for yourself the cause of your own health. Like my patients, you will be forever changed, empowered, and connected to your own source of physical, mental, emotional, and spiritual health, strength, wisdom, and power. You will become less dependent on anyone or anything outside of yourself to experience a new level of health and vitality. Tapping into this source and directing your own course toward health and well-being is the most liberating feeling you can imagine.

Today, we generally give credit to the doctor and his technology for our health, but the awareness of the healing Presence within the body is nothing new; in fact, the idea has been around for centuries. Unfortunately, it has been relatively forgotten.

The Greeks used the term *thymos* to indicate the presence of an inner healing power. The word *thymos* eventually developed into the name for the master control organ of the immune system, the thymus gland.

The Romans followed with the awareness of an inner power they called *vis medicatrix naturae,* or the healing power of nature. This power was recognized in all the healing arts as the ultimate creative force within the human body.

The French continued this lineage of an Internal Intelligence with the term *milieu interior,* which refers to the balanced internal state maintained by the body. In early U.S. history the physiologist Walter Cannon created the term "homeostasis," which represented the ability of the human body to constantly maintain a state of internal balance. The concept of homeostasis is simply a remnant of the understanding provided by this powerful internal healing force.

In modern times the philosophy of chiropractic reintroduced this healing force and called it Innate Intelligence. This powerful internal force is the source of all healing in the human body. Most chiropractors consciously work to release this internal healing power by removing the spinal imbalances that hold it captive.

Regardless of what it is called, it is the acknowledgment of this internal healing Presence that is the cornerstone of any true healing process. Without this acknowledgment we may get some results in treating our symptoms and diseases for a short period of time; however, in the end, these techniques only obscure the real healing process that needs to take place. Treating symptoms and disease do not produce health or encourage healing. Healing is a process, not a one-time event.

Our Intimate Connection with Intelligence

Tuning ourselves to the frequency of our Innate Body Wisdom is remarkably simple, but it does take some awareness and commitment. We must provide space in our lives for an expansive perspective to take place, which can be accomplished in two ways: by directly connecting with nature in the natural world or by establishing a direct connection with the inner Presence of the body. I recommend utilizing both methods as often as possible.

You can activate your connection with your Innate Body Wisdom in a few simple ways:

■ Acknowledge its Presence. This simple acknowledgment opens the door for an intimate relationship of unparalleled proportions. How it develops from there is up to you and depends on your level of interest and response. The more you pay attention to this Presence, the more direct information and inspiration it will give back to you. The more space you create for this Presence in your life, the more of it you will experience.

■ Be thankful. Being thankful for your life exactly the way it is reverses the polarization away from our Inner Intelligence and brings us into alignment with it. This can be a real challenge, especially at first, but with a conscious effort to remain open and curious, you can usually find something to be thankful for, even in the most challenging circumstances.

People with serious health problems are often led to make dramatic changes in their lives. Even though they are overwhelmed initially, they find a way to allow a true attitude of gratitude to be present. They ultimately perceive that their illness or injury was really a blessing in disguise, and one that allowed them to see their life in a totally new way. If you find thankfulness difficult, you can always be thankful for the generous gift of your next breath, without which you would not make it to the following page.

Attaining and maintaining a relationship with the healing Presence of the body also requires listening, understanding, and creating a multidimensional sensitivity to the invisible impulses of your spirit. This is very much like using your intuition, yet with much more focused attention and intent.

■ Adopt a willingness to be guided by this Presence on your life's journey. A spirit of willingness can ultimately result in a conscious union with this healing force. This union with Intelligence occurs by shifting your identification toward your internal abundant Self and away from the external circumstances of your body, mind, and heart.

When you align your identity with your Innate Body Wisdom, you automatically begin to assume some of its qualities and characteristics, which include thankfulness, health, humility, joy, abundance, beauty, truth, the expansiveness of love, and an absolute trust that life will provide you with exactly what you need exactly when you need it.

The qualities and characteristics of this internal force are already present in each one of us and are readily available in each and every moment. To receive them we need only to align ourselves with the experience. This shift in your *perspective* will enhance your *perception* and forever change your life *experience.*

The Healing Process

Usually, by the time we become aware of a problem with the function of our body, our Innate Body Wisdom is already at work finding the solution. For health and healing to occur, we need to become consciously aware of the process that is already underway and of how the body's Intelligence is requesting our participation.

This is accomplished by paying attention to feedback from our bodies on every level of our experience.

Physically, we need to pay attention to our signs and symptoms, and we need to begin connecting those signs and symptoms to changes that are needed in our behavior. It is usually what we are doing or overdoing that causes the symptoms we are currently experiencing.

From the information contained in our symptoms, we can usually ascertain the process that is occurring in our bodies and determine what our bodies are doing to resolve it. We can do this by correlating our symptoms with the body systems that are involved in the process. This will become more and more clear as we go through the book and come to understand how each system works and what symptoms are involved. We can also ask the following questions: How am I currently contributing to the problem, and how can I contribute to the solution?

Am I eating and drinking as best as I can? Is my body functioning at its highest potential? Am I experiencing peace of mind and a joyful heart? Am I consciously connected with my Inner Healing Power in this very moment?"

If the answer to any of these questions is no, you can quickly learn how to change the consequences. This is done by observing how each area of your life directly effects your health and making some important changes right now. You can always enlist the help of someone else, but remember that this is your healing process, not theirs.

Early in my practice, I learned that finding the connection with my patient's Inner Wisdom was my starting point. I would ask myself, "What is this person's body trying to accomplish? What are the signs and symptoms of their disease trying to tell us both about the underlying problem? How can I assist in this process without interfering?" These are the questions that you should ask yourself. When you are aligned with your Internal Intelligence, answers will soon follow.

Most answers come by assisting the body to function more effectively. As a natural health care professional, my job is not to initiate a new healing process or to accomplish any heroic measures, but to assist the body, which is already pursuing health, to function better in the healing process. I realized early on that this healing Presence is much smarter than I am.

This realization intimately connects me with the inner workings of the healing process. Above all else, I began to implicitly trust this healing power to create health in my patients. This experience completely changed my perception about how the body works, and how I could work along with it. I soon realized that I could teach this same process to my patients; it is this same experience that I am now making available to you.

Let's take a look at a fever as an example of how the body works. The old perspective tells us that 98.6 is normal and anything much higher (more than a degree usually) should be quickly controlled by taking drugs. This perspective presents a very stagnant view of life inside the human body. It doesn't take into account that the body constantly undergoes changes; there are cycles of rhythm and experiences in which many internal factors ebb and flow. Body temperature is one of these constantly changing indicators.

When we attune more closely to the Intelligence of the body, we realize that fever signals infection and that an elevated body temperature is our body's way of controlling the growth of harmful bacteria. Our Innate Body Wisdom knows that bacteria can only live in a certain temperature range and that by raising the body temperature only a few degrees most detrimental bacteria will die off. In ancient times, in fact, fevers were thought of as the body's way of cooking out the harmful influences of disease. Actually, this is not far from the truth. Fever is a tool that the body creates for the specific purpose of balancing its internal environment. You see, your body is intelligent, and it knows more about the principles and practices of healing than any doctor or specialist will ever know.

When we take drugs to lower our temperature back to "normal" we inadvertently stop the entire healing process in its tracks. The body temperature may return within normal range, but the detrimental bacteria remain out of control. Before long, this same problem will resurface with even more intensity and will be much more difficult for the body to resolve. This is not to say that high fevers should be ignored, but we must look to correct the underlying cause of the fever and not see fever as our foe.

When we really begin to understand healing as a process that is present before we become aware of it, we can begin to participate in the solution much more effectively and achieve much better results.

Our bodies endlessly give us information about its current state of well-being. Our signs and symptoms provide us with direct information and feedback from our body. Our Inner Intelligence also offers us signs and symptoms of health to indicate that we are on the right track. What are some of the signs and symptoms of health? A high level of physical ability, mental clarity, creativity, strong feelings of love for oneself and for others, love for the world we live in, and an ever-expanding perception of the role that our internal healing Presence plays in our lives.

Signs and Symptoms

Signs of dis-ease, such as a feeling that something is not quite right, actually precede symptoms and are the body's message to us that we are heading off course. Symptoms, such as headache or fever, are more blatant indicators that we have already gone off course.

The way in which we can utilize signs and symptoms can be compared to the way in which we drive our cars. When driving down the road we don't usually lock the steering wheel in one position; instead, we move it from left to right throughout the course of our drive. We are constantly correcting our course. If we kept the wheel in a fixed position we would quickly drive off the road. Try this out next time you drive. Observe how many times you unconsciously correct your course in a matter of a few minutes.

Likewise, these corrections need to occur in relation to your health. If you pay attention to the constant feedback from your body, the signs of dis-ease will signal when you are heading off course. Symptoms are more intense messages, indicating that you have already missed the signs.

The How, Where, and Why of Symptoms

The location and nature of your symptoms will show you the associated organs and systems that are involved. The time of day that the symptom occurs will provide another clue about the problem and your role in it. Your job is to connect all this information together. With a little insight and a willingness to search yourself for the cause, the resolution will soon become obvious.

Upcoming chapters will help you understand how your signs and symptoms point to the cause of your health problems. If you wish, you may go directly to a specific chapter to see how your symptoms connect with different body systems. Remember, a part of you is already aware of the cause and knows the solution.

A quick look at allergies tells us a lot about how the body produces symptoms that must not be mistaken for causes. You can utilize this same basic process to understand your own symptoms.

As a rule, allergies are related to both the immune system and the digestive system. There is usually an overall weakness in the immune system which allows the allergy to be present in the first place, and a digestive or elimination system problem that lies behind that. Allergies to substances such as dust, mold, and grasses occur because of a weakness in the immune system that existed long before any allergic reaction occurs. Correct the weakness in the immune system and the allergies will diminish or in most cases disappear completely. Chapter 9 on the immune system will provide valuable insight and a variety of techniques to help you build your immunity and prevent or minimize your allergies.

A trigger for an allergy frequently can be found in a particular food or environmental substance. Identifying the trigger requires a little more discernment. First, you must notice when an allergy appears. An allergy that appears first thing in the morning, for example, might indicate the effects of something that you ate or drank the night before, or a reaction to a particular environment, such as a smoke-filled room or bar.

Most allergic responses appear soon, if not immediately, after you eat or drink something. In many cases the beginnings of an allergic reaction start even before you finish your meal. Everything in your meal should be evaluated in order to detect the possible trigger. See the Coca pulse test on page 297 for more details.

Likely suspects for triggers are dairy products—such as cheese or milk—wheat, corn, alcohol, or coffee, all of which are difficult for the body to handle. The trigger may also be a matter of eating too much, eating too much of the same type of foods, or a simple thing such as drinking too much liquid with your meal. Drinking with your meal dilutes your digestive juices and adversely effects the function of your entire digestive and elimination systems. This is especially true with ice water served in restaurants, as ice water significantly retards the entire digestive process.

It is important to remember that the ultimate cause of allergic reactions is a weakened immune system. If the trigger were the cause of the reaction, everyone who is exposed to triggers such as wheat, dairy products, dust, and smoke would have allergic reactions to these substances, and that is not the case.

The trigger for an allergy may also be rooted in your inability to eliminate the waste products of normal bodily functions. If you are constipated, for example—which is a rampant problem these days—the Intelligence of your body will start utilizing one or more of the body's backup systems to pick up the slack. A runny nose, for example, can be the body's way of taking the pressure off an already over-loaded elimination system. This is also true for most skin problems.

It is always important to remember that the symptom is actually part of the body's solution to the problem! If you have a runny nose, something else is usually backed up and functioning inefficiently. Shut off these symptoms with suppressants and you are actually hindering your healing process. Correct the cause of the problem, by enhancing your immune system, improving the function of your elimination, and by eliminating refined foods from your diet, and the Intelligence of your body will most likely turn off your symptoms. Your symptoms are not the problem; they are like the fire alarm that alerts us to the dangers of an already existing fire.

Our conscious awareness of the problem, combined with our intuition about its cause, often leads us directly to the solution. Remember to be present and aware during this process, and absolutely honest with yourself about your habits and lifestyle. In later chapters I include several testing methods that help you directly access the Intelligence of your body. These valuable tools add another level of feedback to our already improving perception of reality.

Your Inner Intelligence is always available to assist you in locating the underlying cause of your problems, you just need to be 100 percent honest in the process. No holding out. This process is like learning a new language, and it takes a little time. Be patient with yourself. It can help to remember that this is your native tongue!

Health and Dis-ease

Both lay people and health professionals alike tend to discuss the topic of health in a context of disease. Instead of perceiving health as a dynamic state that is a reflection of our current level of vitality and wholeness, we usually think of health care as a means of eliminating our symptoms and diseases.

This is true in the realm of so-called alternative or natural health care specialties, where getting rid of symptoms and treating disease is still the primary goal. Most natural health specialties simply use herbs and vitamins, instead of drugs and surgeries, to treat symptoms. The mentality remains the same. In most all cases, treating symptoms and disease doesn't get rid of the cause of a problem, it just makes us more comfortable. Generally speaking, our health care system treats the disease within a person, rather than treating the person who has a dis-ease.

Like the mechanistic thinkers of the seventeenth century, we still view the body as a faulty machine that needs technological support in order to function properly. We have accepted the erroneous idea that many of our health problems are due to design flaws in the body, which ultimately equate to design flaws in nature. This perspective leads us to believe that breakthroughs in technology will create for us a better body that won't be so problematic. We believe that the promising new tools of genetic engineering will make us masters of our own fate.

In the process, we have lost our vision of wholeness in which the human body is perceived as an absolutely perfect living organism capable of making any changes necessary to maintain health. This expanded vision includes the perception of the human organism as possessing incredible healing powers that are nothing short of miraculous. The reality behind this expanded perspective of wholeness lies for the most part beyond our comprehension.

Choosing Health

One of the basic laws of nature states that whatever we pay attention to expands. If we focus all our efforts on treating sickness and disease, we end up with more sickness and disease. If we focus our endeavors on building or expanding our health, we ultimately experience beneficial results on all possible levels.

What I am suggesting is an alternative to our current method of thinking about health. Focus on building our health—physically, mentally, emotionally, and spiritually—and we will stay far ahead of the disease process. Try to fight bacteria and treat disease, and we will ultimately lose out.

For our experience of health to change we must shift the way we think and feel about health and disease. Let's look at some of the fundamentals of a healthy perspective:

- The human body is able to heal itself and create vibrant health.
- Both nature and microbes are an essential part of life and our current healing process.
- Health is an active process for which we are ultimately responsible.
- We can always count on our Innate Body Wisdom to provide us with the resolution of our current health crisis.
- Every healing process has a beginning, a middle, and an end, which is yet another beginning.
- Health is the normal natural state of affairs. Disease is totally abnormal.

Shift to the Above-Down Approach

We have tried to resolve our health problems by using a bottom-up perspective, trying to remove one obstacle after another without paying attention to the perspective of the whole. It doesn't work. This is like trying to get a view of a three-story house from the basement. Basically we have kept ourselves busy by putting out the fires of symptoms and disease.

Instead, let's take an above-down approach, which begins with a healthy perspective, the perspective of a whole person, which includes all aspects of our body, mind, heart, and spirit. From this large perspective we can easily work down to the specific details, which is where the term "above-down" comes from. It is like having a view of our house from an airplane: From an airplane we can see the whole house, the neighborhood, and the community in which it sits.

When we understand the perspective of working from above-down, we can comprehend how one thing beneficially or detrimentally effects another and how any change we make effects the whole. Conversely, from a bottom-up perspective, we have a long list of problems to solve that simply never ends.

The Wellness Continuum

I often use a tool called the Wellness Continuum to help my patients embrace the perspective necessary to create health. With a little honest effort and attention, it is easy to locate your current position on the Wellness Continuum and determine your current direction of movement.

The Wellness Continuum includes three distinct areas: an illness side, which illustrates the undesirable path to a premature death; a wellness side, which shows the path to vibrant health; and a neutral point, which represents the symptom-free state of limbo that lies between the two. Because our health care system is primarily focused on relief care and the treatment of symptoms and disease, we have focused our time, energy, and money on the illness side of the continuum, with a return to the neutral point as our goal.

The neutral point represents the stagnant state between wellness and illness: There is no sickness, but there is no vibrant health either. The neutral point represents the final destination of a limited perspective of health.

Signs of Intelligence

On the illness side of the continuum, the pre-symptom category of signs appear like road signs warning us that we are approaching disease and death.

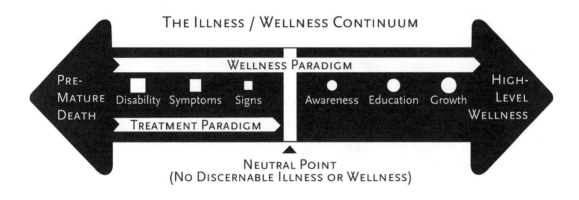

Fig. 2.1: The Wellness Continuum

Signs are not usually spoken of in health care because we don't often recognize them as being important. But our Innate Body Wisdom sends us these signs long before we become ill. We receive this feedback from our movement patterns, our mental attitude, our feelings, and the nature of the spirit that we express. The synthesis of this information will alert us that we are moving in the wrong direction.

Some examples of the signs of dis-ease are feeling tense, anxious, grouchy, depressed, bored, stressed, or a general feeling of unhappiness with your life. Signs also include restlessness, lack of sleep, exhaustion, posture imbalances, temper flares, paleness of skin, a feeling of always being uncomfortable, or the overall realization that something isn't quite right. If you pay attention to what is happening in the present moment, you increase both your awareness of the signs and your ability to resolve the dis-ease.

Symptoms are the natural progression of events when we miss the simple signs of dis-ease. Signs and symptoms present themselves on the physical, mental, emotional, and spiritual levels of our experience, all at the same time. If you become compromised structurally, there is always a corresponding biochemical, mental, emotional, and spiritual counterpart. One level can present more prominently than the others, but as multidimensional beings we always register imbalance on each level simultaneously. Notice this the next time you are demonstrating signs or symptoms.

The Treatment Is Not the Cure

When we don't recognize the signs of dis-ease, and instead treat or obscure our symptoms, we will be led to the next stop on the Wellness Continuum: disability. The word "dis-ability" means to be unable to perform, or to become separate from our natural ability to express health.

Disability manifests with multiple symptom patterns in all forms of named diseases. When functional imbalance exists in the body for a long period of time, several of the body's systems can no longer compensate for the imbalance. Disability occurs when the involved systems become unable to perform their normal functions. When we reach the level of disability, another level of vitality is lost.

Most diseases are diagnosed by the variety of symptoms that are present. The more complex the pattern of symptoms, the more systems in the body are involved. In medicine, the more complex the disease, the more complex the treatment. In my practice, it is not unusual to see a new patient taking anywhere from six to twelve medications at once in an attempt to manage their symptoms and treat their disease.

The progression of disease and the symptoms involved are really evidence of the body's attempt at resolution. When our health degenerates to the level of disability, it indicates that the body has lost much of its vitality, and unless a major shift in perspective occurs, the body is unlikely to recover. Whether the body is expressing a single symptom or a group of symptoms that comprise a syndrome, disability represents unresolved functional problems in the body.

Living on the illness side of the continuum is unfulfilling, dangerous, and extremely expensive. If you find yourself present there, for whatever reason, it is important that you move across the neutral point as quickly as possible into the realm of health.

On the wellness side of the continuum, awareness is the starting point; however, awareness is usually excluded in our current understanding of health. The wellness side of the continuum is not meant to replace the illness portion of the continuum, but to work in conjunction with it. If we are ill, then our priority must be to correct the cause of our functional problems and return to the wellness side of the continuum. You alone have the ability to move in the direction of vibrant health by imple-

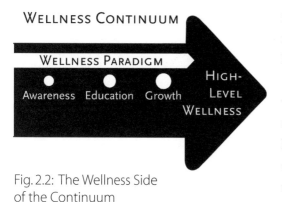

Fig. 2.2: The Wellness Side
of the Continuum

menting the principles and practices of wholeness. Your body is simply waiting for you to lead the way.

The next step on the road to health involves education. With so much to learn about your body, mind, heart, and spirit, hopefully this stage of development remains active for the rest of your life. I have been in the health field for over thirty years and I still find each day a new learning experience.

If you are paying attention and looking in the right direction for health, you will find your education coming from many different sources. Classes and courses, offered through your local community, frequently offer help understanding how your body works and how you can work along with it. Remember: When the student is ready, the teacher will appear. This whole process is much like charting one's course on a sailing ship: To determine where you are and where you are headed , you want to use the stars, the land, the wind, the weather, your instruments, your senses, and your gut feelings.

Make Practical Use of Your Education

This brings us to the last stage on the Wellness Continuum: growth. Growth is the ability to put into practice what you have learned through awareness and education.

Books on diet or nutrition, for example, reflect the experience of the author with his/her particular diet or health system. Each expert has a different story to tell about the ultimate solution to health, and each author has discovered a life-changing method. The funny thing is, few of these experts agree. How can this be? Very simply, each one of these experts has become an expert on themselves. They discovered how to understand the Intelligence of their own body, and they translated that understanding into a way of life. And of course, it worked for them.

In order to grow, you need to do the same thing. You need to become an expert on yourself and your body! It is not up to some doctor, therapist, teacher, parent, or me; it is up to the person who looks back at you in the mirror every day. You need to discover what is right for you.

This is true not only for diet and nutrition but for every aspect of your life, including structural balance, exercise, movement, diet, nutrition, work, personal relationships, your beliefs and feelings, and above all, your relationship with a higher power.

In each and every moment your choice is clear: you can either create health or create dis-ease.

If you choose to create vibrant health, your awareness and participation are required on every level of experience. Physical health includes finding a balance in both the structural and biochemical components of your health. Mental health results from the experience of stillness in the mind and a belief system that reflects a healthy perspective. Emotional health includes your ability to recover from past emotional traumas and be in the present moment with an open heart. Spiritual health allows space for the awareness, perspective, and guidance of a higher power to enter into your everyday life. Your choices will determine your experience.

The Whole Body Scan

The Whole Body Scan is a way for you to get an accurate picture of the working condition of the parts of your body, as well as the whole of your Being.

I discovered this important internal healing process some years ago when it helped me solve a specific problem. I was learning to ski on Telemark skis, and it was a very challenging day to say the least. When it was time for the last run, the sun had gone down and the conditions changed rapidly, as they frequently do in the Rocky Mountains. All of a sudden, I hit a mound of snow that I had gone over several times that day, but it had now turned to solid ice. My skis went in opposite directions, and I heard a loud crack in my lower leg.

I knew this wasn't a good sign. My foot started hurting and felt very strange. I hobbled to my car and headed home. Fortunately it wasn't very far to drive, and in a short time I was sitting in my favorite chair. It was there that I started to direct all of my energy, attention, and awareness into my leg.

Actually, it was more of a natural process, and it began as soon as I closed my eyes. After a few moments I felt incredible heat in the area of my lower leg, which was followed by tingling and a pulsing feeling. In a few minutes I realized that I was less afraid and more at ease. As I continued with this seemingly unstoppable process, the pain in my leg began to diminish. As my sense of peacefulness continued to increase, my level of pain continued to decrease. During this timeless moment, I felt that everything was going to be all right. I relaxed more and more, and the pain proceeded to totally disappear. I had a fractured fibula (the small bone in the lower leg), but throughout the entire time it took to heal—which took two to three weeks less than was originally predicted—I continued using this method and never experienced pain again. While looking at the X-ray, the doctor expressed surprise that the alignment was perfect, particularly with a rotatory fracture. I always wondered what it looked like before I began my little process.

In other words, we can assist our Innate Body Wisdom by consciously directing our attention and energy toward healing. Where our attention might typically be taken up with fear, pain, regret, and blame, feelings which actually siphon energy from our healing process, we can choose to align our intention with this internal healing power and produce amazing results in a very short time.

Another way of utilizing this connection with your Innate Body Wisdom is to take inventory of the conditions throughout your body. This can be accomplished by the Whole Body Scan.

First, close your eyes and get a sense of connection with your breath. Try to sense the state of your breathing as if you were an impartial observer. Notice if your breathing is easy and relaxed, or tense and labored. This simple act of noticing begins to add the quality of ease to the experience. Continue your observations for several breaths, letting your awareness be guided where it will.

Begin to fill your entire body with awareness by slowly filling it with your breath. This inner awareness will soon encompass your skin, and the harsh differentiation between the inner you and the outer will soon get fuzzy and begin to disappear. At this point, you can merge with the healing Presence within your body, especially if you leave your mind at the door.

Notice any areas of your body that seem to feel different, stand out in any way from the rest, or simply grab your attention. Get a sense that in this part of the healing process, your external self is only along for the ride. Let this process happen while you focus on your Inner Being.

At this stage, you can either scan your entire body or focus right away on a particular area of need. You can start where your awareness currently finds itself and allow your healing power to take charge. If your awareness moves to your head, for example, focus all your attention there and let the entire space of your head fill with awareness. Take note of the quality and feeling tone of any area that stands out from the rest, as this will help you recognize any major area that needs your attention. Take one area at a time, focus on being fully present, and allow a state of ease to be present before you move on to the next area.

In most situations, healing requires only that you bring your awareness and attention to a particular part of the body. The healing Presence in your body does the rest. After discovering an area of need, simply remain present with focused attention until the intensity diminishes, the original area energetically blends in with the rest of your body, and the process is complete. In some cases this may take a few sessions. A tremendous amount of healing can happen through this simple healing process.

When we are aligned with the Intelligence of life, anything is possible. The power that guides the movement of the stars and galaxies comes to rest in our body, mind, and heart, with the purpose of uniquely expressing Itself though us. What a miracle to have the source of all life as close to us as our beating heart. Shall we set a limit to our human experience, or shall we chart a new course with our Innate Body Wisdom as our guide, and explore the possibilities of vibrant health and well-being? The choice is yours and the time is now!

Chapter 3

The Nerve System

AS WE BEGIN our journey through the amazing systems of the human body, I would refer to the systems view model located in appendix B. This systems wheel represents a simple understanding of how our Innate Body Wisdom controls and coordinates all body systems to function together in a state of perfect harmony and health.

Our Inner Intelligence uses various body systems to create a constant state of dynamic equilibrium often referred to as homeostasis. This dynamic state depends upon a precise interplay between myriad body systems to create a balance between the internal and external environment for each and every human being.

For this systems wheel to roll smoothly, as in the case of health, all the systems or spokes of the wheel need to be functioning at their own optimal level. If the function of any of these systems declines, the balance within the entire wheel is changed. This will effect the ease with which the wheel rolls and, ultimately, the direction it takes. With the decline in function of any system, ease becomes dis-ease.

As indicated in the accompanying illustrations, the extensive nature of the nerve system in the body is beyond our wildest imaginings. Each year scientists uncover vast new ways in which our nerve system has been functioning. In fact, if all the bones, hair, skin, and muscles were removed from the body, and only nerves remained, we could recognize the facial outline of a person by simply looking at their nerves.

The reason that the brain and nerve system are so extensive, and are the first recognizable structures to develop in the fetus, is because the brain and nerve system control and coordinate the function of every living cell, tissue, organ, and system in the body. The brain and spinal cord, called the central nervous system, are the main switchboard for all communications throughout the body. The central nerve system is the body's communication system, which ferries vital information in the form of electricity and magnetism at alarming speeds across our nerves.

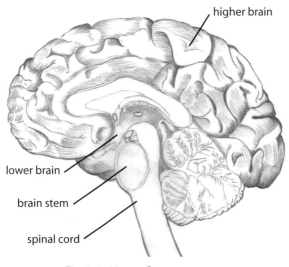

higher brain

lower brain

brain stem

spinal cord

Fig. 3.1: Nerve System

Essentially, it is our nerve system, along with the intimately associated endocrine system, that carries our multidimensional awareness out to each and every cell. This expanded control system allows each cell to share the experience of its current resident. Whatever experience we choose to have is shared instantly with each of our forty quadrillion cells, and each one feels every up and down of our life experience.

This type of extensive communication within the nerve system is the way our Inner Intelligence gets the word out, so to speak, and keeps all parts of the body on the same page. The neuroendocrine system, as it is sometimes called, translates the reality of our consciousness into the neurochemistry of our human form. In fact, it is designed to function at a level of performance we currently are unable to comprehend.

This chapter offers a dozen tips and practices for improving the function of this delicate, marvelous system, as well as a comprehensive summary of its basic operation. Understanding the basics workings of your nerve system will give you many insights about how you were designed to best function. It has been my experience that the better we understand our core technology, the better able we are to take care of it.

The Cerebrum

As you will see in the accompanying illustrations, the central nerve system is composed of three parts: the higher brain, the lower brain, and the spinal cord. These three components contain a variety of nerve cells and fibers that transmit information over an endless array of nerve system pathways.

The first part of the central nerve system, the higher brain, may be compared to the central processing unit or CPU of a computer. It consists mainly of the cerebrum, which is divided by a deep groove into right and left brains, or hemispheres. The two sides are connected by thick bundles of nerves called the corpus callosum. The cerebrum represents the largest portion of the nerve system, yet it is the portion of the brain that we understand the least. Our brains are so complex that we have only begun to scratch the surface.

Our right and left brains function differently. The left brain is linear, masculine, and analytical in nature, while the right brain is more spatial, feminine, and expansive in nature. Fortunately for us, they function together as one whole brain with an endless stream of integrated connections.

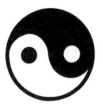

Fig. 3.2: Yin Yang Symbol

This integration of the masculine and feminine energies is not unique to the human brain; it is found everywhere in nature and in every aspect of the human body. The yin and yang symbol pictured here illustrates how the masculine and feminine are always intimately connected and functionally complementary.

HEALTH TIP #1: The Cross Crawl Exercise

Crawling is not merely a step toward walking. Infants learn to crawl because crawling actually helps strengthen the communication between the two hemispheres of the brain. Many of us either did not have sufficient experience in the crawling mode, were made to walk too early, or have developed a brain imbalance by overperforming one-sided activities, such as golfing, hammering or shoveling, checking groceries, or vacuuming. Rebalancing offers tremendous benefits.

The following Cross Crawl Exercise is the easiest and best exercise I know for improving that cross patterning in the brain. It is extremely helpful in improving problems with coordination, erratic body movements, an overall sense of confusion, attention deficit disorders, disorientation, problems involving sense of direction, and an inability to perform tasks well on both sides of the body. The exercise can also be helpful with vision problems, including reading difficulties, when both eyes do not work well together, or in instances when eye-hand coordination is impaired.

Some people will find this exercise extremely simple, while others will find it extremely confusing and difficult. The more confusing it is, the more important it is to do.

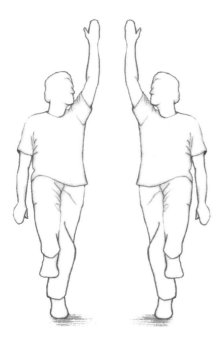

Fig. 3.3: The Cross Crawl Exercise

The Cross Crawl can be done lying on your back or standing in place, but I would suggest you start out lying down. Lie on your back with both arms resting comfortably at your sides and the palms of your hands facing downward. Begin by raising your right arm straight over head, bending your left knee toward your chest at the exact same time.

As you raise your right arm overhead, turn your head to look at your right arm. Simultaneously perform the arm, leg, and head motions, and then move back to the starting position.

Next, raise your left arm overhead, bend your right knee toward your chest, and turn your head to look at your left arm. Remember: Perform all movements quickly and simultaneously. Do 25 repetitions for both the right and left sides.

As this exercise gets easier, you can add the motion of your eyes to the sequence. Begin by raising your arm, following the motion of your hand with your eyes. When that becomes second nature, move your eyes in the opposite direction of your hand without moving your head. For example, as your head turns to face your right arm, move your eyes to the far left. As your head and arm turn back to the left, move your eyes to the far right. The more permutations you add, the better your brain will like it.

This exercise introduces myriad possibilities into the nerve system. It allows you to improve the communication between your right and left brains, as well as to improve the ability of your nerve system to handle multiple tasks. Cross-country skiing and swimming also use cross patterning and can help improve left-brain–right-brain communication.

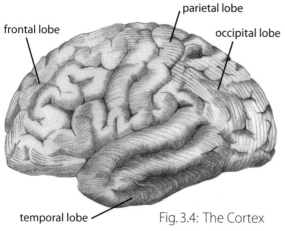

parietal lobe

frontal lobe

occipital lobe

temporal lobe　　Fig. 3.4: The Cortex

The Cortex

Back to the cerebrum. The outer layer of the cerebrum is called the cerebral cortex. The cortex is packed with gray matter, and integrates our sensory ability to see, hear, touch, taste, and smell, as well as our ability to move in various patterns and complexities of movement. Three quarters of all the nerve cells in the body are located in the cerebral cortex.

The cortex is also home to a vast information storage area for past memories. The cortex integrates our ability to learn, to think, to use languages, and to feel emotions and feelings. All this information is located in one neat little package from which information can be instantly recalled.

Nerve impulses travel at an incredible speed of one hundred yards (the length of a football field) per second, which is why human beings are such quick thinkers and have such lightening fast reflexes.

Imagine for a moment what happens when we play the piano. Our eyes look at the sheet music, creating nerve impulses that go directly to the area of the brain that has learned how to read music.

Our brain then sends messages to each finger about how to press down just the right keys with just the right amount of pressure. The brain also tells our fingers how long to hold that pressure with sensitivity and feeling to create the exact intonations that are so important in playing music. We then rapidly move to the next series of notes and phrases until the piece is finished. When you think about it, what occurs within the nerve system is nothing short of astonishing.

Our nerve system takes sounds and connects them to the movement of our fingers, providing just the right interplay between feeling, sound, and movement. Playing the piano involves the integration of both the sensory and motor portions of the cerebral cortex.

Even more amazing, an accomplished pianist can perform a piece from memory after playing a score once or twice. Some musicians have developed the ability to listen to a piece of music once and connect that listening directly to their fingers, bypassing the written score entirely. They are said to play by ear. In reality they play by the sensory and motor portions of their cerebral cortex.

You can improve the integrative function of your nerve system by learning techniques that integrate sensory and motor functions together. These include any-thing that improves your hand-eye coordination, including playing a musical instru-ment, typing, playing ball-related sports, learning new dance steps, playing video games, or even driving home using a different route.

The key here is to integrate something new into your brain and nerve system on a regular basis. The more foreign the activity, the better it is for your brain. Health problems arise when we perform the same actions over and over again, and this applies to routines with food, exercise, thoughts, feelings, and the spirit we choose to carry. To keep your cerebral cortex on its toes, keep trying something new.

The Lower Brain

Much of what we call unconscious or automatic activities occurs in our lower brain. This portion of the nerve system automatically carries out a multitude of functions that are necessary for human life, and offers another example of how the Intelligence of our body regulates and balances its own internal environment. The work of the lower brain includes the function of all our organ systems, the regulation of our body temperature and body weight, the control of blood pressure, respiration, equilibrium, and the coordination of movement for the entire body, especially the eyes. As we will discover later, the eyes play an important part in both our movement patterns and our overall health.

Feeding reflexes in response to the smell and taste of food, such as salivation or licking our lips, are additional functions that originate in our lower brain. Feel-ings and emotional patterns, such as anger and excitement, sexual activities, pain and pleasure responses, are also attributed to this rudimentary portion of our brain.

These lower brain structures are intimately associated with the cranial bones of the skull and the upper portion of the cervical spine. Any misalignments in the cranial bones or upper cervical vertebrae will have a significant effect on the func-tion of this vital part of the central nerve system.

The structures that comprise the lower brain, the most important of which is the hypothalamus, are shown in the figure 6.3 on page 150. The hypothalamus is part of the nerve system, but it is also an important part of the endocrine system.

An example of hypothalamus function includes the regulation and conservation of water in the body. Using information gathered from specialized receptors throughout the body, the hypothalamus can detect the amount of water present anywhere in the body.

The next time we reach for a glass of water, we may be responding to thirst commands from our hypothalamus. In this case, the Intelligence of our body knows that the water levels in the body are too low, and it directs the hypothalamus to produce the sensation of thirst. This sensation causes our mouth to go dry and motivates us to get something to drink.

The hypothalamus also controls the amount of water that is released from the kidneys, as well as the amount that is recycled by our large intestine. When we have taken in enough water, either directly or indirectly, the sensation of thirst goes away and the body returns to its normal pattern of water use.

If you listen to the feedback that your Innate Body Wisdom gives you, in this case to drink more water, you can assist your body immeasurably in its job of maintaining a balanced internal environment, which is an essential component of health.

Furthermore, your Inner Intelligence will tell you when to eat or drink, when to stop eating, when you have eaten too much, when you have eaten a meal that it doesn't like, when it is time to sleep, when it is time to slow down, and when it is time to get yourself in gear.

Your Inner Intelligence will give you cues about how and when to be sensitive to others, how to find the solutions to your problems, and how to find your own path to health and happiness. If you learn how to listen to what the your Inner Body Wisdom is telling you, you can make the necessary changes. The more you take action on this vital information, the stronger and clearer your intuition becomes.

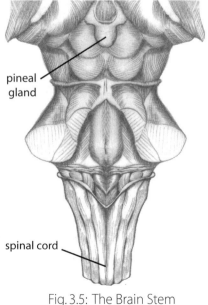

pineal gland

spinal cord

Fig. 3.5: The Brain Stem

The Switchboard

The third level of the nerve system is the level of the spinal cord. The spinal cord functions as the transfer station for all incoming or sensory information from the body to the brain, and for outgoing motor messages from the brain, which make the body move. The spinal cord is comparable to a relay station or switchboard, where incoming and outgoing messages are instantaneously exchanged utilizing thirty-one pairs of spinal nerves.

Sensory information becomes integrated at all three levels of the nerve system—the higher brain, the lower brain, and spinal cord—creating an integrated feedback system throughout the body. This feedback system covers the relatively simple reflexes of the spinal cord, the more complex responses of the brain stem, and the very complex communications of the cerebral cortex.

In the cortex of the higher brain, we finally become aware of how we feel, sense, and think about the incoming information from all of our senses. It is at this point that we evaluate the information that our Intelligence is sending us, and choose the appropriate course of action we wish to take.

The necessary information for that action is then transferred from our conscious higher brain, through the lower brain and spinal cord, and to our muscles, where that action is carried out in the form of movement and behavior.

Too Much and Too Little

There are also two types of nerve responses in the nerve system that function to speed up or slow down activity in the body. Sympathetic nerves speed up our internal reactions, while parasympathetic nerves slow them down. This is an important consideration in both health and dis-ease, as our nerve system frequently gets stuck in a mode that is either too fast or too slow.

When our nerves get stuck in a mode that is too fast, many organs and systems begin to elicit a wide variety of symptoms and dis-ease as a result of the body wearing itself out. When the body gets stuck in a mode that is too slow, organs become sluggish and ineffective, causing symptoms and dis-ease that relate to underactivity.

This principle is a valuable premise of chiropractic philosophy, which attributes all dis-ease to either too much or too little function, resulting from structural interference in the nerve system. This perspective can simplify our understanding of both health and dis-ease, and assist us in finding the functional causes of our physical problems.

Understanding these principles begins to change the way we think about health and dis-ease. By thinking in terms of correcting functional problems instead of treating symptoms and disease, we can expand our perspective of health. As we align ourselves with the purpose of creating health rather than fighting disease, we move out of the realm of effects and into the realm of cause. This enlightening perspective takes the fear and mystery out of disease and empowers us to co-create health with the power of our Inner Intelligence.

In nerve system terminology, facilitation means to increase the flow of nerve system function, and inhibition means to slow it down. Facilitation and inhibition are both important aspects of normal nerve function that can be applied to all levels of our physical, mental, emotional, and spiritual experience. Functional problems arise when we become fixed or stuck in a perspective that is either too much or too little of the right thing.

The following exercise will enhance the biomechanics of your spine, which in turn beneficially effects the function of your brain, spinal cord, and peripheral nerves.

Let the Intelligence of your body guide you through this exercise, and notice specific areas of your spine where interference may exist. This exercise takes only one minute, yet it will keep your spine flexible and happy for many years to come. Practice it daily for the best results.

HEALTH TIP #2: The Twist and Towel Exercise

This Twist and Towel Exercise improves the blood supply to the spine and increases the lymphatic drainage of waste products. The Twist and Towel Exercise also enhances the natural curves in the spine, which are vitally important in maintaining the strength and stability of our structural core. In my practice I have found that the loss of the forward curves in the cervical (neck) and the lumbar (lower back) areas contributes to many functional health problems throughout the body.

I recommend doing the Twist Exercise first thing in the morning while sitting on the edge of your bed. The Twist will limber up your spine, increase the blood supply to your vertebrae, help remove unwanted waste products, and better prepare you for the activities of your day.

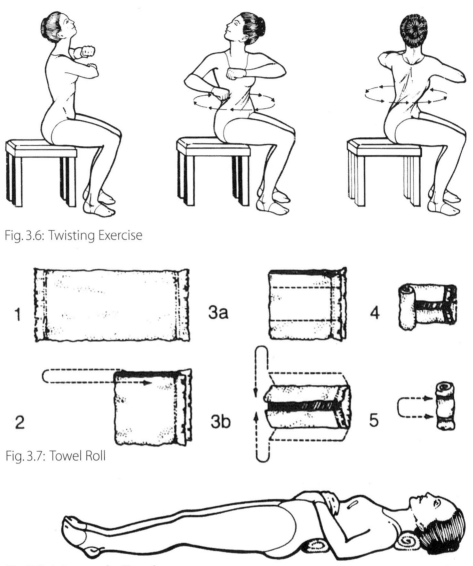

Fig. 3.6: Twisting Exercise

Fig. 3.7: Towel Roll

Fig. 3.8: Lying on the Towels

Sit near the edge of your chair or on the edge of your bed with your feet flat on the floor. Rock your pelvis forward to increase the lumbar or lower back curve, and elevate your chin slightly to bring your neck curve into a neutral position. Sit with your spine erect as in the illustration. Raise your arms in front of you, at chest height, joining your hands if you wish. You are now ready for the Twist Exercise.

Begin with a twisting motion to the left, initiated by turning your head, then your torso, and follow by swinging your arms and elbows behind you. All this is accomplished in one smooth, continuous motion. This movement will also mobilize your pelvis, lower back, midback, neck and shoulders. Twist your torso to the left side until you reach the end of your range of motion.

Move directly into the next twist by turning your head to the right, followed by your torso, arms and elbows, until you reach the end of your range of motion. With a continuous back-and-forth motion from left to right, performed at a fairly brisk tempo, count each twist until you have reached a total of 50 revolutions, 25 twists on each side.

During this exercise, your spine will begin to mobilize, and you might hear some popping and cracking noises, which are normal for this exercise. There should be no pain; if there is, slow down the exercise or discontinue it.

Introducing this amount of motion into the spine changes the center, or nucleus, of our spinal discs from a gel state to a liquid one. This is an important factor in improving your spinal curves, which is accomplished by lying on your back over two towel rolls for approximately 20 minutes. The two towels directly support the forward curves of the spine as illustrated. This is the easy part of this exercise and is best done on the floor or in your bed prior to sleep.

The neck curve is actually larger than the lower back curve, so the rolled towel for the neck should be slightly larger than the one for the lower back. For the neck roll, use a small bath towel, and a hand towel is usually perfect for the lower back roll. Follow the instructions for rolling the towels in the accompanying illustration.

Place the neck towel under the lower portion of your neck, making sure that your head is touching the surface of the floor or bed on which you are lying. If your head doesn't touch, your neck towel is too large. The smaller lower back towel is placed under your back in the area opposite your navel. Just lie there for 20 minutes with these two important curves supported by the towels. You should not feel any pain while lying on these towels. If you do, make the towels smaller. This portion of the exercise should feel really good.

In the evening, prior to sleep, perform the Twist Exercise again, followed by the Towel Exercise for 20 minutes. These exercises are a great preparation for sleep or rest, and can be used anytime throughout the day to relieve spinal tension or ease pain. Under normal conditions, the twist is done in the morning and evening, while the towel rolls are used only in the evening.

To insure spinal health, establish a spinal exercise program at home and incorporate regular spinal checkups with a chiropractor.

HEALTH TIP #3: Regular Spinal Checkups

Because the normal function of the nerve system is so vital to the entire body, I recommend regular chiropractic checkups to insure that your nerve system is functioning at optimal levels. After an initial period of corrective care, maintenance chiropractic helps to keep your spine and nerve system free of interference. Information on selecting a chiropractor is provided in appendix A.

Make No Bones About It

Note the different areas of the cerebrum in figure 3.4 on page 38, and the function designated to each one. Each named area, or lobe, corresponds to the cranial bones that cover them. The four lobes of the cerebrum include the frontal lobe, which is related to speech, behavior, skilled movements, memory, and thought; the parietal lobe, which is associated with basic movements, speech, sensations of touch, and body position; the temporal lobe, which relates primarily to hearing, speech, emotions, and feelings; and the occipital lobe, which is primarily associated with functions of vision. The function of a fifth lobe, relating to feelings and emotions, and containing the limbic system, still remains much of a mystery. By design, our brains are truly integrated structures at every level of operation.

The fact that each area of the brain is covered by a specific cranial bone is particularly relevant, as each cranial bone directly connects areas of the skull to areas of sensory and motor function. This emphasizes the importance of maintaining the alignment of our cranial system.

When stress and tension increases in the cranial membranes, which are directly attached to the inside of our skull bones, the individual cranial bones begin to misalign, creating structural stress, interference, and myriad functional problems directly associated with related portions of the nerve system.

A misaligned cranial system creates structural stress and functional problems that lead to disability and dis-ease, quite literally affecting us deep within the core of our brain. A balanced cranial system, on the other hand, helps to improve sensory and motor function throughout the body.

Mem-Brains

The key to understanding the function of the cranial bones lies in the system of membranes that connect the cranial bones to the brain. The brain is connected to the skull by three layers of tough membranes, the external layer of which connects directly to the inside of the skull and is called the dura mater or "tough mother." The dura mater connects the cranial bones together, while guiding, limiting, and synchronizing the collective expansion and contraction of all the bones in the skull.

In essence, the inner layer of membranes is the external covering of the brain, while the middle layer provides space for the cerebral spinal fluid to travel in and around the central nerve system. Although I will describe the three layers of meningies separately, in reality they are intimately connected together and function as a single unit.

Most medical texts do not recognize the fact that this core movement exists at all in the cranial bones, much less acknowledge its vital significance to the health of the entire body. In my experience, these cranial movements are an essential component to the life and health of all human beings.

The integrated movement of the cranial bones pump cerebral spinal fluid throughout our vast system of nerves. This fluid provides essential nutrients for our nerves and conducts electricity through the magnetic field of the brain. The pumping mechanism of the cranial bones provides the same natural respiratory rhythm for us now as it did inside of our mother's womb.

The meningies travel the entire length of the spine and attach to the base of the spine at the sacrum to form a durable membrane network that helps to guide the motion of our spinal vertebrae.

The reciprocal tension membrane system, as this series of membranes is called, helps our body to accommodate for structural imbalances caused by a variety of structural traumas, many originating from the trauma of the birth process. The condition of these membranes echo the state of balance that exists within the body's structural system and reflect the level of flexibility in the entire nerve system.

In a healthy nerve system, these membranes join the skeletal and nerve systems together. In dis-ease, the tension of these membranes can increase to the point where they misalign the bones of the skull and the vertebrae of the spine, causing numerous imbalances and dis-ease conditions to appear.

These important membranes help to maintain the integrity of the nerve system and are an essential component of structural balance throughout the body. For most people, unfortunately, both the significance and condition of these structural membranes remains unknown.

Initially, it is important to recognize that tension exists in the cranial system. The next step is to reduce that tension by practicing the Tennis Ball Exercise shown below. From a biochemical standpoint, alcohol (especially red wine) generally increases the tension on these important membranes.

It is also wise to establish a relationship with a trained cranial therapist who can occasionally check the condition of your cranial system. Most often the gentle treatment utilized in this cranial work is administered by a doctor of osteopathy trained in the Sutherland method. Specific resources for osteopathic cranial practitioners are listed in appendix A.

HEALTH TIP #4: Cranial Balls

The following exercise is extremely easy and effective for resetting your cranial system. This technique is not intended to replace cranial treatment, but it is a good way to keep your cranial membrane system in balance.

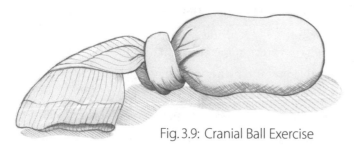

Fig. 3.9: Cranial Ball Exercise

Three common household items are all you need for this exercise: two tennis balls and an athletic tube sock. Place the tennis balls into the sock, and tie a knot in the sock to keep the balls as close together as possible. If you prefer, you can also purchase an apparatus that serves the same purpose (see appendix A).

Lie on your back and place the knotted sock under the base of your skull just above your neck. The tennis balls should be positioned on either side of the base of your occiput. To reset you cranial system, keep the tennis balls on the base of the skull and away from your upper neck. Lie on the tennis balls for 5 minutes. This simple technique resets your cranial mechanism, enabling you to experience what is called a still point. When a still point is reached, your breath will change slightly and your cranial system will be reset. You can also use the tennis ball/sock combination to release tension from your spine. Simply center the tennis balls on either side of your spine and gradually move the balls from the base of your spine to the base of your skull.

Our Sensory System

Our nerve system includes a vast array of sensory nerves that help us orient ourselves to the world around us. Sensory function primarily includes our special senses of sight, hearing, smell, taste, and equilibrium. Additional body senses also collect information from the body's mechanical and temperature receptors. These receptors are located throughout the body and sense environmental conditions both outside and inside the body. Mechanical receptors bring us our sense of touch, including the ability to sense different frequencies of vibration. Our nerve endings have the ability to receive more than a thousand impulses per second, which make our bodies super sensitive to both vibration and sound.

This is significant in understanding how sound vibration and tone positively or negatively effect our health. When we embrace certain negative emotional states, we create a vibrational feeling tone that can create dis-ease and dis-harmony in the body. When we embrace positive feelings or emotions, we create feeling tones that enhance our health. Chapters 12 and 13 give several practical methods for tuning in to health-producing frequencies.

Information about the relative position and movement of different parts of our body, involved in proprioception and kinesthetics, is also managed by our sensory system. These two senses allow us to know the present location of our arms and legs, both in relationship to each other and to the gravitational field of the earth, which permits us to move gracefully through space with one flowing motion after another. Without these special senses, graceful movement would be an impossibility.

We receive additional sensations from the system of organs located throughout the body, which give us feedback in the form of pressure and pain. We also receive a tremendous amount of feedback from our skin, including tickling and itching sensations, and the deep sensations of pressure and pain from bones, muscles, and fascia. Fascia is like a slipcover designed for every muscle: It helps to contain a muscle, isolate its function, and conduct electricity throughout the body.

Our elaborate system of sensory feedback is designed to give us a complete picture of exactly where we find ourselves in space relative to the outside world. Our senses give us information about the condition of every square inch of our body, both inside and outside of our skin.

The input from all of our special senses is so detailed that it is far beyond our ability to actually utilize. For that reason, 99 percent of the sensory information we receive from our special senses gets filtered out. We are only consciously aware of 1 percent of what our senses have the ability to feel!

Our Innate Body Wisdom provides every opportunity to understand what is happening within and around us. The following exercise will help develop your awareness to the sensory feedback your body is giving you.

HEALTH TIP #5: The Whole Body Scan

To heighten your awareness of your sensory system, you can use the Whole Body Scan I introduced at the end of chapter 2. The more you practice the scan, the more you will understand the information that your Inner Intelligence is trying to communicate to you.

Movement

Located in the cerebrum, the motor cortex is the area responsible for all motor responses or movement created by the human body. It is here that the pathways for familiar movements are remembered and actions connected to our thoughts and feelings are initiated.

To see how the sensory and motor systems work together, let us look at an illustration of a simple reflex arc.

A reflex arc is a complete circuit of communication that is established to and from the brain between every organ, tissue, muscle, gland, and cell in the body. I use this reflex arc to illustrate how communication works in your nerve system.

The reflex arc is a feedback loop that lets the brain know what the rest of the body is doing in order to initiate appropriate action. The accompanying diagram is a simplistic representation of how this process works, but provides an understanding of the nature of communication within a healthy nerve system. The actual communication between all these structures is so complex that it boggles the mind.

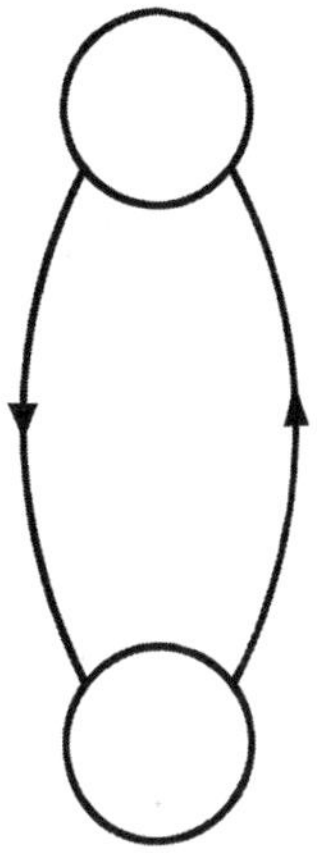

Fig. 3.10: Simple Reflex Arc

Communication

Did you ever notice that your senses are located in the front of your body? That is because our senses are designed to gather information as we move forward in the world and to help us perceive what is going on in our immediate environment. Our senses collect information and relay that information to the cerebral cortex to be evaluated before any action or movement takes place. All this occurs in the blink of an eye.

Sensory information moves across sensory nerves from our organs of sight, hearing, smell, taste, and touch, and goes directly to our spinal cord, where some information is instantly transformed into reflex actions, and other impulses travel through to the midbrain and on to the cerebral cortex. In the cortex, information is evaluated, discarded, or acted upon in the appropriate manner. Some information triggers automatic responses from the Intelligence of our body, while other information is subject to conscious action based on our view of the world, filtered through our sense of perception.

Depending on the decisions made, nerve impulses then move from the motor cortex of the brain to specific organs of locomotion (movement) that are responsible for carrying out our desired actions.

The communication circuit is a pretty simple thing, but sometimes interference exists in the nerve system that keeps this communication arc from completing itself. If a misalignment exists in a spinal vertebra, for example, instructions from the brain will not get through properly. If any interference exists in this communication circuit, then a state of dis-ease is present in the nerve system, which will show up as a functional problem in the body and an aberration in our pattern of movement. This is the essence of chiropractic.

This type of interference is extremely common in our culture and is the cause of much structural dis-ease in the body. When interference is present anywhere in the motor portion of our nerve system, our movement patterns and our behavior are adversely affected. The body is designed to express itself through movement, and when this movement is compromised in any way, so is our expression. No health care program can ever fully succeed without taking into account the importance of an unimpeded communication circuit.

When practiced on a regular basis, the following exercise creates a cycle of balanced movements that will enhance your ability to move in an integrated fashion. This exercise demands balance throughout the full range of motion. It is an excellent exercise to perform daily, as it is both quick and comprehensive. When doing this exercise you are not only exercising your body, but all three levels of your brain as well.

HEALTH TIP #6: The Roundabout

Begin this exercise by standing tall with your weight evenly distributed on both feet. Slowly transfer all of your weight to your left leg, paying close attention to keeping your body erect. Slowly bring your right knee toward your head while bending your head toward your knee. Straighten your right leg out in front of you while returning your upper body to an upright position. Make sure that your left leg is energized and not hyperextended. As illustrated in position 1, you are now balancing on your left leg, and your right leg is straight out in front of you at an angle of 90 degrees.

The idea is to keep your balance while slowly rotating your extended leg 180 degrees from the front to the side and finally around to the back. Keep your torso

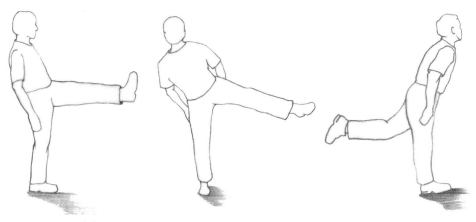

Fig. 3.11: Roundabout

facing in the same direction. If you are standing on your left leg, for example, slowly rotate your right leg (position 2) all the way to the side, and finally around to your back (position 3). Try to keep both legs straight and to maintain the height of your extended leg at 90 degrees throughout the rotation. You will find that there are areas in the rotation that are more difficult than others. For best results, move slowly and steadily through these restricted areas.

Complete the rotation on one side, and then switch legs for rotation on the opposite side.

I'm sure you will quickly discover that this exercise requires a heightened sense of balance and muscle control. The Roundabout works to integrate the various levels of your central and peripheral nerve systems.

At first this exercise may seem difficult; as you continue practicing, however, you will quickly get the hang of it.

Electricity and the Brain

Our brain generates enough electricity to activate the nerve system that is connected to all our cells tissues, organs, and systems throughout the body. In fact, the brain actually generates enough electricity to run a small appliance!

Electrical activity in the brain occurs as brain waves of various frequencies, and can be measured and recorded by an electroencephalograph machine, or EEG for short. Most likely you have heard about the different types of waves generated by the brain during wakefulness, sleep, and deep sleep. They are classified by their Greek names: alpha, beta, delta, and theta.

Even when these classic brain waves are absent, there is always electrical activity in the brain in the form of low-voltage electrical waves. Electricity constantly moves through the entire nerve system, activating myriad brain and endocrine system structures to perform their assigned tasks. Electricity is also generated directly from our nerve cells. Meditation generates coherent brain waves in the delta and theta ranges of 1–12 hertz, which just happens to be the same frequency range that attunes the body to the frequency pattern of the earth! Meditation has also been found to reduce mental and physical stress, focus brain waves into a more coherent pattern, and synchronize the function of the right and left brains.

The ability of nerves to transmit electrical impulses depends on their ability to regulate the movement of sodium and potassium ions in the body, and to a lesser degree, chloride and calcium ions.

Collectively, these ions are called electrolytes and exist as salts that are vital to the electrical function of our nerve system and to the survival of the human body. These ions can become depleted in the body, causing fatigue and a cascade of electrical problems.

Nutritionally, it is vital to establish the proper balance of these important mineral ions in order for the nerve system to be energized enough to transmit electricity and to attract the accompanying magnetic field. Sources of these vital salts are listed in the section on nerve chemistry at the end of this chapter.

The interplay between these ions creates within the nerve cell the equivalent of a microscopic battery. The average nerve cell generates the electrical power of 100 microvolts or about 1/10th the power of a penlight battery. If we multiply this by the 100 billion nerve cells in our brain, we can see why the brain is a dynamo of power.

HEALTH TIP #7: B&E Acupuncture Points

There are several acupuncture points that can improve the efficiency of your nerve system and help to relieve pain in the body. On the illustration below, each point marked "B&E" (for "beginning" and "end") is the beginning or end point of a particular acupuncture meridian.

Tap a tender B&E point on your head while you hold a painful area of your body. Try to correlate a tapping point on your head with its related organ, and hold your hand over that organ while you tap. To locate related organs, you can use the Organ Map Chart in chapter 7 or an anatomy book. Tender or painful areas of the body often correlate with the name of the B&E point. When you find a tender B&E point, tap it for a period of 30 seconds.

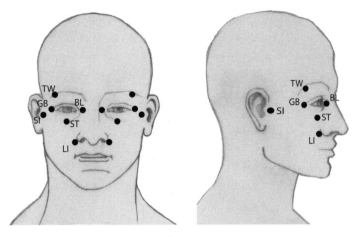

Fig. 3.12: B&E Acupuncture Points

SI = Small Intestine
BL = Bladder
TW = Triple Warmer
GB = Gall Bladder
LI = Large Intestine
ST = Stomach

HEALTH TIP #8: Chapman Reflex Points

The following points represent the connection between the nerve system and the lymphatic system. These points help to improve the flow of stagnant lymph in the body, especially in relation to our organ systems.

To treat these points, rub them in a circular, clockwise direction for approximately 30 seconds. Soreness at these locations indicates that a point needs to be stimulated and that the associated lymphatic system is congested. See page 128 in chapter 5 for the chart.

Nerve Chemistry

While impulses along a nerve are transmitted electrically, transmission of information from nerve to nerve is accomplished purely by electrochemical means. The biochemical portion of nerve transmission occurs in the spaces between nerves, called the synapse, which is a Greek word meaning "to connect together."

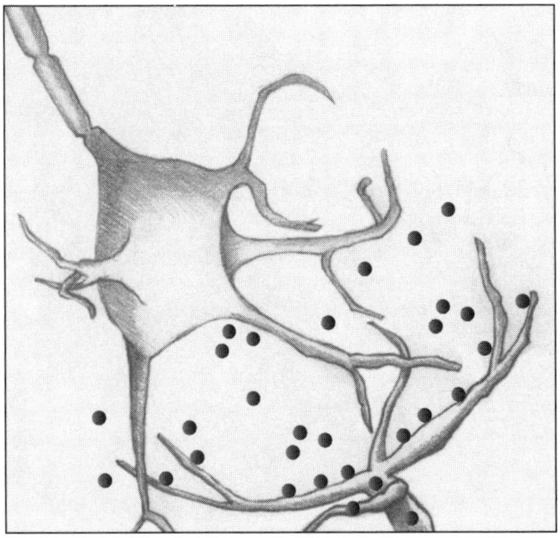

Fig. 3.13: Neurotransmitter

Within these spaces, the body produces chemical messengers called neurotransmitters that transmit impulses between adjoining nerve cells. When an impulse comes to the end of a nerve cell, the neurotransmitters determine whether the signal continues on to the next nerve or is terminated at that point. In the cerebral cortex alone there are some sixty trillion of these synaptic spaces. Cells communicate with each other through neurotransmitters.

Our thoughts and feelings actually influence the formation of these neurotransmitters, which have the ability to transmit subtle information from one nerve cell to another. Neurotransmitters not only carry chemical information but somehow are able to convey our intentions and feelings to every cell in the body.

Through examining the different aspects of our nerve system, I hope to illustrate the magnitude of possibilities that are available to us. In fact, one of the great contributing factors to our uniqueness as individuals is our complex network of nerves and brain biochemistry. Some aspects of this network are inherited, and some are learned.

The more we use certain nerve pathways, the easier it is for our nerve system to connect, for as we develop skills and habits, so do our nerves. Our choices in life not only determine which nerve pathways we develop; they also help to determine our patterns of movement and behavior.

HEALTH TIP #9: Nutrition for Your Nerves

The nerve system is fed by a number of nutritional and biochemical factors that are essential for normal function to occur. Specific whole foods, vitamins and minerals derived from whole food sources, and a variety of herbs assist the nerve system to function normally in the body. These important nutrients include minerals and vitamins.

▇ Essential Minerals for the Nerve System

The essential minerals necessary for the healthy function of the nerve system are sodium, potassium, calcium, magnesium, phosphorus, sulfur, manganese, silicon, and iodine.

For human consumption, minerals normally need to be transformed into organic forms by plants. Inorganic minerals, which are present in most nutritional supplements and refined foods, make absorption difficult for the body. All mineral supplements referred to here are from concentrated whole food sources whenever possible. Suppliers for concentrated whole food supplements are listed in appendix A.

Sodium is necessary for nerve conduction, nerve stimulation, and muscle contraction. Food sources include okra, celery, carrots, beets, cucumber, asparagus, poultry, strawberry, eggs, spinach, peas, cheese, whey, fish, oysters, lentil beans, kelp, and Celtic sea salt.

Potassium is essential for nerve conduction, sympathetic nerve stimulation, and muscle contraction. Food sources include green leafy vegetables, bananas, whole grains, sunflower seeds, potato skins, parsley, blueberries, dill, peaches, coconut, cabbage, figs, and almonds.

Calcium is necessary for nerve transmission and muscle contraction. Food sources include dairy products, tofu, eggs, leafy green vegetables, onions, cauliflower, figs, prunes, dates, sesame seeds, bonemeal, salmon, and sardines.

Magnesium is necessary for nerve system relaxation. Food sources include grapefruit, oranges, green leafy vegetables, wheat germ, seafood, nuts, garlic, figs, yellow cornmeal, raw goat milk, eggs, and kelp.

Phosphorus is essential for nerve transmission, parasympathetic nerve stimulation, and muscle contraction. Sources include seafood, poultry, meat, whole grains, raw goat milk, eggs, yellow corn, nuts, seeds, and garlic.

Sulfur is abundant in the brain and nerve system. Food sources include eggs, cabbage, cauliflower, onions, asparagus, carrots, horseradish, shrimp, spinach, garlic, and melons.

Manganese feeds the brain and nerve system. Food sources include eggs, whole grains, almonds, black walnuts, green vegetables, mint, and parsley.

▮ Vitamins for the Nerve System

Vitamins are essential to the function of a healthy body. They are not manufactured in the body, so they need to be ingested in the form of food.

Due to the poor conditions of our soil and the amount of processed foods consumed by Americans, it is essential to take a whole food multiple vitamin and mineral supplement to provide general support for the body. My recommendation is to take a low potency, full spectrum, concentrated whole food vitamin. Source for all these supplements are listed in appendix A.

Vitamin B is a complex of different vitamins that support the overall function of the body in general and the nerve system in particular. The B-complex vitamins naturally divide themselves into two groups: one group that stimulates the function of the nerve system, and one that relaxes the function of nerve system.

In most B vitamin supplements, all the B vitamins are lumped together in one product that stimulates and inhibits the nerve system at the same time. This combination may be beneficial for some, but it is detrimental for most. Bottled B vitamins are also usually synthetic in nature and contain unusually high doses of all the B vitamins.

If your first or second urination after taking vitamins tends to be bright yellow in color, you'll know that you are taking more B vitamins than your body can handle. The bright color indicates that your money is going directly down the drain.

If your nerve system is already stressed and overstimulated, you don't want to stimulate it even more by taking high-potency synthetic B vitamins. In that case, eat a variety of whole foods containing the relaxing portion of the B-complex vitamins. These foods include brewer's yeast, eggs, tuna, wild salmon, almonds, sunflower seeds, dark green leafy vegetables, peas, and beans.

If a lack of energy is your problem, eat a variety of whole foods containing the stimulating portion of the vitamin B complex. These foods include brewer's yeast, wheat germ, black strap molasses, brown rice, whole grains, nuts, and seeds.

Before any B vitamin supplementation is attempted, eat an abundance of organic whole foods that contain the B-complex vitamins. Much of the time eating the related whole foods is all that is required. It is only in cases of long-standing nutritional deficiencies that supplementation is usually necessary. Sources for whole food, low-potency vitamin B supplements, and its biochemical complement vitamin G, are listed in appendix A.

Vitamin C, a very misunderstood vitamin, is important for the normal function of every system in the human body. Even in our health food stores, the vitamin C complex has, for the most part, been replaced by the fractionated chemical known as ascorbic acid.

In reality, ascorbic acid is an antioxidant found as a protective coating surrounding the vitamin C complex. Ascorbic acid is helpful as an antioxidant and for lowering the pH of the body, but it is not vitamin C. The vitamin C complex naturally includes the following: vitamin P—or bioflavonoid; vitamin K and vitamin J; rutin; and organic copper in the form of the enzyme tyrosinase, which helps us to make certain neurotransmitters and other unknown factors that have yet to be discovered. Natural whole food supplements that contain the whole vitamin C complex are listed in appendix A.

Whole foods that contain the vitamin C complex include the following fruits: oranges, lemons, limes, tangerines, grapefruits, berries, and melons. Vegetables that contain the vitamin C complex include green and red peppers, spinach, tomatoes, asparagus, and onions.

Essential fatty acids (EFAs), also called vitamin F, are vital to the function of our brain, nerve system, and endocrine system. EFAs are composed primarily of omega-3, omega-6, and omega-9 fatty acids. These oils are essential for the body, which uses them to make the sheaths that surround and insulate our nerves.

Due to the amount of altered fats consumed by Americans, supplementation with essential fatty acids has become an important component for nutritional health.

Omega-3 fatty acids are contained in fish oils and flaxseed oil, and a combination of the two seems to work best. Fish oil, which includes the chemical names EPA and DHA, is essential for developing healthy brain and nerve-system tissue in the body. Fish oils are associated with improving mental development and brain function, and are important for the healthy motor function of our nerves. Like omega-3 oils from vegetable sources, fish oils are anti-inflammatory in nature. When taking fish oils, it is important to make sure that they are guaranteed to be mercury free.

Omega-6 fatty acids are contained in extra virgin olive oil, and cold-processed sesame oil. Black currant seed, borage, and evening primrose oils also contain a combination of omega-3 and omega-6 oils.

Americans are most deficient in high-quality omega-3 fatty acids. Quality sources of omega-3 oils include fish, beans, flaxseeds, marine algae, and nuts—especially walnuts. The EFA content of any oil is destroyed when heated, so be sure to consume oils in their raw form.

Ribonucleic acid, or RNA, is an essential nutrient for brain function and memory. RNA will enhance the overall function of your brain and nerve system. Sources for RNA supplementation are located in appendix A.

Lecithin makes fats more utilizable in the body. It is also an important nutrient for the health of the membranes and nerves throughout the brain and nerve system. Lecithin granules can usually be found in your local health food store.

▓ Herbs for the Nerve System

The function of the brain and nerve system are supported by the following herbs:

Chamomile soothes and relaxes the brain and nerve system. It is a great herb tea to prepare the body for a good night's sleep.

Feverfew supports overall nerve system function and helps to normalize the contraction and relaxation of blood vessels in the brain. It can often be helpful with migraine headaches.

Gotu kola is great brain food. It improves circulation to the brain and is helpful in conditions of memory loss, agitation, anxiety, insomnia, and hyperactivity.

Hops relax the nerve system by promoting sleep and alleviating restlessness.

Passion Flower has a sedative effect on the nerve system. It is the preferred relaxant for the nerve-system, as its beneficial effects are not usually accompanied by any side effects.

Skullcap is known as a calmative for stress and nervous excitability, and it helps improve the overall function of the nerve system.

Valerian root is called nature's tranquilizer because its action depresses the sympathetic nerve system. Valerian is effective as a sleep aid but may have some side effects.

These herbs can be taken in tea, capsules, or in the form of herbal tinctures. These herbs can be purchased at your local health food store and should only be taken as directed.

Fractionated Foods

It is important to note that certain food sources adversely affect the function of the brain and nerve system. Some of these substances can inhibit the beneficial effects of whole foods, essential fats, vitamins, and minerals.

These foods include refined carbohydrates, which leach essential B vitamins and minerals from the body. Our internal Intelligence actually tries to make whole foods out of these refined carbohydrates by using up the body's valuable reserves of vitamins and minerals.

Coffee and other caffeine stimulants, such as soda, push the sympathetic nerve system into overdrive, which increases our stress levels and helps to wear out the body.

Refined sugar has a two-fold effect in the body: It not only leeches out valuable B vitamins and minerals, but it also acts as a stimulant, overworking the nerve system, increasing stress in the body, and weakening the endocrine system.

Hydrogenated oils and other altered or trans fats (look also for the words "partially hydrogenated vegetable oil") are heated and processed to the point of being unusable in the body. Trans fats actually block the absorption and utilization of essential fatty acids throughout the body, and they are a detriment to your health. You can find these altered fats hiding out in baked goods with a long shelf life, especially those on supermarket shelves, because trans fats do not go rancid. These fats also tend to be solid and/or opaque at room temperature.

Feeling and Thinking Nerves

Feelings and emotions are generated in two places: in the brain, within a structure called the limbic system, and in our solar plexus, in what is called the enteric nerve system.

The limbic system is a cluster of central brain structures centered around the thalamus and hypothalamus, and surrounded by a layer of the cerebral cortex. These deep structures located at the core of the brain are directly associated with our feelings, emotions, and behavior. Electrical stimulation of these brain areas produce feelings of relaxation and pleasure, as well as feelings of extreme pain, anxiety and fear.

When these emotions and feelings are activated, they become reflected throughout our body in numerous ways—most notably in our movement patterns and physical posture. Associated with every feeling and emotion, physical postures run the gamut from defensive to receptive. When certain areas of the limbic system are stimulated, a laboratory animal assumes the posture and attitude of rage, and attacks at the slightest provocation.

Stimulating different areas of the limbic system in humans produces excitement, wakefulness, alertness, sleep, increased respiration and heart rate, licking, chewing, swallowing, vocalization, sexual activity, and an overall increase in gastrointestinal and glandular activity.

The limbic system is directly connected to the sensory and motor portions of our nerve systems. This important connection explains how the sensory system of the body can produces feelings in the brain, and how feelings initiated in the limbic system can cause a sensory response that is felt throughout the body. The limbic system establishes the important connection between our physical body, our emotions and feelings, and our behavior.

We often use these overall body sensations and feelings to help us determine what is true in the present moment, and what action is appropriate for us to take. With a little practice you can learn to trust your feelings and to see them as important feedback, guidance, and direction from your Inner Intelligence.

The limbic system as a whole is a subjective system, which limits our ability to mentally evaluate and understand its function. This fact only adds to the importance of using your capacities of heart and spirit to guide you through the unknown.

Our Gut Feelings

Before an important event, have you ever felt as if you had butterflies in the pit your stomach? These feelings, located throughout our solar plexus, are caused by a little-known portion of our nerve system called the enteric nerve system. Often referred to as "gut feelings," this aspect of our nerve system is located throughout our esophagus, stomach, and intestines.

When we experience deep-seated feelings and emotions, or even a sense of impending doom, we may experience a lump in our throat and a pain in our gut.

When these feelings remain unresolved for any period of time, they can cause ulcers, chronic abdominal pain, problems with swallowing, digestion, or assimilation and elimination problems, such as colitis and irritable bowel syndrome.

When feelings and emotions run freely in and out of our body, we tend to have few emotional problems. If we have trouble expressing our feelings or letting our emotions go, a multitude of problems quickly arise.

When we look at the anatomy of the nerve system within the gut, we find many of the same structures and substances that are located deep within our brains. For instance, there are over 100 million neurons in the gut, which is more than is found in the entire spinal cord! This is an unusually large number of neurons to be dedicated solely to digestion.

Ninety percent of all neurotransmitters are produced in the gut, and they are the same ones that control many of our intricate brain functions. The only plausible explanation is that the gut—an integral part of our nerve system—is another brain. No one really knows why, but neuropeptides, psychoactive drugs, and opiates are also produced in the gut.

Researchers are currently espousing the two-brain theory, which suggests that part of our feeling brain is located in our limbic system, and another part is located in the gut. In reality, there is one feeling brain with two aspects connected together by what is called the vagus nerve. The vagus nerve seems to control the volume and the degree of interconnection between these two mysterious systems, the enteric nervous system and the limbic system.

This information becomes useful when you pay attention to your gut feelings. As a culture, we have so many digestive problems that are directly related to our emotions, and we need to sort them out. When we learn to handle our emotions responsibly, and to resolve our own emotional transactions and relationships, our digestive problems will substantially decrease.

We can also use our gut feelings as a barometer to evaluate our interactions with others. The enteric nerve system will immediately let you know when an emotional storm is approaching, when it has subsided, and when you are emotionally incomplete. We must also learn how to protect our gut when we are in abusive situations. Chapter 12 is dedicated to the health of our emotions and feelings.

HEALTH TIP #10: Emotional Holding Points

The following diagram illustrates a series of emotional holding points that can be used to help balance your emotions and feelings. There are two sets of points, one on each side of the body, located in four different quadrants on the head.

These points are to be held with very light pressure under the fingertips, usually for a period of one minute or until a symmetrical, beating pulse is felt under your fingers. Using both hands, hold the points in the same quadrant at the same time. Initially, erratic pulses will be felt under each hand, but they will synchronize themselves in a short time.

Use these points whenever emotions have gotten the best of you. You may need to pulse only one quadrant, or you may need to pulse each of the four quadrants, depending on how much your feelings get out of control.

When you use these points, you will most likely find a sense of relief by untangling yourself from your emotions. As a bonus, you will find that releasing these emotional holding points will help synchronize your right and left brains. When holding these points, it is helpful to consciously replay any relevant emotional experience; this often completes the emotional process, both in your body and in your heart.

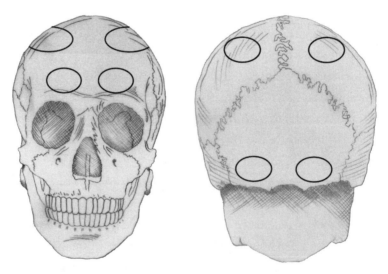

Fig. 3.14: Emotional Holding Points

HEALTH TIP #11: Exercise Your Mind and Emotions

The consequences of the constant ramble of the mind and chaotic emotions create havoc in the brain and nerve system, which is why exercises for the heart and mind are as important as exercises for the body. I have found that the combination of sound, breath, movement, and light provide healing effects for both mind and emotions. Healing music reverberating throughout the body helps bring about healing in the body, mind, and heart. Breathing, singing, and chanting, combined with free-form movements, are a great recipe for health. Check out the health tips in chapters 11, 12, and 13 for more details.

The following exercise will help to quiet the mind and nourish the heart and body.

HEALTH TIP #12: The Slant Board Exercise

This is perhaps the easiest exercise you will ever do. To perform the exercise you will need a board, about five or six feet long and about eighteen inches wide. A strong ironing board will usually do the job. Place one end of the board securely on the seat of a sturdy chair while the other end of the board rests on the floor. You can also see appendix A for slant board resources.

The Slant Board Exercise is done while lying on your back with your arms resting comfortably at your sides, palms facing up. Your head is placed at the lower end of the board while your legs and feet are at the end nearest the chair.

Gently ease on to the board and rest there with your feet higher than your head. This allows some of the effects of gravity to be reversed. Think about it: We are always standing upright, sitting, or lying flat on our beds with our heads elevated by a pillow. The Slant Board Exercise passively improves the circulation to your brain and vital abdominal organs at the same time.

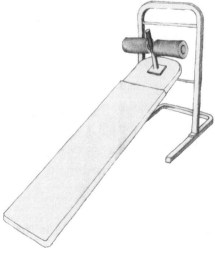

Fig. 3.15: Slant Board

Perform this exercise for a minute or two at first, slowly building up to a maximum of 10 minutes.

Keep the area on both sides of the slant board clear of any debris or obstacles so you can easily get yourself on and off. After sliding off the board, lie with your back on the floor for a few minutes before slowly standing up again. This exercise enriches the brain with oxygen and other important brain fluids. If performing other exercises, perform the slant board exercise last. It will energize you in the middle of the day, but may overstimulate you at night. This exercise should be performed on a daily basis.

The Spirit of Health

Our understanding of how the brain performs complex intellectual functions and abstract thinking remains one of the great mysteries in the human body. We have some scientific theories about how these complex functions may occur, but we do not even know how such complex functions exist.

Scientifically, we have learned where many specific functions are located in the brain, but we are pretty sketchy about the hows and whys of the functions. Although we know a great deal about memory and learning, we have yet to fully understand their true meaning. What is thought, awareness, feeling, consciousness, or spirit? The answers remain a mystery.

We do know, however, that the spirit we express is a precursor to the health that we experience. This makes it important to be aware of the spirit that you embrace in each and every moment. If that spirit is one of complaint, anger, resentment, or jealousy, it will invariably lead you to the experience of dis-satisfaction and dis-ease. On the other hand, if you embrace the spirit of wholeness, love, truth, peace, and tranquility, it will lead you to the experience of health and well-being. In order to create multidimensional health in our lives, we must first create the space for it to exist.

HEALTH TIP #13: The Space Between Activities

Immediately after performing a few minutes of focused breathing, or in the quiet moments following exercise, sit quietly with your eyes closed. Here you may find the essential components to the spirit of wholeness residing in the background (especially if you don't re-engage your mind and rush off somewhere). Whenever there is a break in the action, take a moment to be present in a space you create. Just as the space between the notes defines the music, the space between activities is teeming with spirit. Breathe it in. The big idea here is to bring this spirit from the background of your life into the foreground.

In this regard, you will find the meditation practices offered in chapters 12 and 13 to be of great service. Relax and enjoy!

Chapter 4

The Musculoskeletal System

OUR MUSCULOSKELETAL SYSTEM is primarily responsible for all body movement and comprises over 60 percent of our total body mass. Our muscular system not only allows us to move from place to place, utilizing skeletal muscle contractions, but it includes all of the tissues, organs, and blood vessels throughout the body.

The contraction and relaxation of muscle tissue is responsible for the beating of our hearts, the circulation of blood, the movement of lymph and urine through the body, and for the movement of food and waste products through our intestines. The key word for muscle is movement. The word "muscle," derived from the Greek word for mouse, describes how a muscle contraction looks like a mouse trapped beneath our skin.

Skeletal muscle comprises the majority of the tissues in our arms, legs, abdomen, back, chest, neck and face, and is directly interconnected to a variety of functions throughout our body. This integration is directly reflected in our posture and movement patterns, which—if we know how to interpret what we see—reveal the current state of the entire body. Even the contraction and relaxation of our facial muscles reflect the true nature of our feelings and emotions, regardless of what we say or think we feel. The design of the body always reveals our true, multidimensional state of health through our posture and movement patterns.

Skeletal muscles help preserve the shape of the body by holding all our bones and joints in just the right place. Muscular action also creates the heat that regulates our body temperature. Shivering, for example, is a natural function of muscles that quickly builds up body heat.

Movement constantly occurs throughout the body, even when we are asleep. The continuous expansion and contraction of our breath, the purposeful micro-movements of our bones, organs, and tissues not only helps circulate cerebral spinal fluid throughout the body, but helps synchronize and integrate all the separate parts of the human organism into one organized living whole.

In the skeletal system, this synchronization is accomplished by the subtle movement of the cranial bones of our skull in concert with the sacrum and coccyx at the base of our spine. This intimate connection establishes what is called the "core link," which links together the micro-movements of every bone in our body. When the base of the cranium moves, the sacrum and coccyx do likewise. In a healthy body, all of our bones dance to the internal rhythm of this core expansion and contraction pattern.

Amazingly enough, every system, organ, tissue, and cell throughout the human body, including the central nerve system, moves in response to this expansion and contraction motion. This steady unifying rhythm can be called the breath of life, and is one of the most amazing miracles found in nature.

Whenever the rhythm of this internal movement is synchronized, health is present. Whenever this motion is disturbed, dis-ease is the end result.

Alignment with Gravity

Our neuromusculoskeletal system is truly interconnected and interdependent with all the other systems of the body. This is especially true for the vast system of connective tissue that unites our biomechanical structures together.

These same principles of wholeness and interconnectedness also come together in one of the simplest geometric forms: the triangle. Structurally speaking, the triangle is one of the most stable geometric structures, and has been utilized in myriad building structures, including the tipi, the tent, the mast of a ship, the geodesic dome, and the ultimate triangular structure—the great pyramids.

I have always been impressed at how a big top tent is erected, and how it is able to stand on its own. Its basic triangular shape is suspended in midair like a suspension bridge. The big top seems to defy gravity, and the secret of its success is due to a series of guy wires that support its central pole. Regardless of the exact shape of the tent, a triangle shape exists from its very top, continuing to the points where the guy wires anchor to the earth.

Tensegrity, a term coined by Buckminster Fuller and his associates, describes this inner tension that allows a structure to hold itself up. By utilizing the principle of "creative inner tension," tensegrity actually creates an inner force that counters the effects of gravity. In a geodesic dome, this "creative inner tension" pushes in on itself as it lifts the structure of the dome up from the ground.

As it turns out, the body is constructed in just the same way. All the muscles, tendons, ligaments, bones, organs, fascia, and connective tissues join together to create the push and pull of "creative inner tension" that holds the human body together and upright against the force of gravity.

Just as the center pole of a circus tent doesn't support the entire weight of the big top, our bones really don't directly support the entire weight of our body. The ligaments, tendons, fascia, and connective tissue actually support our body weight. The central pole can be compared to the bones of our spine, while our ligaments, tendons, fascia and connective tissue can be compared to the guy wires. All these supportive structures combine to form an internal communication network that assists the body in maintaining the best level of balance possible.

Just as gravity plays an essential role in the design of the big top, it also does so in the structural design of the human body: It is the constant force to which they both align. The central pole needs to align itself directly under the tip of the big top, and the spine needs to align itself directly under the center of our skull.

A body that is in alignment with the force of gravity creates less structural stress and elicits more ease and fluidity of movement. The more our structural system falls out of alignment with gravity, the more structural stress is created, and the more difficult and inefficient movement becomes.

A misaligned structural system creates myriad problems for the integrated systems of the body, especially in the normal function of the nerve system. Interference in the nerve system presents itself in the form of misalignments of the spinal vertebra, the bones of the cranium, and the bones of the extremities. This interference creates confusion, disorganization, and inefficiency in the sensory and motor pathways to and from the brain, and it wreaks havoc throughout the neuromusculoskeletal system. In the philosophy of chiropractic, this interference is viewed as the underlying cause of all disease.

Incorporating the alignments and exercises presented in this chapter—along with chiropractic care of the spine and alignment of the cranial bones—insures a healthy neuromusculoskeletal system that is optimally aligned with gravity and free of interference.

Flexibility

Along with movement and alignment, flexibility is another important characteristic of a healthy neuromusculoskeletal system. Believe it or not, this flexibility starts in our bones. The way bones look inside of the body is very different from how they appear outside of it. Inside, they are soft and supple, and have the ability to flex and bend. Outside the body, bones become hard and brittle.

There are two different types of bone tissue that combine together to provide just the right combination of strength and flexibility. Compact bone is the dense outer layer of bone that provides more strength, while cancellous bone is the more porous inner layer that provides flexibility. This same combination of strength and flexibility is present in trees. The strength of the outside layer allows the tree to stand tall, while the more porous inside layer allows the tree to flex in the wind.

Our Inner Intelligence creates just the right amount of strength and flexibility in our bones based upon how we use them. If you are a big football player who needs to block and tackle, you will develop bones that are much stronger and much less flexible than someone who practices yoga. Someone who stands on concrete eight hours a day at work needs more strength and less flexibility than someone who bends constantly in their garden.

The amazing truth here is that our Inner Intelligence creates exactly the type of bones we need to perform the work we choose to perform. And, if we change the way we move, the body will change the bone structure's amount of flexibility and strength to suit our new lifestyle. Pretty amazing, I'd say.

Obviously, it would be better to retain the flexibility that we were born with as children than to lose it and try to get it back. But it is never too late to develop flexibility, especially since the body completely recycles the chemical structure of our bones every seven years or so.

Flexibility also relates to the way we develop our muscles in the first place, as muscles respond to the quality and quantity of stress that we place upon them. Exercise is actually a stress to the body, and breaks down muscle tissue. In the days following exercise, the Intelligence of our body responds to the increased stress load by making our muscles grow in size to handle it.

This is why bodybuilders constantly increase their muscle mass by lifting weights. For most body-builders, unfortunately, the more muscle mass they develop, the less flexibility they have in their neuromusculoskeletal system, and the more difficult it is for them to move easily and gracefully.

Conversely, if the stress load on our muscles decreases, our muscles will become smaller. Remember, our Inner Intelligence creates muscles that are just the right size for the amount of work or exercise contained in our lifestyle. If we don't use our muscles, they become smaller.

This is evidenced when a broken limb is placed in a cast. After six to eight weeks of relatively no muscle use, the muscles become so weak that, until creative stress in the form of exercise and movement are reintroduced, they are almost useless. After a period of time, the muscle usually returns to its normal size and strength. The body's muscular system is truly responsive and alive.

Flexibility of movement is also an important factor in determining how well our nerve system functions, as it equates with our ability to bounce back or recover from previous traumas. The flexibility exercises described in the Flexibility Techniques in Health Tip #11 on page 99 are an excellent starting point and are well worth cultivating on a daily basis.

Flexibility also reflects health at other levels of our experience. For example, physical flexibility often represents emotional and mental flexibility. Stiffness of movement may be an important manifestation of inflexibility on the mental and emotional levels.

It is important to remember that, initially, our nerve system is extremely pliable and flexible. Observing the movement and flexibility of young children, people often say, "I wish I could bend like that." But we all once had the flexibility of a child, as flexibility is essential for moving through the birth canal. As time moves on, however, our body reflects the nature and condition of the road we travel.

Physically, our body has compensated for whatever injuries and traumas we have experienced, especially those encountered in the first moments of life. Birth trauma is often the beginning of a long road to structural and postural misalignment.

In many cases, the drama and trauma of our birth experience is instrumental in setting the tone for our entire life story. In thirty years of working with children and adults, I have seen countless examples of birth trauma, which people can carry with them their entire lives. This includes structural imbalances reflected in posture, as well as imbalances in emotional and mental posture.

As we grow older, our body adapts to the consequences of our life experience. Structurally, our system begins to lose its flexibility, alignment, and normal ranges of motion. This changes the way our nerve system functions, as well as the way we move and live on planet Earth.

Our body posture and movement patterns reflect the sum total of our physical, mental, emotional, and spiritual life experience. We can compare our physical life to the rings of a tree. When a tree is cut down, we can observe, by the size and condition of its internal rings, what has happened to the tree in each year of its life. And structurally, our body changes each year according to the climate and conditions of our life. These conditions determine how straight and tall our tree will grow and move, and how flexible we will become in response to the winds of time.

Core Alignment

In order to maintain a healthy, functioning neuromusculoskeletal system, the alignment of the central core of the body with the invisible force of gravity is absolutely essential. Every living thing has a central core to which all its other parts orient themselves. In the human body, the brain and spinal cord are the central core from which all other parts of the body receive essential instructions. Optimal levels of human function and performance depend on the structural alignment of our central core to the gravitational field of earth.

Alignment of the core necessitates alignment of the spine, the cranium, and the supportive structures of bones, muscles, fascia, and connective tissue. This alignment can be attained and maintained through the variety of techniques, insights, exercises, and alignments presented in the first section of this book.

Core alignment is greatly enhanced by utilizing optimal sitting and standing postures throughout the course of a day. The descriptions presented below for optimal sitting and standing postures are an integral part of basic core alignment process. Awareness of core alignment, and your ability to maintain it throughout everyday movement patterns, will greatly benefit the function of your entire body.

The results of maintaining core alignment show up as ease of movement, optimal levels of neuromusculoskeletal system performance, and an uninterrupted flow of life-force energy through our brain and spinal cord.

Of the many indicators of core alignment, posture is perhaps the most significant. Any imbalances or distortions in your posture are a direct indication of the presence of structural misalignments. Misalignments can be present in the spine, pelvis, cranium, or extremities. Postural alignment is a key factor in maintaining structural integrity, and can be used to point us toward the need for beneficial changes in our lifestyle.

Optimal Postural Alignment

Whether you are sitting or standing, walking, running, or sleeping, a balanced posture will greatly enhance your structural stability, while an imbalanced posture will bring out your structural weaknesses. Learning the basics of how to align your posture is an initial step in developing the body awareness of core alignment.

The experience of postural alignment necessitates bringing your awareness and understanding to the unique aspects of your own body. Postural alignment will assist you in all of your activities and reduce the amount of stress on your spine and structural system.

Structural problems usually arise when too much or too little curve is present in the spine, so the first thing we are looking for in both optimal standing and sitting postures is the balance point between too much and too little curve.

Too much curve in any of the three curves of the spine creates weakness in the spinal support muscles and inefficient mechanics for spinal movement. Too little curve in the spine makes the spinal muscles bear too much weight, making them unnecessarily tense and tight.

The accompanying illustrations indicate normal and abnormal posture.

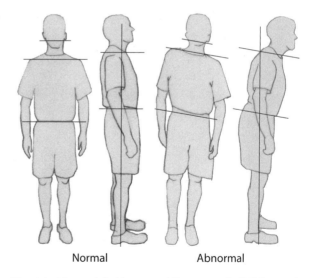

Normal   Abnormal

Fig. 4.1: Normal & Abnormal Postures, A–P & Lateral

HEALTH TIP #1: Evaluate Your Posture

The first step in evaluating posture involves honing your perception skills to notice the difference in the details. This shift in perception can be developed by closely observing the posture of friends and family, as well as your own.

Observe your own posture in a full-length mirror to determine whether you are carrying abnormal postural stress. You will want to observe both the front and side views of your body. When looking at your posture, consider several areas of the body, including the head, shoulders, hips, knees, feet, and hands. In the illustration of normal posture viewed from the front, the head and ears are level, the shoulders and hips are level, the knees and legs are aligned in the center of the body, and the hands and feet are in a neutral position. The normal posture from the side view indicates the position of normal spinal curves.

The illustration of abnormal posture from both the front and side view indicates the postural distortions that go hand in hand with structural misalignments. In the front view, note that the head and ears are tilted, the shoulders are uneven, the pelvis is lower on one side, one knee is out of alignment, the arches of the feet are dropped, and one hand is rotated inward. The side view illustrates a head forward position, an accentuated midback curve, a tipped pelvis, and hyperextended knees.

Evaluate your own posture in the mirror and compare it to the illustrations of normal posture. From the front view, note any distortions or tilting of your head, shoulders, and hips. Also observe the position of your feet: Are the arches dropped down (pronation)? In the neutral position (normal)? Or are they elevated (supination)? Observe your knees and legs. Are they straight, or rotated to either side? Check your hands. Is one hand rotated to the inside or outside compared with the other?

Drawing straight lines and arrows as indicated, record any distortions in your posture on the posture record sheet provided in appendix B. Make copies of this sheet in order to chart your progress.

Compare the side view of your posture with the normal illustrations. This can be a little difficult, as it is hard to see your head and neck from the side, but you can get a good indication by looking in the mirror. If you can, have someone take pictures of you facing the side and the front while you are in your normal standing posture. These pictures are often a big eye-opener.

When reviewing the photographs, observe the alignment of your head, legs, knees, and hands as you did when looking in the mirror.

If you can arrange to have photos taken of your posture, compare your gravitational weight line (GWL) with the normal one provided in the illustrations. Note the body structures that the GWL normally passes through, and whether or not these structures are the same for you. This evaluation will give you a good idea of how well your body is standing up to the constant stress of gravity.

Paying attention to the details of your own posture is an important way to determine the overall condition of your structural system. Once you get an initial baseline of information, you can evaluate how well the exercises and alignments are working for you over a period of a few months.

HEALTH TIP #2: Find Your Optimal Standing Posture

Stand comfortably with your weight equally distributed on both feet. Accentuate your lower back curve by tipping your pelvis back and your belly forward, reaching the maximum range of forward motion for the pelvis and the maximum lumbar curve.

Now find the minimum lumbar curve by rocking the pelvis backward, moving your navel as near the spine as possible to reach the end range of motion for the pelvis, the place where the lumbar curve is completely lost.

It is important to find these two end ranges of the rocking motion, as the optimum lower back curve lies actively balanced between the two.

You know that you have reached the balance point in the lumbar spine when your abdominal muscles feel engaged, activated, or slightly contracted. In this state, the abdominals, trunk muscles, and connective tissue structures that support

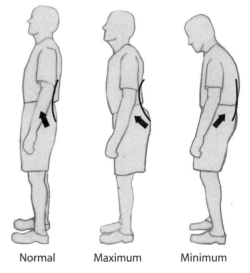

Normal   Maximum   Minimum

Fig. 4.2: Maximum, Minimum, & Normal Lumbar Standing Curves

your lower spine actually begin to accomplish the work for which they were designed. Utilizing the principles of tensegrity, these structures combine together to uplift the human form.

When this balance point is reached in the lumbar spine, and the trunk muscles are actively engaged, the remainder of the components of optimal standing posture naturally follow.

For optimal posture, it is also important to have the neck aligned directly over the rest of the spine. This is done by finding the balance point between jutting your chin forward and tucking the chin back as far as it will go without straining.

While maintaining this balanced curve in the lumbar spine, locate the maximum neck curve by comfortably raising your chin to the ceiling. Next, find the minimum neck curve by lowering the chin as far as it will go without straining. The balance point for the neck curve lies midway between these two ranges of motion.

When you attain this position of balance in the lower back and the neck, gravity—which frequently works against us—becomes neutralized by the forces of tensegrity. Effortlessly supporting the body, these forces rise up from the muscles, connective tissues, and skeleton to create an uplifting feeling of ease and balance throughout the body, which is evidenced by your ease of movement.

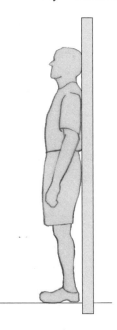

Check in with your standing posture throughout the day by utilizing the following simple method. Standing erect, back yourself against a wall or a closed door. The wall gives you a baseline for your core alignment, and is already aligned with gravity. Once you are at the wall, locate the balance points for your lower back and neck curves, activate your core abdominal and trunk muscles, and find the position of balance and ease. Standing at the wall takes only a moment, yet helps to calibrate your optimal standing posture. Try to retain this posture as you move away from the wall and into the activities of your day.

Fig. 4.3: Standing Posture
against a Wall

Optimal Sitting Posture

The same principles that help to determine optimal standing posture hold true for sitting posture as well. Whether at a desk, dinner table, or in your automobile, your sitting posture is the most stressful. Some of us sit for hours at a time, creating structural stress that can overwhelm our structural integrity.

The key to sitting with the least amount of stress is to maintain the right amount of lower back curve, as it is responsible for keeping our body sitting upright in an active position. Just the right amount of lumbar curve will bring ease to the entire spine, activate your core abdominal and trunk muscles, relax the shoulders, and effortlessly balance your head over your shoulders.

Too much curve in the lower back can jam the joints of your lumbar spine, strain your midback, tighten up your shoulder muscles, and cause neck strain and pain by causing too much curve to in your neck.

Too little curve in your lower back increases the strain on your entire structural system, overworks your muscles, ligaments and tendons, and reduces the fluid movements that are inherently present when your spinal curves are in tact.

HEALTH TIP #3: Find Your Optimal Sitting Posture

To achieve the optimal sitting posture begin by sitting comfortably in a straight-back chair or on a stool with your thighs parallel to the floor, your legs bent at a 90-degree angle, and your feet flat on the floor.

Rock your pelvis forward until you reach the area of maximum lower back curve as you did in the optimal standing posture. In most cases involving lower back pain, people usually rest in a position of maximum lumbar curve without even realizing it. This position jams the joints in the lumbar spine and strains the muscles of the lower back, especially when the arms are raised, as when doing computer work or washing dishes. So, locate the point of maximum lumbar curve, but only for a moment.

Next, find the minimum lumbar curve by rocking the pelvis backward, reaching the position where the lumbar curve is completely lost. The optimal lower

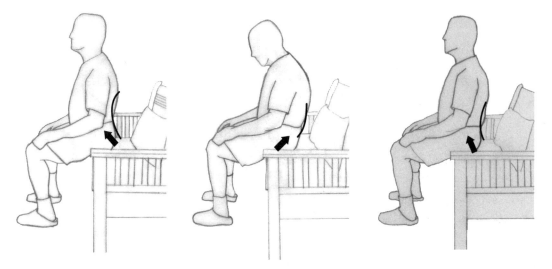

Fig. 4.4: Maximum, Minimum, & Normal Sitting Lumbar Curves

back curve is attained by reaching a balanced position that lies between the maximum and minimum curves.

When this balance point is attained, the abdominals and trunk muscles become actively engaged, the neck becomes relaxed, and the structural stress on the spine is greatly reduced or eliminated completely.

At this point, move your awareness up to your neck, and proceed with the same process used when finding your optimal standing posture: Raise and lower your chin, jut out and tuck in your jaw. Find the balance point between these two extreme neck movements and arrive at the position of ease that lies between them. Gently engage the muscles on the front side of the neck as you did with your abdominal muscles.

Become aware of the ease that results from this aligned sitting posture compared with the stress and tension that are usually produced by sitting. Check in with your sitting posture several times throughout the day and make the appropriate changes. With practice, the correct sitting posture will soon become second nature.

HEALTH TIP #4: Use a Lumbar Sitting Cushion

The use of a lumbar sitting cushion is often necessary for those who spend a great deal of time sitting. This is especially true for those who experience an increase in pain or discomfort immediately after sitting for long periods of time. The use of this type of sitting cushion allows movement of the sacrum and lumbar spine to occur while you are sitting. This is often a big help for those who experience lower back, pelvic, or leg pain. Sources for the sitting cushion are located in appendix A. For those who have spinal pain while sitting, it is often necessary to receive help from a chiropractor to reestablish normal spinal function in the lumbar spine. Once this is achieved, the cushion can help to maintain that balance.

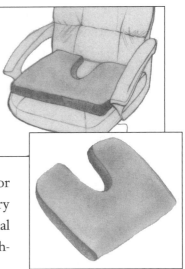

Fig. 4.5: Sitting Lumbar Cushion

Our Posture of Heart

The beneficial feelings experienced by assuming optimal postures are emotional as well as physical. Posture and feelings go hand and hand, and the posture that you naturally assume has associated feelings. To illustrate this point, let us try a little experiment.

Stand in the posture of maximum lumbar curve. Now, assume this same hyperextended posture throughout your entire body: Stick out your chest, raise your head, and point your chin upward, putting your nose in the air. Walk around in this funny position for a minute or two.

Notice how this posture makes you feel. Some may feel assertive, aggressive, proud, or even cocky. Others may feel extremely vulnerable or embarrassed. Notice that your feelings have changed right along with your posture.

Associated feelings are especially true in the converse posture of flexion. Again, while standing, reach the position of minimum lumbar curve, and let your entire body assume this contracted position. This includes slumping your shoulders, letting your head drop, and gazing down at the floor.

Walk around in this posture for a minute or two. If you are like most people, you will immediately begin to feel some sadness and grief, as this is an accentuated version of the posture of depression. In this posture, your breathing is closed off, as is your vital connection with life. If you feel depressed in this posture, quickly change back to the optimal standing or sitting posture and observe how quickly your feelings change. This is a great example of how your posture corresponds to your moods, and how your moods and feelings are directly reflected in your posture.

Because a person's physical posture also reflects the feelings of that person, I refer to the feeling posture as the posture of heart.

Activating Your Body

Activating your body is an important part of both optimal standing and sitting postures. Actively engaging your abdominal and trunk muscles, aligning your head and neck, and slightly energizing your body's musculature brings along with it a heightened sense of tone that energizes and activates the entire body.

Energizing the body in this manner opens up the body's healing energy channels, wakes up areas of the body that tend to be shut down, and connects all the parts of the body into an interconnected functioning whole. In this heightened state of physical awareness, you can easily become more consciously connected to your own Internal Intelligence.

The feeling of connectedness that results from assuming this active posture can be transferred to all types of exercise and movement. Moving with this sense of active awareness adds a whole new dimension to movement. I designed all the exercises and alignments you will find in this chapter with the goal of active awareness.

HEALTH TIP #5: Activate Your Body

Whenever you are involved in any exercise, alignment procedure, or conscious movement pattern, it is essential to actively engage your body in the process. This is accomplished by slightly contracting or energizing the entire musculature of the body during the movement. The activation of your entire muscular system will stimulate the release of lymph fluids from the tissues, increase the supply of fresh blood to the muscles and organs, activate bone structures, and facilitate a heightened level of function in the nerve system.

Actively engaging your body integrates the function of a wide variety of systems, increases the power of healing throughout the body, and encourages structural alignment.

Active and Passive Stretching and Exercise

Aligning the structural components of your posture while activating your skeletal muscles is another aspect of structural alignment that can be applied to all forms of stretching, exercise, and movement.

The word "active" applies to the way in which your musculoskeletal system supports and protects your body. When this occurs, the whole body becomes engaged in the process of exercise and movement. Active stretching involves engaging the muscles of the whole body to help align skeletal structure.

Passive stretching or exercise, on the other hand, is the process in which one part of the body passively participates in a movement pattern or exercise at the expense of the whole. Instead of being part of the action, the passive part does not engage in the movement; in essence, it is being acted upon.

This common form of stretching and exercise frequently allows a joint to exceed its normal range of motion, which can easily cause injury to the joints. Overstretching or overextending the range of motion of a joint is a common cause of injury.

Activating the stretch reflex is another downside of passive stretching. The stretch reflex signals the body that movement is taking the joint past its normal range of motion. Your body's Intelligence hits the brakes to prevent injury to muscles, ligaments, tendons, and joints.

Most runners and other athletes passively stretch their legs in preparation for a run. Unknowingly, they are activating the stretch reflex, which drastically lowers their muscle performance. Passive stretching actually sets up an athlete for injury. Even though the intent is to make muscles work more effectively, passive stretching shuts down muscle function. As a result, many of today's runners are advised not to stretch before a run, as it can be a precursor to injury.

When performed properly, active stretching or exercise does not trigger the stretch reflex, nor will it allow the joint to move past its normal range of motion. For the sake of your musculoskeletal health, the components of active stretching and exercise should be implemented into every stretching exercise and movement program.

All of the alignments, exercises, stretches, or movements presented in this book are of the active variety. Although passive stretching is an extremely common practice, I do not recommend it.

Range of Motion

Evaluating a joint's range of motion is a great indicator as to how well the joint functions. This is true whether you are isolating the movement of a single joint in an extremity, or the motion of hundreds of joints throughout your spine.

Whenever I evaluate the function of any area of the body, I often begin by evaluating its range of motion. In creating a structural health care program for yourself, you can do the same thing. You can evaluate the movement of any area and compare it to the opposite side of your body. A balanced range of motion in a joint on both sides of the body usually indicates the normal position of skeletal structures.

Perform a range of motion study on both sides of your body, and compare them to the appropriate illustration. Performing any range of motion should not elicit pain or discomfort in the process. Any discomfort, pain, or restriction in movement indicates a potential problem.

Be aware that joint motion occurs in a cone of motion. These motion cones stack up to allow for maximum movement and protection in the body. Because the structure of a joint determines its function, normal joint function, optimal alignment, and a balanced range of motion all go hand in hand. Think of it this way: Structure=Function=Range of Movement.

HEALTH TIP #6: Evaluate Your Range of Motion

You can easily evaluate the range of motion in any joint, and determine if there is any restriction, by evaluating how well it moves through its entire range. You can also begin to change an altered range of motion by using a simple method of correction.

Let us use the wrist as an example. Stabilize your elbow by placing it on a tabletop, or stabilize it with your opposite hand to prevent the movement of the elbow. Once the joint is stabilized, slowly move the wrist through the largest motion cone possible without forcing it. Notice any area of restriction, and be sure to compare the motion of a joint on one side of the body to the motion of the same joint on the other side, observing any differences.

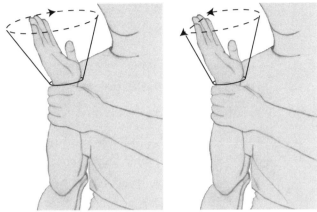

Fig. 4.6: Normal & Abnormal Motion, Cone of Wrist

HEALTH TIP #7: Improve Your Range of Motion

If you find an area of restriction in the range, you can begin to work on improving its motion. By noting discomfort and a flattening of one side of the motion cone, you can find the exact area of restriction in the range of motion.

After identifying the area of restriction, move your wrist (or any joint) to the range of motion that is exactly opposite the restriction. If this position creates more ease, gently stretch the joint in that direction for a few seconds. This procedure usually brings relief to the joint and helps to balance its range of motion. Perform this procedure two or three times in succession, repeating it several times throughout the day, until the discomfort is relieved and the range of motion is improved. This simple yet effective exercise can be utilized to improve the range of motion (ROM) for any joint in the body, including the vertebrae of the spine.

Care should be taken with any joint that elicits severe pain when the range of motion is performed. Pay atten-

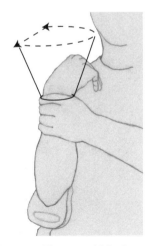

Fig. 4.7: Abnormal Motion, Cone & Correction

tion to what the Intelligence of your body is telling you. If chronic joint pain persists, have the area checked by a doctor of chiropractic.

HEALTH TIP #8: Range of Motion Exercises (ROME)

■ The Clock

I use this exercise in my practice to enhance the function of the sacrum, pelvis, and lower back regions of the spine. The exercise has two different positions that are performed while lying on your back. As with all active awareness exercises in this section, the exercise is performed by engaging your awareness, focusing your attention, and activating your musculature.

THE CLOCK #1

Lie on your back with your knees bent and your feet flat on the floor. As if someone were looking down upon you from above, superimpose the image of a clock over your lower back and pelvis.

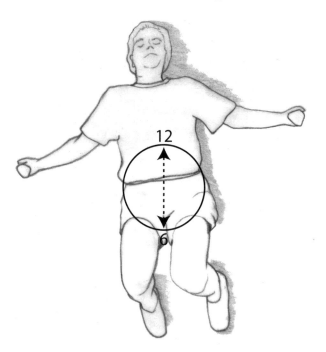

Fig. 4.8: The Clock #1, 12–6

The twelve o'clock position is located above the navel, which represents the center of the clock. The six o'clock position is superimposed over the lower tip of your tailbone.

Engage the muscles of your abdomen, trunk, and lower back, rocking the lower back and pelvis until the point of minimal lower back curve is reached. This can also be accomplished by raising the tailbone until the twelve o'clock position on the clock touches the floor. Hold this position for several controlled breaths.

Rock the pelvis again, this time increasing the curve until the tailbone, which represents the six o'clock position, is closest to the floor. Hold this position for several controlled breaths.

The complete exercise is performed by rocking the pelvis back and forth between twelve o'clock and six o'clock several times in succession. Perform this movement slowly and purposefully, while activating all associated muscles. Take a full 10 seconds to move from twelve o'clock to six o'clock and back again.

CLOCK #2

Assume the same starting position as in the first Clock Exercise. This time, instead of switching from twelve to six on the clock, move your pelvis in a circular motion, bringing each number of the clock, one by one, to meet the floor. Move all the way around the clock, slowly and purposefully, from one to twelve o'clock, maintaining your active awareness throughout the movement. Make sure that you actively and uniquely engage each muscle for every number on the clock.

If you are like most people, there will be a few positions on the clock for which it will be difficult to control the movement of your muscles. These places represent areas in which the normal motion pattern is breaking down, and structural misalignments are most likely present. Complete the exercise by moving all the way around the clock in both a clockwise and counterclockwise direction.

This exercise is wonderful for reestablishing the normal movement pattern in the pelvis and the lower back. It is an excellent recipe for easing lower back pain, and can be used whenever the movement of your lower body is restricted in any way. Do not wait for abnormal motion or pain to occur before you use this potent Range of Motion Exercise

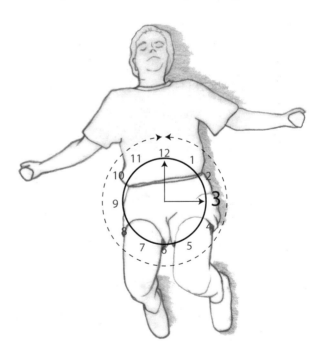

Fig. 4.9: The Clock #2, All Numbers

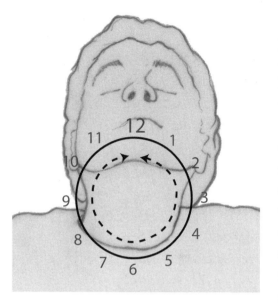

Fig. 4.10: The Clock Illustration, Over the Chin

(ROME). Use it now to help repattern your pelvis and improve your health. The exercise can also be done lying on your back with your legs outstretched. The version illustrated here, with the legs bent, should be attempted first.

After you have mastered the Clock Exercises, you will find it helpful to add the movement of your chin. Let your chin move around the clock in the same movement pattern as your pelvis. The chin up position is at twelve o'clock, and the chin down position is at six o'clock. The addition of the chin beneficially effects movement of the head and neck, and helps to synchronize movement in the upper and lower body. For information and resources on the Feldenkrais method, see appendix A.

HEALTH TIP #9: Series of Range of Motion Exercises (ROME)

In the musculoskeletal system, active movement throughout the full range of motion of a joint or group of joints creates an endless variety of beneficial exercises. The same basic principles presented in the Clock Exercises can also be applied to other areas of the body.

Your Eyes

Because our musculoskeletal system aligns itself visually, the eyes are a natural starting point for Range of Motion Exercises (ROME). Amazingly, structural imbalances throughout the body are usually connected to structural imbalances in the eyes. Using ROME to improve the range of motion of the eyes not only helps to improve your eyesight by activating lazy muscles, but it can have a beneficial effect on interconnected areas of function in the body. Utilize the same clock principles in all ROME.

Begin by sitting in the optimal sitting position. As far as you can without straining, and without moving your head, look up at your forehead with your eyes. In this exercise, your face is considered to be the clock: Three o'clock is your right ear, and nine o'clock your left. Move your eyes toward the end range of motion as you did with your pelvis. However, move your eyes even more slowly and purposefully than you did with your pelvis, and try to touch each of the 360 degrees of motion around the clock with your eyes.

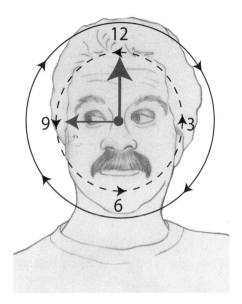

Notice the places where your eyes want to pass through the exercise quickly. Very slowly move your eyes back and forth in these areas of imbalance. Areas of muscle weakness in the eyes correspond to areas of visual disturbance and muscular weakness in the body.

Fig. 4.11: ROME for the Eyes

ROME your eyes in both a clockwise and counterclockwise direction. Begin ROME with both eyes, and then concentrate on one eye at a time by closing the other. Two or three slow yet purposeful repetitions in both directions are usually sufficient to produce significant results. To further improve your vision, use the Tibetan eye chart located in appendix B, which is surprisingly challenging and beneficial.

■ Your Neck

Begin by moving your head and neck easily from side to side and front and back several times. This will warm up your neck muscles and prepare your neck for ROME. It is especially important to activate and energize the muscles of your neck, and I do not recommend using the full cone or circle of motion right away, as some people may experience dizziness or pain when the entire motion cone is exercised at once. This dizziness and pain is usually caused by structural misalignments and/or degeneration in the cervical spine. Initially, I recommend that this ROME be split into two separate parts. If severe dizziness is encountered, discontinue the exercise and visit your doctor of chiropractic.

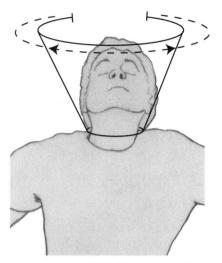

Fig. 4.12: Side to Side Neck
ROME, 90%

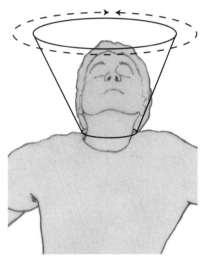

Fig. 4.13: Full Neck
ROME

Begin to ROME your neck by using only the left side. Slowly, with your chin down and centered, rotate your head gently to the left, moving toward the end range of motion until you reach resistance at the back of your neck. Stop at this point and retrace your movements over the left side of the motion cone, returning to your starting point at the midline of your body with your chin in the lowered position.

Next, ROME on the right side of your neck. Be purposeful, and always bring your full awareness to the exercise. Go slowly, and remember to activate and energize your entire body in the process, especially your neck muscles. If you use the accompanying illustrations as a guide during the exercise, please do so without allowing your head to jut forward.

As you progress, you can connect your individual left and right movement patterns into one continuous motion by slowly and gently swinging your neck from side to side, still limiting the full range of the motion cone. Perform the ROME several times from side to side. If restrictions are found in the neck area that are not painful, you can work at improving your range by utilizing the correction offered in health tip #7.

Eventually, if no pain or discomfort is experienced in the split exercise, you can cautiously connect both halves of the exercise together and utilize the full cone of motion for the neck. Proceed slowly and purposefully around the clock in both directions.

■ Your Trunk

The muscles of the trunk are utilized by the Intelligence of the body to maintain an upright and balanced position in the body throughout all movement patterns.

In order to maintain a healthy structural system, it is especially important to have these muscles actively engaged whenever we sit, stand upright, or exercise.

ROME for the trunk can be accomplished by sitting on a backless stool or bench, the edge of your chair, an exercise ball, or on the floor. Interlace your fingers, and lightly place your hands on the top of your head. Bend forward at the waist, engaging your abdominal and trunk muscles. Proceed around the motion cone for the trunk, moving slowly and purposefully, activating and engaging the muscles of the trunk as you rotate. See the accompanying illustration for details.

Proceed around the cone of motion for the trunk, moving clockwise several times and counterclockwise several times. Feel the muscles engage as you rotate around the clock or motion cone. For anyone with lower back strain or pain, these muscles will usually be extremely weak or drastically overworked. Proceed with care, and go very slowly. If this exercise seems too difficult to perform, try keeping your hands at your sides. If severe pain is elicited, it usually indicates the presence of structural misalignments in the lumbar spine and the need to see a doctor of chiropractic.

Fig. 4.14: Trunk ROME

▇ Your Pelvis

As with trunk rotations, this exercise is performed while sitting. To initiate pelvic ROME, rock your pelvis back until you reach the point of minimum lumbar curve. From this point, proceed slowly around the clock, finding the end range of motion for the pelvis. The face of the clock for this exercise is now on the seat of your chair. Actively move your awareness around the entire motion cone for the pelvis.

Alternately push each portion of the pelvis down toward the seat of the chair as you rotate around the clock. Visualize the location of twelve o'clock at your pubic bone and six o'clock at your tailbone. For help in guiding your movements, place your hands on your hips or lightly on your knees.

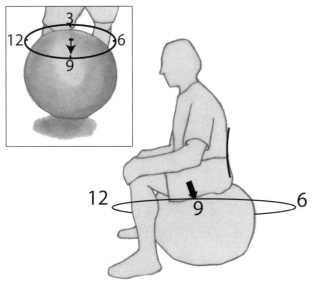

Fig. 4.15: Pelvic ROME

Actively engage all the muscles of your body as you move around the motion cone, taking care to push your pelvis down and touch each number on the bottom of your chair. Rotate your pelvis several times in each direction. Check the accompanying illustration for details. For the most fun, try this exercise on an exercise ball. ROME for the pelvis is an excellent remedy for lower back pain and morning stiffness, and can be performed several times throughout the day. If you sit all day at work, make sure your chair is up to snuff, and use the pelvic ROME.

■ Your Extremities

You can also utilize ROME to improve the function of your extremities. The ankles, knees, hips, shoulders, elbows, and wrists can all be exercised with the same active awareness.

Reach the end of the range of motion for each particular joint, and slowly proceed around its motion cone, activating and energizing the associated muscles as you go. As always, maintain an active awareness throughout your entire body.

ROME are especially good for the wrists and ankles. I find that when these exercises are performed on a regular basis, the flexibility and range of motion of these joints increase significantly. Movement is a sign of life; as we move, so do we live.

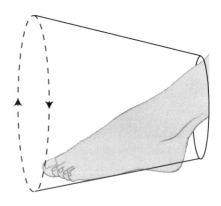

Fig. 4.16: Ankle ROME

HEALTH TIP #10: The Alignment Series

I have provided several alignment techniques in this chapter, including the concept of core alignment, optimal sitting and standing postures, and other tips on posture.

Alignment with gravity is a key component to health. The following Alignment Series, which is based on the principles of yoga, helps the body to attain and maintain proper alignment of the spine and extremities. I have used this Alignment Series for many years to help my patients and myself to align skeletal structures.

The Alignment Series is a combination of three separate postures that are utilized in the discipline of yoga. I have found that connecting these postures together provides the most effective combination for aligning the spine and increasing one's health and well-being.

Before describing the poses, I want to share a few thoughts about yoga. Standing yoga postures incorporate many aspects of triangles with angles of 30 degrees, 60 degrees, and 90 degrees, angles which also provide the strength and stability in many common building structures. If performed properly, yoga is the most scientific practice available today, as it uses these geometric forms as a guide for aligning the structure of the body. Yoga postures are not actually considered exercises, as they are designed to integrate the body, mind, heart, and spirit of a person. The word "yoga," which translates most accurately as "union," naturally evokes a heightened state of awareness, and brings with it a true sense of the sacred.

Before you begin the triad, you will need the secure footing provided by your bare feet, and a thin sticky mat. Sometimes these postures can be performed on a wooden floor, but a sticky mat is really your best bet. Sticky mat distributors are listed in the appendix A.

When performing any standing yoga pose, it is important to activate your legs by contracting your leg muscles as much as possible throughout the series. Maintaining this active state in the legs insures that the pose will be safe and effective.

I recommend that you learn each of the postures separately before joining them together into a flowing series, using the accompanying illustrations as your guide. To insure stability, you may initially wish to support your body in the postures by stabilizing yourself with one hand on a countertop, railing, stable piece of furniture,

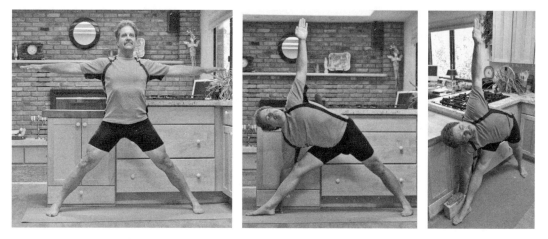

Fig. 4.17: The Triangle Pose

or a wall. Using a means of support allows you to experience the benefits of the posture without being totally dependent on your balance. Do not worry: Eventually you will be able to stand on your own two feet. For now, it is much better to achieve the proper alignment with support rather than assume improper alignment without it.

The First Position: Triangle Pose

1. Assume the optimal standing posture (described on page 77) on a sticky mat.
2. From this position step your feet 3 to 4 feet apart, and face forward as in the first series of illustrations. Raise your arms straight out from your sides, and keep the palms of your hands facing the floor. In this position, turn your right foot lengthwise along the mat at a 90-degree angle, and turn your left foot slightly inward.
3. On an exhalation breath, extend your right arm straight out to the side while bending the trunk of your body. Bring your right hand as close to the outside of your right ankle as possible. While some people will be able to touch their right hand to the floor—only do so without straining—many people need a small block to lean on. Remember to keep your legs actively engaged and energized throughout the posture. Until you are able to maintain your balance, you can support yourself with your left hand against a counter, railing, or wall.

4. Gently rotate your head to look up at the ceiling.

> **Note: If there is any discomfort in the neck, do not look toward the ceiling but keep your head facing forward.**

Lengthen the trunk of the body while you energize and activate your legs. As indicated in the illustration, make sure that your hips, legs, and back are all in a straight line. Hold this position for one to three controlled breaths, using the last inhale to return back to the optimal standing posture. Perform the Triangle on both sides of the body.

> **Note: To assure balance, always perform alignments and yoga postures on both sides of the body in the same session.**

▨ The Second Posture: Extended Side Angle Pose

The second posture in the triad is the Extended Side Angle Pose. For now, I want you to think of this as a separate posture; after you learn it, however, you can initiate it directly from Triangle Pose.

1. Assume the optimal standing posture on your sticky mat.
2. From this position step your feet 3 to 4 feet apart, and face forward as in the Triangle Pose.
3. Raise your arms straight out from your sides. The palms of your hands should be facing the floor.
4. Turn your right foot lengthwise along the mat at a 90-degree angle, and turn your left foot slightly inward.
5. On an exhalation breath, bend the right knee as close to a 90-degree angle as possible between your upper and lower leg as illustrated. For this pose, your right hand should remain slightly to the outside of your right foot, in approximately the same position as in the Triangle Pose.
6. Place the palm of your right hand as flat on the floor as possible without straining. Use a yoga block for support, or use a railing, countertop, or wall.
7. Stretch out and energize the left leg as much as possible while keeping your left foot flat on the mat. Activate your leg muscles by elevating your kneecaps.
8. Stretch your left arm out over your left ear and head, keeping in alignment with your outstretched and energized left leg as indicated. You can support yourself

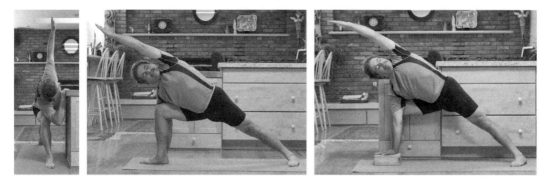

Fig. 4.18: The Extended Side Angle Pose

in this position by using your left hand on a countertop, railing, or wall. (An illustration is worth a thousand words!)

Allow this position to actively stretch every part of your body. Hold the posture for three controlled breaths, activating and aligning your entire body in the process. In the midst of activating your body, learn to relax!

On an inhalation breath, return back to the optimal standing posture. When linking the poses together, always return back to the Triangle Pose. Practice each of the first two postures separately on both sides of your body before combining them.

▋ The Third Posture: Half Moon Pose

When you feel comfortable performing the first two poses of the series, you may introduce the final posture in the Alignment Series, the Half Moon Pose. Initially, you can begin this pose by supporting yourself with your hand as illustrated, and then drop down into the Half Moon Pose. After the pose becomes more familiar, you can move directly into this pose from the Extended Side Angle (ESA) Pose.

1. From the ESA Pose, balance yourself on your right leg while extending your right hand about 12 inches in front of your toes.
2. Align your right thumb with the little toe of your right foot. As you lean over, allow your left leg to rise, becoming parallel to the floor.
3. Straighten your right standing leg completely, and use your newly positioned right hand and arm to balance yourself. With your left arm, you can use a coun-

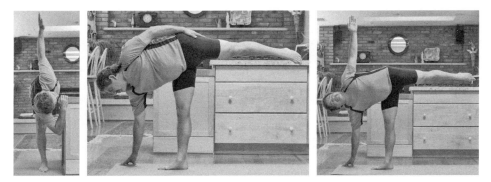

Fig.4.19: Three Photos of the Half Moon Pose

tertop, railing, or wall for balance. Your left leg should now be parallel to the floor, your left foot pointing straight out in front of you.

4. If you're not holding on for balance, raise your left arm straight over your head. If possible, turn your head to look up at the ceiling. Hold this illustrated posture for several controlled breaths.

> **Note: Use the illustrations to get the big picture, and the written words to refine the pose.**

Once you are ready to join the three poses together, you'll want to go from Triangle (1) to ESA (2) and on to Half Moon (3). From Half Moon (1), return back to ESA (2) for a moment or two, and then move back to Triangle (1) for a moment. Complete the series by returning to the optimal standing posture.

> **Note: In all three alignment postures, it is important keep your neck aligned with your body as indicated.**

Perform all three poses on one side of the body, returning to the optimal standing posture before repeating the series on the opposite side of the body. Always begin and end in optimal standing posture.

The Alignment Series is much easier then it sounds. You should utilize the illustrations as much as possible to simplify the poses.

The Alignment Series helps to align your structural system, energize and recharge your muscles, mobilize all body fluids, clear the heart of stagnant emotions, and quiet the mind.

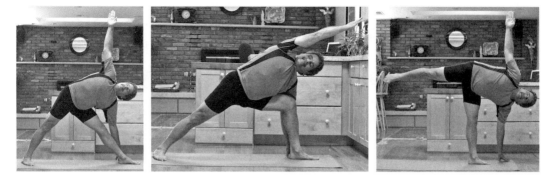

Fig. 4.20: The Triad

The Alignment Series is the best possible way that I have found to prepare yourself and your structural system for the activities of your day. For the most beneficial results, practice the Alignment Series on a daily basis. Once you learn the triad, it only takes a few minutes to practice. Enjoy!

HEALTH TIP #11: Flexibility Techniques

Along with movement and alignment with gravity, flexibility is another characteristic of a healthy neuromusculoskeletal system. Flexibility is the ability of your body to be elastic and flexible, which relates to your neuromusculoskeletal system's ability to recover from trauma. Elasticity specifically refers to the body's ability to bounce back after any form of multidimensional stress.

Children often provide a clear reference point for the normal function of the neuromusculoskeletal system, much of which has been lost in the adult. Young children are especially envied for their elasticity, adaptability, and flexibility.

Fortunately, flexibility can improve without causing injury to the body when the principles of active stretching and exercise are applied. In order to regain some of your inherent flexibility, you must take care not to exceed the active range of motion of your joints. In other words, don't overstretch! You will know when you are overstretching if you elicit any type of pain response, or if your whole body is not consciously engaged in the activity. It is nearly impossible to actively overstretch.

This is particularly hard for Americans, who subscribe to the ideas that "if a little is good, a lot must be better" or "if there's no pain, there's no gain." These perspectives produce a plethora of bad results.

The following flexibility exercises have been extremely helpful in caring for my own structural system and for countless numbers of patients. These are excellent exercises to perform each morning and evening, producing quick and obvious results. Performing these exercises on a regular basis helps to improve both the flexibility and the efficiency of your neuromusculoskeletal system.

As is true with all other alignments and exercises, the absolute essential starting point is to maintain an active awareness. Let the body's Intelligence guide you through these exercises and help you recognize which are of particular benefit for you. Continue to create your own structural health program by feeling the results and taking note of what does and doesn't work for you.

The Twist and Towel Exercise presented in the previous chapter is a great way to improve flexibility. For best results, perform the Twist Exercise first thing in the morning. To prepare your spine for sleep, perform the Twist again in the evening, and include the Towel Exercise.

▇ Wringing Out the Spine

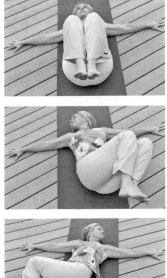

This is another "feel good" exercise that introduces movement into the spine and encourages flexibility. It is especially beneficial for the lower back. Perform this exercise while lying on a carpet or mat as indicted in the illustration.

1. Lie flat on your back with your arms stretched out at your sides for stability. Let the palms of your hands touch the floor.
2. Bend your knees to your chest, and elevate your feet a foot or so above the floor. Maintain the relative position of your knees throughout the exercise.
3. Move your knees as far as you can to one side without straining, and simultaneously turn your head to the opposite side.
4. Return to the original starting point, and repeat the exercise on the other side.

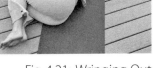

Fig. 4.21: Wringing Out the Spine

Maintain the image of wringing out a towel throughout the exercise, your spine representing the towel. Repeat the exercise several times on each side. If you wish, you may pause for a moment or two with your knees on the floor before proceeding to the other side.

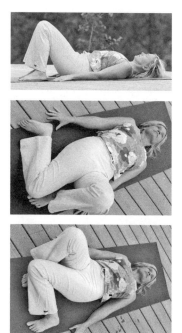

Fig. 4.22: Knee Drops

Knee Drops

Knee Drops are another exercise particularly helpful for the sacrum and the lower back.

1. The exercise is done while lying on your back with your knees bent and your feet flat on the floor. Maintain hip distance between your feet and knees.
2. While in this position, drop your right knee toward the approximate location occupied by your left foot. Return the knee to its starting point, and proceed to drop your left knee to the position of your right foot. It is important to drop your knees: Do not push or force them.
3. Continue to drop one knee, followed by the other, alternating your knees with the location of the opposite foot. This simple yet effective exercise can be performed several times on each side. As in the previous exercise, you may pause on each side for a moment or two for added benefits.

The Cat and the Camel

This yoga warm-up is actually a combination of two different yoga poses: the Cat Stretch and the Camel.

The Cat Stretch has long been utilized to elongate and stretch the spine. If you have a cat, you already should have a good idea about this exercise, as cats usually do this exercise at the beginning of each day. Let your cat show you how to really get into the spirit of this pose.

1. Begin the Cat portion of the stretch by kneeling on all fours, placing your hands directly under your shoulders, and your knees directly under your hips as indicated in the illustration.

2. In this position, slowly let your head drop toward the floor. At the same time, elevate your back and shoulders as high as possible without bending your arms. Hold this position for a brief moment, letting the movement push your breath out as much as possible.

3. As you begin to inhale, move directly into the Camel portion of the exercise. The image of the camel is a bit of stretch, but try to visualize two humps, represented by your hips and shoulders, and a big saddle in the middle of your back. As a camel, let your belly hang down as low as possible while elevating your chin, head, hips, and buttocks. The accompanying illustration will give you the general idea.

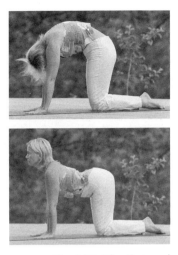

Fig. 4.23: The Cat and the Camel

Your breath is the key to connecting these two postures together. When you are the cat, fully exhale while letting your back rise up and your head and hips descend. As the camel, let the breath rush in to fill your belly and your lungs while you lift your head and hips. The Cat position contracts the spine; the Camel position extends it.

4. To experience a full range of motion throughout your spine, create a back-and-forth motion between the Cat and the Camel. Continue this back-and-forth motion for several repetitions. Use this exercise when you notice restricted movement anywhere in your spine or in your breathing. Take it from your cat: This is an excellent way to start the day.

■ Hip Elevator

This yoga warm-up is great for your whole body and has the same starting position as the Knee Drop Exercise.

1. Begin by lying on your back with your knees bent and your feet flat on the floor.

2. With your feet and knees hip distance apart, elevate your pelvis off the ground as high as possible without straining. In this elevated position, activate your whole body, especially your legs, and relax your neck. Hold this pelvic elevation for at least three controlled breaths.

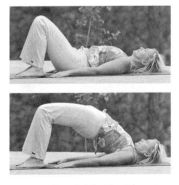

Fig. 4.24: Hip Elevator

3. As shown in the first illustration, slowly let your pelvis down to the floor. Repeat the exercise two or three times. This is an excellent exercise for the spine, pelvis, legs, and shoulders.

▪ Two Psoas Stretches

In an attempt to accommodate various forms of trauma in your lower body, the psoas muscle frequently tightens. This can be evidenced by a short stride length on one side of the body while walking. The psoas muscle is an important stabilizer for the lower back, trunk, and pelvis. The following two psoas-muscle stretches both work very well. If you have an extreme lumbar curve (your buttocks seem to stick out a lot), try the active psoas stretch, which can help reduce your lumbar curve.

THE RUNNER'S STRETCH

1. As indicated in the illustration, this stretch is accomplished by lunging forward with your right leg bent at the knee, keeping your left leg perfectly straight behind you. Align your straight leg with your body and spine, and don't let your knee sag down. Keep your back foot straight—as it will tend to twist—and stand upright on the ball of your foot.

2. Place your hands on the floor, keeping your arms on either side of your front foot. Your hands and arms help with balance and activate your upper body by supporting some of your body weight. Your head is relaxed with your neck in the neutral position.

3. With your right leg forward, you are stretching your left psoas muscle. This is a very active stretch. Hold this stretch for several controlled breaths before gracefully switching legs.

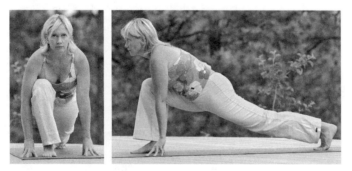

Fig. 4.25: The Runner's Stretch

Yoga Psoas Stretch

This posture is similar to the Runner's Stretch and is great for both the psoas muscle in your back and the gluteus maximus muscle in your buttocks.

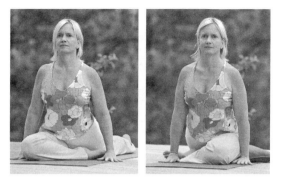

1. Begin the pose by kneeling on all fours.
2. Bring your right knee to the floor between your hands, leaving your right heel a few inches from the crotch of your legs. Sit back a little in this position.

Fig. 4.26: Yoga Stretch with One Pillow

3. Move your left leg straight behind you. The bottom of your foot should face the ceiling. As in the runner's stretch, your arms support some of your body weight and help with balance. Your spine should be as erect as possible in this position.

For many people, it will be necessary to place a small pillow or blanket under the sitting bone of the bent leg. This will help to keep the hips level and reduce the amount of strain on your hip and buttocks muscles. The Psoas Stretch is an active stretch for the psoas muscle on the side of the extended leg, and for the muscles of the buttocks and hip on the bent leg side. Hold the posture for several controlled breaths before switching legs and directions.

■ The Dancer's Stretch

Practiced in the standing position, this is a great side stretch for the entire body.

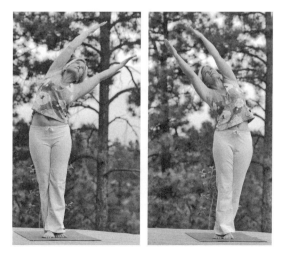

1. Begin the stretch by placing your right foot over your left foot, and bending your body to the right side as far as you can without straining.
2. Complete the stretch by elevating your left forearm directly over the top of your head to a position that is parallel to the floor.

Fig. 4.27: The Dancer's Stretch

3. With the right foot crossed over the left, you will be stretching the left side of your body. Maintain the stretch and a steady breath for 5–10 seconds before proceeding to the opposite side.

Dancers often use this stretch to limber up their spine, legs, and arms prior to movement or exercise. Even if you are not a great dancer, this is a great exercise.

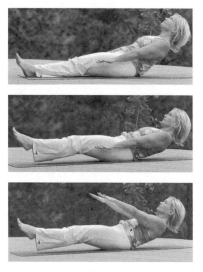

Fig. 4.28: Two the Core #1

Two the Core

The following two exercises activate and strengthen the core muscles of the body that are vital to muscular balance and structural stability.

In the Tuck and Strengthen Exercise, begin each repetition by lying on your back with your arms extended at your sides. There are four distinct steps, which can be followed by looking at the accompanying diagrams.

1. Do a partial sit-up, and remain in this position throughout the first three steps. Your legs remain on the floor while your arms extend and elevate four to six inches, as if you are trying to touch your toes.
2. Now elevate your legs four to six inches off the floor
3. Move your arms up to a 45-degree angle, but hold everything else in the same position.
4. Return to the resting position on the floor.

These four steps can be counted out in a steady cadence and will eventually blend into one continuous movement with four distinct steps. Continue to increase the number of reps until you reach at least fifty sets.

In the Knees to Chest Exercise, lie flat on your back and assume the same position as the first core exercise. Begin each repetition lying flat on the floor. This exercise also has four steps.

1. Bring your knees to your chest, keeping your arms extended four to six inches off the floor.
2. Straighten and elevate your legs until you reach a 90-degree angle to the floor while maintaining the position of your arms.

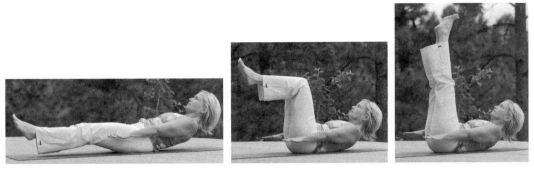

Fig. 4.29: Two the Core #2

3. Return your knees to your chest as in step one of this exercise.
4. Return to the resting position.

Use these two exercises on a daily basis to strengthen your core abdominal muscles. These exercises will help increase your core awareness in all your movements, which anchor all movement patterns. Continue to increase the number of reps until you reach at least 35 sets.

Two Foot Stretches

These are two wonderful exercises for your feet, ankles, and legs. The exercises can be rather painful at first, especially if you have foot or ankle problems, but don't let that stop you. You may need to go very slowly at first, spending only a few moments in each position. Gradually increase the time you spend in each posture.

1. **a.** Begin the first exercise by kneeling on the floor with your buttocks touching the back of your heels (if possible).

    b. Make sure that your feet are as close together as possible and that the bottoms of your feet are facing the ceiling.

    c. Sit back and relax on your heels.

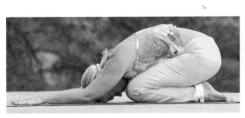

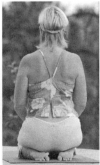

Fig. 4.30: Foot Stretch #1

If this position is painful to your knees, place a small hand towel behind your knee(s). This opens up the joint and helps make this exercise work much better. Breathe during the posture, and activate the muscles in your legs. If possible, spend several controlled breaths in this position. If this posture is still painful, sit back on a pillow to elevate your pelvis until the pain is diminished. Use as large a pillow as you need to eliminate the pain, but smaller is better. Slowly come out of this position, and go right into the next one.

2. The basic position for the second Foot Stretch is the same as the first. This time, however, you will need to tuck your toes under you when sitting back on your heels.

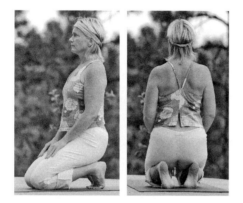

Fig. 4.31: Foot Stretch #2

This stretch can be downright painful after a while, but it provides tremendous results. At first you may be able to spend only a few short moments in this position, but as you keep at it, the stretch will definitely get easier. The work in this position comes from sitting on your heels with your toes tucked and your spine erect. Remember to breathe in this position and to *activate* your legs. Work up to the point where you can hold both stretches for at least 30 seconds each.

HEALTH TIP #12: Energy Exercises

Here is a series of three squatting poses that benefit the body energetically, and that build flexibility and strength. The Energy Exercises also energize the organs of digestion and elimination.

■ The Squat

1. As indicated in the illustration, this exercise is performed by squatting down, keeping your feet flat on the floor and your knees tucked into your

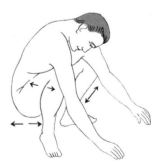

Fig. 4.32: Squat #1

armpits. Your arms are pointing out in front of you, and will actually help with your balance if positioned properly.

Initially, this position may be difficult, but several intermediate steps can be taken until you can assume the full position.

2. If you find it difficult to squat with your feet flat on the floor, you can place a small, rolled towel or sticky mat under your heels.

3. If you cannot balance yourself in this position, you may lean against a wall or hold on to a stable piece of furniture with your hands to stay upright.

4. If you use any of these intermediate steps, keep working to reach the full posture. When you do, the benefits will increase dramatically.

At whatever stage of the posture you find yourself, continue your controlled breathing for 30 seconds. At that point, begin to add a gentle rocking motion to the equation. Begin rocking forward and backward, then side to side. Finally, rock in a small circular motion both clockwise and counterclockwise. Remember to breathe throughout all the movements.

Keep working at the exercise until you have added all the elements: feet flat on the floor, arms straight out in front, and all three of the rocking motions. The benefits of this exercise are absolutely wonderful.

◾ Squat with Wrapped Arms

This is a variation of the Squat, with the additional component of wrapping your arms around your knees as illustrated. For some people this may make the pose much easier.

In the final position of the pose, the same three rocking movements are added.

Another addition includes the action of pushing out against your wrapped arms with both of your knees. This pushing produces creative abdominal tension, which is beneficial for both digestion and elimination. Remember to breathe during the pose, and hold the position for 30 seconds.

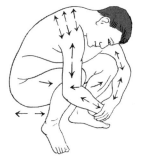

Fig. 4.33: Squat #2

■ The Youthful Pose

This is also a variation of the initial Squat. Your feet are a little wider apart, however, and your toes are slightly wider apart than your heels.

1. Another significant difference involves your elbows, which are placed against the inner knees. To support the weight of your head, your fingers are interlaced, thumbs resting on either side of the bridge of your nose as illustrated.

2. Push your knees inward and your elbows outward to create a dynamic tension. This creative tension engages an entirely different set of muscles, energizes the body, and helps to drain your sinuses.

3. Continue the rocking motion as with the other poses. If you have time for only one energy exercise, this is the one!

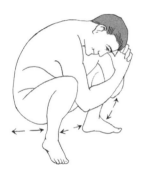

The Energy Exercises are great for preparing yourself and your structural system for the activities of the day. For the most beneficial results, practice all three on a daily basis. Once you learn them, it only takes a few minutes a day to improve your attitude and your structural balance.

Fig. 4.34: The Youthful Pose

Chapter 5

The Care and Feeding of the Human Frame

THE VAST MAJORITY of the physical body is composed of bones, muscles, connective tissue, and joints. It is therefore in our best interest to know how to keep these structures vibrantly healthy and alive.

Throughout this chapter, I provide practical solutions to common structural health problems and important insights to accompany them. These insights offer clues about why these problems occur in the first place, and why they reoccur. Insight facilitates important connections with your multidimensional self, which keeps you looking in the right direction for health. In this way, the idea of wholeness becomes practical.

Bones

Let us begin by taking a practical look at our bones. Our bones serve us in numerous ways: they help support us against the force of gravity, they enable us to be flexible yet strong, they protect important organs from injury, they store our minerals, they create new blood cells, they act as an integral part of our immune system, and they conduct electricity and magnetism throughout the body.

There are 206 bones in the human skeleton, including twenty-two in the skull, three in each middle ear, one in the throat, twenty-six in the spine, thirty-two in each upper extremity, thirty-one in each lower extremity, one sternum bone, and twelve pairs of ribs.

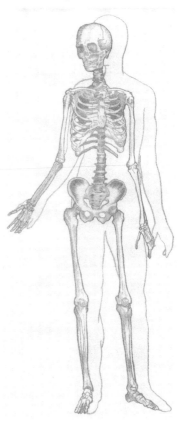

Fig. 5.1: The Skeleton

We have long bones in our arms and legs designed for strength and for the production of both red and white blood cells; short bones in our hands and feet designed to allow for intricate movements; flat bones, like our sternum, scapulae, and skull bones, which produce large amounts of circulating red and white blood cells; and irregular-shaped bones, like the vertebrae in our spines that help support the weight of our body.

Bone is an amazing structure, and although we tend to think of it as hard, dense, and dead, bone is flexible and alive in a living body. Think of the wishbone at your last Thanksgiving Day meal: you had to wait a few days for it to dry out enough before you could make a wish. That is exactly how living bone acts in the human body, or in any body for that matter.

Bone is composed of a tough organic *matrix,* a word derived from the Latin for "mother," which describes the substance inherent in all parts of the body. Compact bone matrix is approximately 25 percent matrix and 75 percent mineral salts. Bone matrix is composed primarily of collagen fibers that provide the tensile strength required for bones to support our body weight and to perform all the extraordinary feats the human body is capable of performing.

Bones are constructed much like reinforced concrete. The collagen fibers contained in bones, tendons, and muscles are similar to the steel rebar that provides concrete's tensile strength. Calcium and other bone salts, which provide compression strength in bone, are similar to the cement, sand, and rock that provide compression strength in concrete. It has been estimated that the strength of bone is superior to even the latest reinforced concrete.

Bones Renew Themselves

Like every other part of the body, living bone constantly renews itself by replacing its old, worn-out parts. If only my car could do this! There are two different types of bone cells involved in this renewal process: osteoclasts, which actually eat old bone, and osteoblasts, which create new bone.

As a side note, every living process has three different components to its function. There is the breaking-down portion, the building-up portion, and the maintaining portion. In relation to bone, the breaking-down portion is accomplished by osteoclasts, which are present in large masses throughout our bone tissue. Masses of osteocytes eat holes in our bones, in an "out with the old, in with the new" sort of process.

As a matter of fact, scientists are discovering that drilling holes in bones actually stimulates new bone growth, and they are utilizing this method in bone repair. It seems to me the best medical technologies are successful when they copy the infinite wisdom of the body. As you will see, these hole-eating bone cells are essential for new bone growth to occur.

The eating process in our bones continues for about three weeks, or until a little tunnel is formed, often as big as a millimeter. At this point, nothing short of a miracle occurs. The Intelligence of the body transforms osteoclasts into osteoblasts on the spot. Osteoblasts immediately begin to fill the tunnel with strong new bone, working for several months to counteract the tunneling of their former selves. Another amazing inside story!

In children, where bone growth is constantly occurring, osteoblasts greatly outnumber osteoclasts. In adults, where bones are already formed and already the right size, maintenance predominates with osteoclasts and osteoblasts, whose activities are about equal. This breaking down and building up of bone is a constant activity that occurs in every bone in our body throughout our entire lifetime.

For the health of our bones, it is important to keep these bone cells happy and healthy. Outside influences like pesticides, radiation, toxic chemicals, and toxic metals interfere with energy flow in the body and consequently interfere with the process of bone renewal and repair. Inside influences like structural misalignments, emotional upsets, mental stress, and physical exhaustion also interfere. These influences can result in myriad bone-related health problems.

HEALTH TIP #1: Eat Whole Foods for Healthy Bones

Provide your bones with the whole food nutrition they need to continue the process of bone repair. Include as many of the following foods as possible: brewer's yeast, wheat germ, black strap molasses, brown rice, whole grains, raw almonds, black walnuts, raw sunflower seeds, eggs, tuna, wild salmon, seafood, organic meat and poultry, whole grains, organic green leafy vegetables, peas, beans, raw dairy products, tofu, onions, garlic, cauliflower, figs, prunes, dates, sesame seeds, grapefruit, oranges, yellow cornmeal, and kelp.

Bone Acts as a Conduit for Electricity and Magnetism

Because the body is responsive to electricity and magnetism, we encounter another phenomenon of particular interest called the piezo-electric effect. The piezo-electric effect describes the way that our body's Intelligence adds new bone to areas that need it the most and removes it from areas that don't.

When the stress load on a bone increases—often due to long-term misalignments—the body builds more compact bone to accommodate for the additional stress load. The Intelligence of body will build up our bones according to the amount of weight that bears down on them.

For example, if a bone is slightly offset after a fracture, our Internal Intelligence actually moves part of the bone to line up directly under the stress.

Conversely, the portion of the bone that is not bearing as much weight will slowly be removed. When a limb is broken and placed in a cast, the opposite limb usually becomes stronger and larger. The broken limb atrophies from little use and a reduced stress load.

This principle became crystal clear when NASA's astronauts first went into space for extended periods of time. Due to the absence of stress on their bones caused by the weightlessness of space, many of the minerals in their bones showed up in their urine bags. When astronauts came back to earth and started walking around again, the density of their bones quickly returned. This not only says a lot about our amazing Internal Intelligence, but it also says a lot about how important movement and exercise are in keeping our bones dense, strong, and healthy.

Positively and negatively charged electrical currents constantly pass through our bones, attracting positively and negatively charged minerals, such as calcium, magnesium, and phosphorus. If these charges are out of balance, a variety of bone conditions can occur, including degenerative arthritis.

It is interesting to note that the electrical current flowing through bones allows osteoblasts to form at the negative end of a current, and osteoclasts to form at the positive end. The Intelligence within our body has the ability to transform the most inert material on earth, rock, into one of the most alive tissues in the human body.

HEALTH TIP #2: Keep Your Structural System in Alignment

Just as reinforced concrete needs to align with the stress load placed upon it, so does our structural system. For optimal results, perform the Alignment Series in chapter 4 at least three times per week, and utilize regular chiropractic care at least on a monthly basis.

Bones Provide a Storage Unit for Minerals

Minerals can be quickly mobilized by the body whenever they are needed anywhere in the body. If there is a lack of minerals in our tissues, the body will mobilize calcium and other minerals from our bones and move them into our tissues as needed. Problems arise when we are unable to utilize the minerals from our foods and return them to our bones. The pH of the body is perhaps the single most important factor for this process to be successful.

As you may know, pH relates to the acid/alkaline balance of a substance. In the body, pH is also a measure of electrical activity. The pH scale runs from 0–14, with 0 being the most acidic, 7 being neutral, and 14 being the most alkaline. The ideal pH of human blood is 7.4. The ideal pH of water is 7.

Numerous problems arise throughout the body when the pH fluctuates in either direction. This is especially true for our bones. Unfortunately, these fluctuations occur on a regular basis due to the acids that are produced by the body, and by our predominately acid-producing diets.

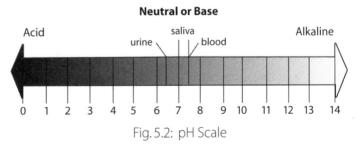

Fig. 5.2: pH Scale

Today's diet consists primarily of acid-forming foods, which can really swing the pH into the acid zone. In my opinion, this acidic condition is a major precursor for all degenerative disease.

In fact, an overly acidic condition in the body can be the key factor for a host of dis-ease conditions. Some of the surprising symptoms of acidity in the body include the following: decreased bone density, as in osteoporosis; predisposition to bone fractures and arthritis; fatigue, muscle pain or weakness, loss of muscle mass; cramping, restrictions in breathing, loss of breath; bloating of the stomach; difficulty of movement, joint stiffness upon rising; excessive sighing, insomnia, and difficulty in holding one's breath. If these symptoms are left unresolved, they may lead to degenerative diseases such as diabetes, heart disease, and possibly cancer. Excessive acidity in the system is a major obstacle to creating vibrant health and should be monitored on a regular basis.

The pH of blood is difficult for the average person to test, and the slightest variation is extremely significant. Fortunately, the pH of saliva is similar to that of blood and is easily tested. Nitrozine paper, or pH sticks, can be obtained at your local drugstore.

The pH of urine is also a good indicator of acid/alkaline balance, and can also be tested with pH paper. The normal pH of urine is 6.4. Anything lower indicates the need for a more alkaline diet.

Surprisingly enough, checking your ability to hold your breath can give you a quick indication of your pH. In most cases, difficulty holding the breath more than 20 seconds is indicative of an overly acidic condition.

Some researchers suggest that the normal pH of saliva is 7.4, others say it's between 6.5 and 7.0. I find that anything below 7 is too acidic. I mentioned earlier that water pH is normally 7.0. If you check your tap water you may find it far below 7, and more in the 5+ range. Filtering it usually improves the situation. Make sure you are drinking sufficient amounts of water, and that it is pH-balanced and free of harmful chemicals, such as chlorine and fluoride. More details about water later.

A more complete list of acid offenders is located in appendix B, but the short list includes all meats, poultry, and fish; all cheeses, especially the sharp ones; popcorn and most condiments; most grains, including rice; alcoholic drinks, coffee, and soft drinks.

A short list of alkaline foods begins and ends with vegetables and fruits; grains such as millet, quinoa, amaranth, and flax; and walnuts, almonds, eggs, and plain yogurt. The short list may help, but make a copy of the full list in appendix B to put on your refrigerator.

The ideal pH balanced diet contains 75 percent alkaline-forming foods and 25 percent acid-forming foods. The idea here is not to avoid acidic foods completely, but to balance them over the course of a few days. Eat protein one meal, and follow it with veggies and salads for the next two meals. Drink coffee one day, and follow it with fruit juices or smoothies for a few days. If you consistently experience any of the symptoms mentioned earlier, it indicates the need for a prolonged alkaline diet. When your acid/alkaline balance comes within the normal range, the Intelligence of your body will shut off your symptoms, and your ability to hold your breath will increase.

HEALTH TIP #3: Check Your pH on a Regular Basis

Using pH sticks, nitrozine paper, or Hydrion test strips, make sure the pH scale you use spans from 5.0 to 7.5. After you discover what's going on with you pH, a weekly check will be sufficient. Just touch the paper or stick to your tongue and compare it to the scale on the package. It is more accurate to take at least eight pH readings. To determine your average pH, divide the total pH numbers by the number of tests you take. To help balance your pH, utilize the acid/alkaline diet sheets in appendix B and the nutritional products in appendix A. For best results, check your pH first thing in the morning before eating or drinking. It would also be interesting to check your pH when you are feeling under the weather and compare it to your normal pH value.

Time your ability to hold your breath, and continue timing it as you change to a more alkaline diet. Keep track of how it improves as your pH normalizes. Avoid sodas and soft drinks that leach calcium from your bones!

Bone Salts are Crystals

Bone salts are an integral component of bones, and are primarily composed of crystals. That's right, our bones are made of crystals! These tiny crystals measure some 200–400 angstrom units. An angstrom unit is used to measure wavelengths of small objects, and represents one ten-billionth of a meter—these are very small crystals.

Bone salt crystals are mostly composed of calcium and phosphorus and are shaped like a long, flat dinner plate. Other salts like magnesium, sodium, potassium, and carbonate ions are attracted to and absorbed on the surface of these crystal plates to add strength to our bones.

Unfortunately, this attraction also presents a major problem whenever radioactive materials or toxic metals are present in the surrounding environment, as they too become attracted to the surface plates of our bone crystals.

Frequent contact with substances in our environment like strontium, uranium, lead, gold, mercury, or other common heavy metals allows them to become part of our bone structure. Toxic metal poisoning initiates many environmental sensitivities, and can result in a permanently weakened immune system and myriad modern-day disease processes.

Heavy metal toxicity is much more common than one might imagine. In my practice I find a large percentage of my patients have at least some level of heavy metal poisoning. A variety of sources for these metals includes our water, food, salt, galvanized or copper pipes in our homes, aluminum cookware, tin or aluminum cans, synthetic vitamin and mineral supplements, outdated dental procedures, and a host of other common sources. See chapter 9 for a list of toxic metals and their abundant sources.

These foreign metals have a strong attraction to our bones, more so than many of the important salts normally found in bone tissue. Toxic metals also lodge themselves in organs, such as the kidney or liver, and can cause permanent weaknesses and chronic disease in many body systems.

HEALTH TIP #4: Have Your Toxic Metal Load Evaluated

Have your toxic metal load evaluated by a chiropractor or other health care practitioner trained in toxic metal testing. Testing can be done by hair analysis or through muscle testing procedures. Finding toxic metals in the body is only half of the problem; finding a healthy way to remove them is the other half. Removing toxic metals incorrectly can cause more complications than leaving them alone. Look to chapter 7 for more details on how to handle toxic metals.

Bones and the Immune System

The hollow core of long bones provides an efficient production site for a wide variety of white blood cells, which compose an essential part of our immune system by attacking and neutralizing foreign invaders in the body. White blood cells are responsible for our white blood count, which, when elevated on a blood test, indicates that our body's Intelligence is waging a war somewhere in the body. Medically, an elevated white blood cell count is an indication of infection.

The hollow core of long bones is also a manufacturing site for new red blood cells. These red blood cells carry the vital component of oxygen to each cell and carry away the acid waste-product carbon dioxide. More functions of the red blood cell are included in chapter 8 on the cardiovascular system.

HEALTH TIP #5: Build a Healthier Immune System

Basically, whatever level of immune system health you are currently experiencing isn't good enough. In today's environment, you need to stay one step ahead of the next wave of bacterial and viral mutations. Chapter 7 on the immune system indicates what you can do now to build superimmunity and prevent problems in the future.

The exercises offered in chapter 4 will help to strengthen your bones and improve the circulation of red blood cells to your bones and joints. These exercises are a great way to keep your bones healthy and alive.

Other Bone-Related Factors

As we will see in chapter 6, the endocrine system has a major influence on mineral balance throughout the body. The endocrine system directs hormones to conserve and balance our water and mineral levels, which has an immediate effect on the health of our bones.

Today, hormone replacement therapy is viewed as the answer in our society to the ever-expanding problem of loss of bone density. Hormone replacement therapy causes a plethora of serious side effects and is only marginally effective.

Hormones do prevent bone loss. The problem is that some hormones also prevent osteoclasts from breaking down our bone tissue, which we know is an essential part of the bone repair process. If these little guys cannot break down our bones, osteoblasts cannot rebuild them; the result is brittle bones that break at the drop of a hat. This condition is now running rampant throughout our elder communities. As you will see in chapter 7, another reason for brittle bones is fluoride, which is added to our water source.

Sunlight is another necessary component for healthy bones. In the presence of vitamin D (sunlight), our bones and teeth absorb calcium and phosphorus according to the demands placed on the body. Getting at least a half hour a day of sunlight is as important to your bones as taking a calcium or magnesium supplement.

Exercise is another essential component of healthy bones, and it works because it is a healthy stressor to the body. The body will build up our muscles in response to that stress. Up to a point, bones creatively respond to stress, but there is a necessary interplay between exercise and rest, which allows the body and its bones enough time to recuperate.

Many people make the mistake of overexercising or overstressing the body—bones and all—every day. Since exercise essentially breaks down the body, overexercising never gives bones and soft tissue an opportunity to rebuild themselves. Make sure to give your body the rest it needs by using this formula: Exercise one day, rest the next.

You can keep bones healthy by mineralizing the body on a daily basis. Bones like to assimilate minerals in certain forms, and human beings need plants to transform minerals from rocks into a form that we can utilize. For this reason, it is important to take organic mineral supplements from whole food sources, as minerals that have been transformed by plants are much more effectively utilized in to the body. Please avoid synthetic nutritional supplements!

HEALTH TIP #6: Exercise and Move Your Body

Exercise and move your body every other day. If you want to get outside every day, go for a walk or short bike ride. Explore a combination of several different types of exercise in order to vary the type of stress your body experiences. Explore movements such as dance, yoga, or Tai Chi, which involve more of your multidimensional being. Also remember to include the flexibility series in chapter 4.

HEALTH TIP #7: Take Whole Food Vitamin and Mineral Supplements

Take whole food vitamin and mineral supplements on a daily basis, but make certain they are not synthetically manufactured. Synthetic vitamins and minerals can adversely affect your bones and compromise other areas of your body. Sources for whole food vitamins and mineral supplements are listed in appendix A.

Whole food vitamins for bones include vitamins B, C, D, vitamin F/essential fatty acids, and are responsible for mobilizing calcium from your tissues and into your cells. Vitamin T, contained in tahini and sesame oil, is an important nutrient to allow for continued production of red and white blood cells.

Organic minerals for bones include absorbable calcium, preferably calcium lactate or citrate; sufficient amounts of magnesium; phosphorus; natural iron from natural sources, such as red meat, poultry, salmon, tuna, and spinach. Most sources of iron are inorganic metals, which are not readily absorbable and therefore toxic to the body. You may also want to include a nontoxic bonemeal supplement, such as the one I use in my breakfast drink. See page 214 for my breakfast drink recipe.

Muscles

Our body flesh is composed primarily of muscles, over 625 pairs of them, which act together as one functional unit. The contraction and relaxation action of our muscular system actually helps us integrate all the separate functions of the body.

Muscles not only allow us to move, but they reflect the state of corresponding internal organs. If a muscle is weak, for example, it may be due to weakness of corresponding internal organs, which are also muscles. Muscle action helps us move waste products out of our tissues and into our elimination system, and facilitates breathing by contracting our ribs and expanding our lungs. Muscle contraction and relaxation even helps us to express our feelings, which are written all over our faces.

There are three distinct layers of muscles in the body that get connected by a thin layer of fibrous tissue called fascia. Muscle fibers in these layers usually run in opposing directions, allowing for movement to take place in every possible direction. Our muscular system is truly a work of art.

Fascia allows these layers of muscle to glide over each other, creating a beautiful array of intricate movements coordinated by the brain and nerve system.

These three layers also contribute to an overall support system, consistent with the tensegrity model outlined in the previous chapter, that helps maintain the upright integrity of our spine and our skeleton.

Tensegrity is particularly evident in the trunk of the body, which is responsible for maintaining our upright integrity and the lumbar curve in the lower spine. When activated, all the layers of our abdominal muscles, back muscles, and muscles along our sides contribute to the appealing curvature of the waist, the absence of which indicates weakened muscles and an unsupported spine.

The abdominal muscles assist the body with exhalation, and work in tandem with the diaphragm, which is one of the primary muscles of respiration.

Gait Patterns

An important mechanism in the body that integrates much of our movement patterns is called the gait mechanism. Gait mechanics help to organize groups of muscles to move and function together. Gait literally means our manner and style of walking. Medically, there are different types of gait patterns according to a variety of disabilities. You may be familiar with gait patterns related to horses, such as a gallop or trot. Understanding the importance of gait patterns in the human body gives us insight and information about how effectively our muscular system is integrated.

Whenever we move, muscle action needs to be coordinated throughout the entire body. In order for a muscle to turn on or contract, the opposing muscle needs to be shut off or relaxed in order to allow room for movement to occur. The more refined our movements, the more complicated the process.

A simple example is demonstrated by flexing your arm. In order for your arm to flex (your hand moves toward your shoulder), the biceps muscle in the front of your arm needs to contract or get shorter. At the same time, the triceps muscle on the back of your upper arm must be turned off so it can lengthen. As you flex, use your free hand to feel your relaxed triceps and your contracted biceps muscles.

This pattern of turning muscles on and off is true for individual muscles and for groups of muscles as well. The muscle patterns involved in getting up from a chair while reaching for something on a shelf are amazingly complex. Imagine the complex movements necessary for playing basketball!

Thankfully, the coordination for switching muscles on and off is under the control of our lightening fast nerve system. In turn, the nerve system utilizes information from movement sensors located in every muscle of the body. Healthy muscles are essential for these sensors to work properly and for harmonious movement patterns.

A simple movement pattern involving large muscle groups is demonstrated in walking. As we take a step with our right leg, our left arm swings forward automatically, and the muscles on the front of the body for both muscle groups contract and shorten. At the same instant, the muscles in the back of the right arm and left leg are inhibited in order to lengthen and create space for the movement of walking to occur. Because muscles are attached to bones, the whole body moves forward.

Normal gait patterns involve muscle groups from the top of our heads to the bottoms of our feet. Our muscles usually act with such amazing grace and coordination: When they are working properly, these switching movements are undetectable.

As it turns out, a large portion of the switching mechanism for these coordinated actions is located in our feet. If structural interference occurs either in our feet, our spine, or in the cerebellum of our brain, our gait mechanism can be significantly altered, which is indicative of confusion, disorganization, and dysfunction in the nerve and muscular systems.

HEALTH TIP #8: Use Range of Motion Exercises and Foot Exercises

Use the ROME series outlined in chapter 4 to evaluate and improve the function of your feet. Regular use of the Cross Crawl Exercise, located in chapter 3, will help to coordinate muscle action throughout the body. To improve the stability of your feet, use this powerful foot stability exercise. The Foot Stability Exercise is performed while standing barefoot, your arms hanging comfortably at your sides.

Stand near a wall or strong railing, as you may initially need help with your balance. Try to keep the arches of your feet in a neutral position. Slowly shift your weight to your right leg, and then bend the left leg slightly at the knee so that you

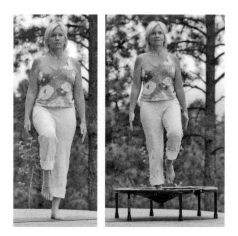

Fig. 5.3: The Foot Stability Exercise

are now standing on one leg. Notice how your right foot is now moving rapidly in several directions just to keep you standing.

The quick small movements that you are seeing in your foot is the Foot Stability Exercise you are looking for. This exercise strengthens the small stabilizing muscles in the foot and lower leg, and most forms of exercise ignore them. To insure foot and ankle stability, these small muscles need to be energized and strong. If your foot is wobbling a lot in this stage, it indicates that you need this exercise on a daily basis to stabilize your feet. Perform the exercise on both feet for 15–30 seconds before moving on to phase two.

Phase two incorporates the exact same exercise, only this time close your eyes. Holding on for stability may be a real necessity here. Notice how much more movement there is in your foot now that your eyes are not helping you with balance. This exercise increases the strength and stability of the feet, ankles, and knees. If you can, do this exercise for at least 15 seconds on each side.

For phase three, perform the same exercise on a mini trampoline. Try it first with your eyes open, and then with your eyes closed. *Make sure you have mastered phases one and two of this exercise before you attempt phase three.* When using a mini tramp, keep it close to a wall for stability. I also find it better to wear athletic shoes rather than go barefoot while on the trampoline.

The Stretch Reflex

There are several aspects of muscle function that have enormous practical value. The stretch reflex in the body is one of those aspects. Throughout the body, reflexes generally represent the interface between the nerve and muscular systems. Reflexes have been used in health care to evaluate the health of our nerve system, and are a normal part of an extensive system of automatic nerve system responses.

We are most likely familiar with the withdrawal reflex, triggered when we inadvertently touch a hot stove. In order to avoid injury, this involuntary reflex is designed to quickly pull the involved body part away from the source of pain. The reflex is accomplished without any conscious effort or control on our part, and usually occurs before we even realize what has happened. The knee-jerk reflex is another familiar example.

Reflexes have what is called an all-or-none response, and provide an example of how muscle contraction works. Before we even know it, our Internal Intelligence has taken over, specific muscle groups have contracted, and our body is out of danger. Many reflexes happen on a regular basis without our awareness and certainly without our consent.

The stretch reflex acts as an internal braking system for a muscle when rapid changes in muscle length occur. Like other reflexes, the stretch reflex helps to keep the muscle from being damaged. The stretch reflex keeps us from tearing muscle fibers completely away from the bone. Gradual stretching of a muscle elicits a mild form of the stretch reflex, while sudden stretching elicits a strong muscle-stretch reflex.

When a muscle is stretched suddenly, a specialized muscle cell—called a spindle cell—is activated. This spindle-shaped muscle cell is a sensor for changes in muscle length. Spindle cells trigger the stretch reflex, which shuts down the action of related muscle groups.

The stretch reflex indicates two important things in relationship to our health. The stretch reflex is not only an indicator of the health of our muscular system; it also indicates the level of stress that is present in the body, notably in the function of the adrenal glands.

Instead of the stretch reflex being triggered by the presence of a potentially damaging situation, the stretch reflex often gets triggered by normal muscular actions, such as passive stretching. When this occurs, the body shuts down the function of some of the muscle groups that we were hoping to improve. It is an unfortunate reality that overstretching, which is often the result of passive stretching, activates the stretch reflex and sets us up for injury. For that reason, many top-level running authorities are now suggesting that runners stretch after they run.

The stretch reflex also relates to the overall accumulation of stress in the body. In my office, I often use the stretch or stress reflex to evaluate the health of the adrenal glands. A simple use of the reflex will immediately reveal overstressed adrenal glands. Chiropractors across the country have found adrenal stress to be present in over 75 percent of their patients.

HEALTH TIP #9: Utilize the Principles of Active Stretching

As outlined in the previous chapter, active stretching prevents the stretch reflex from weakening muscles that can set you up for injury.

HEALTH TIP #10: Evaluate the Function of Your Adrenal Glands

Try to think of your adrenal glands as indicators of how well your body is handling the stress created by your lifestyle. You can also utilize the information provided in chapter 6 to create healthy adrenal glands. If you are currently a chiropractic patient, have your chiropractor evaluate the function of your adrenals. This may be the most important test you can ever take.

Trigger Points

Under normal circumstances, muscles receive instructions from the nerve system before they contract. When they contract, muscles are governed by a principle called the all-or-none effect. If a nerve impulse is strong enough, the entire muscle will fire. This same principle is true for nerves as well.

Frequently, a muscle develops what are called trigger points, which are located in a muscle at the point where the nerve and muscle fibers meet. The trigger point is actually a buildup of muscle toxins at the junction that gradually increases in size, reaching a point where it causes pain and begins to trigger the contraction of the muscle without the approval of the nerve system. Trigger points are usually found in muscles that have been overused or injured, or they occur in a nerve system that has been compromised by the presence of spinal misalignments.

HEALTH TIP #11: Treat Your Trigger Points

Use the Muscle Trigger Point Chart to treat your own trigger points, or better yet, have someone stimulate them for you. Trigger points can be released by holding

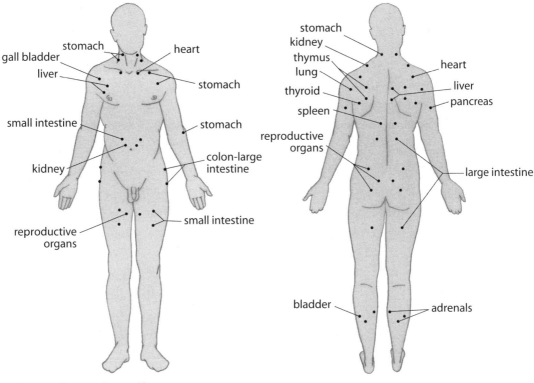

Fig. 5.4: Trigger Point Chart

fairly consistent pressure, about 5–10 pounds as indicated on a bathroom scale. Hold each point for 15–30 seconds if possible. You can use your thumb, a therapeutic massager, or a tennis ball to reduce them in size. Try not to overtreat your trigger points, and only work a few points during the same session. The Stick is specifically designed to release trigger points, and you can get more details about it in appendix A.

After just one or two sessions, your trigger points will be noticeably less tender, and the related areas of muscle will also be less painful. If painful or sensitive trigger points persist, you will most likely need the related areas of your spine aligned by a doctor of chiropractic.

Research has shown that trigger points have a nutritional component that relates to a deficiency of vitamin B12 and folic acid. If trigger points are commonplace for you, check the resources for B12 and folic acid in appendix A.

Muscle Cells

There are several different kinds of muscle cells in the body, most of which are designed to contract or shorten muscles. Each muscle is composed of thousands of muscle cells called muscle fibers, which are controlled by a single nerve and bound together by connective tissue in units.

Besides the scant sensory receptors for pain and deep pressure in the muscle, each skeletal muscle has an abundance of two special receptors called muscle spindle cells, and Golgi tendon organs (GTOs). Spindle cells detect the length of a muscle and are primarily located in the muscle belly. Golgi tendon organs, on the other hand, are designed to detect muscle tension and are located at both ends of muscle tendons. Golgi tendon organs complement the action of spindle cells; if the spindle cell acts as the gas, the GTO is the brake.

GTOs in a tendon are arranged in a series of folds that unravel as the tension on a muscle increases. There is one GTO for approximately every ten to fifteen muscle fibers. The GTO is also a protective mechanism that keeps us from damaging our muscles. When tension on a muscle increases, GTOs activate, slowing down muscle contraction. If it were not for the GTOs, we could easily tear a muscle right off the bone.

It is our GTOs that allow our muscles to act smoothly, whether we are carrying an empty glass or a bowling ball, and to achieve the grace and beauty of movement that characterize the human body.

When an infant is developing motor skills, they can appear awkward, hitting themselves in the head while trying to get something into their mouths.

At this particular developmental stage, their nerve system is setting the normal limits for spindle cell and GTO function. We all are very uncoordinated until our body learns how to get the movement patterns right. And when we do, our movements become simple and automatic.

With practice, some arm wrestlers can actually override the GTO mechanism to improve their technique. When a muscle finally does give out during a match, it is not unusual for a muscle to completely tear from the bone or, in some cases, to break the bone itself.

HEALTH TIP #12: Improve the Function of Painful Muscles

Utilize these two simple techniques to improve the function of tender or painful muscles.

a. Locate the ends of the muscle, where the muscle attaches to the bone, using an anatomy book if needed. If this area is involved, there will be tenderness or pain. Massage the area with 5–10 pounds of deep pressure at the attachment points, using your thumb and fingertips for 30–60 seconds.

b. Locate the belly or middle of the muscle, and search for any areas of pain or discomfort. Contact the belly of the muscle using a broader finger contact, and massage the tender area across the muscle belly. The Stick, a tennis ball, or an electric massager can also be used.

Muscle-Organ Relationships

Another practical aspect of muscles is their direct relationship to our organs. In applied kinesiology, for instance, every major muscle corresponds to a specific organ. When that organ is in a weakened state, the associated muscles will be weak as a consequence.

Let's use the adrenal glands as an example. When the adrenal glands are in a weakened state, muscles that stabilize the knee and support the arch of the foot demonstrate significant weakness when tested. Conversely, when the adrenal glands are strengthened, the muscles supporting the knee strengthen, along with those associated with the arch of the foot.

The correction is much more than simply exercising a weak muscle; as a matter of fact, if an organ weakness is present, exercising the associated weak muscle will have little or no beneficial effect until the problem in the organ is resolved.

An organ-muscle relationship chart is included in Health Tip #13 below. This chart is a valuable means of connecting organ weakness with muscle dysfunction and pain. If you know the location of a weakened organ, which is usually indicated by your symptoms, you can begin to strengthen that organ and the associated muscles at the same time. Organ-muscle relationships are directly associated with acupuncture meridians and often include more then one muscle.

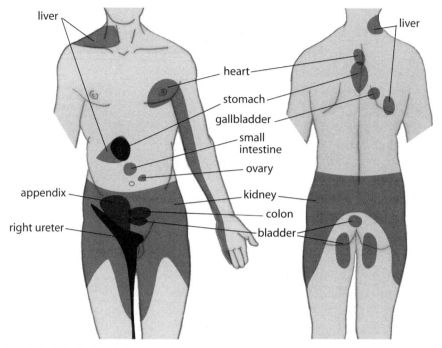

Fig. 5.5: Pain Referral Chart

I also include here a pain referral chart showing the location of pain and its related organs. These two charts are very helpful in tracking down suspected weaknesses in our organ systems, which should be a major concern in your health care endeavors.

HEALTH TIP #13: Use the Muscle-Organ Relationship & the Pain Referral Charts

Both charts are invaluable in correlating common muscle and body pains to specific organs.

■ Aerobic and Anaerobic Muscles

Another characteristic of muscle contraction is a muscle's ability to twitch. This twitch can be initiated by small electrical impulses either from within the body or from an external electrical source.

There are two basic types of twitches that muscles elicit: isotonic and isometric. Isotonic twitches are those that make a muscle twitch fast, while isometric twitches make a muscle twitch slower.

Slow-twitching muscles help to stabilize our movements, while fast-twitching muscles are the muscles that make us move. Fast-twitch muscles are classically smaller in size (like those in the eye), and contract or twitch at a rate of 1/100th of a second. Slow-twitch muscles are usually larger (like the stabilizer muscles in the lower leg), and twitch at a rate of 1/10th of a second.

Organ	Muscle	Acup. Meridian
Pituitary	Upper Trapezius	Kidney
Thyroid	Teres Minor	Triple Warmer
Thymus	Infraspinatus	Triple Warmer
Heart	Subscapularis	Heart
Lung	Deltoid	Lung
Pancreas	Triceps (blood sugar)	Spleen/Pancreas
	Latissimus Dorsi (digestion)	Spleen/Pancreas
Stomach	Pertoralis Major Clavicular	Stomach
Liver	Pertoralis Major Sternal	Liver
Gall bladder	Popleteus	Gall Bladder
Spleen	Lower Trapezius	Spleen/Pancreas
Adrenal Cortex	Gracillis (parasympathetic)	Circulation/Sex
Adrenal Medulla	Sartorius (sympathetic)	Circulation/Sex
Small intestine	Quadraceps, Abdominals	Small Intestine
Colon	Tensor Fascia Lata	Large Intestine
Ileo cecal valve	Iliacus	Kidney
Kidney	Psoas	Kidney
Ovaries/Testes	Piriformis	Circulation/Sex
Uterus/Prostate	Gluteus Medius	Circulation/Sex

Fig. 5.6: Muscle-Organ Relationship Chart

Although most muscles are capable of both types of twitches, they usually have a predominance of either fast- or slow-twitch muscle fibers. The type of twitching that is present in a muscle is determined by its function in the body, and is yet another example of how structure follows function.

Oddly enough, both types of muscles also relate to our Thanksgiving dinner. Fast-twitch fibers that allow for quick movements relate to the white meat of the turkey. These muscles are less elastic, more dense, fatigue quickly, and require large glycogen (sugar) storage within the muscle. These muscles are also referred to as anaerobic muscles and are primarily located in the upper extremities of the body.

Anaerobic refers to the ability of muscles to function without oxygen, and to their primary dependence on sugar metabolism, which requires sufficient quantities of the B vitamin pantothenic acid. Anaerobic muscles contract or twitch rapidly but are less able to sustain that contraction for a long time.

Aerobic, isometric, or slow-twitch muscles, on the other hand, relate to the dark meat of the turkey. They are much more elastic in nature, are more capable of sustaining a muscle contraction, and depend on oxidation of fats for their fuel. To sustain their function, aerobic muscles require sufficient quantities of the mineral iron, which is necessary for endurance. Slow-twitch aerobic muscles are primarily located in the lower extremities of the body.

For optimal muscle function to occur, both isometric/aerobic/slow-twitch muscles and isotonic/anaerobic/fast-twitch muscles require essential fatty acids (high-quality fats) in sufficient quantities. Aerobic and anaerobic muscle problems are suspected when a person is initially able to perform at the desired level but is unable to repeat the performance a second or third time. Fatigue, weakness, or cramping at the end of the day is also a possible indication of aerobic/anaerobic dysfunction.

HEALTH TIP #14: Use High-Quality Essential Fatty Acids

To improve aerobic and anaerobic muscle function, EFAs should be an essential component in any health or exercise program. The B vitamin pantothenic acid is recommended when quick movements of the upper extremities are found to be lacking, and an absorbable form of iron is recommended when low endurance or fatigue results from reduced amounts of energy and/or oxygen in the legs. Sources for all muscle-related supplements are listed in appendix A.

Neurolymphatic Treatment Points

As the name suggests, neurolymphatic treatment points allow a person access to the connection between the nerve and lymphatic systems. These valuable points allow us to effectively assist lymphatic drainage in a muscle, which greatly assists muscle function and repair.

Rubbing a tender neurolymphatic reflex point has an immediate strengthening effect on its associated muscle. When tenderness exists in these points, it is assumed that the lymphatic system related to that muscle is not performing its job of removing the waste products of normal muscle activity. Stimulating these tender points helps the lymph system to drain these waste products and quickly strengthen a weakened muscle. A chart of the neurolymphatic reflex points is included below.

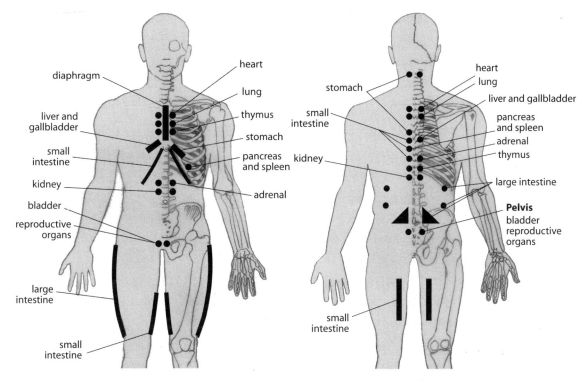

Fig. 5.7: Neurolymphatic Reflex Chart

Muscles and Feelings

Every part of the body works like a hologram by representing the condition of the body as a whole. This is especially evident throughout our musculoskeletal system, our posture, and in our muscles of facial expression.

Think about how intricately our neuromusculoskeletal system must be designed to be able to express our every feeling, not only with our posture but also with our muscles of facial expression. In working with patients for over thirty years, I have found the information projected by the muscles of facial expression to be extremely telling about the inner state of a person.

Whether we like it or not, our inner state of depression, sadness, resentment, hatred, happiness, joy, or contentment is written all over our faces.

Connective Tissue

Connective tissue comprises a vast portion of the human body and includes fascia, ligaments, tendons, cartilage, and bone. Cartilage, which is translucent elastic tissue, is present in large amounts, especially throughout a developing skeleton. With the exception of our joints, cartilage changes to bone in the adult skeleton.

Ligaments are composed of strong fibrous tissue that stretches very little and connects bones together. Tendons are strong, white, glistening bands of inelastic fibers that attach muscles to bone.

Fascia is the most amazing tissue in the body and varies in thickness according to the body's functional needs. In its most common form, it is like a thick membrane unifying all muscle function throughout the body. Fascia separates muscles and sections of muscles, allowing them to glide through a membranous sheath as they contract. Fascia is one continuous sheet throughout the body and acts like a slipcover for muscle contraction. Fascia is also a major conductor of electricity throughout the body.

HEALTH TIP #15: Support Your Connective Tissue Nutritionally

Nutritional support for connective tissue includes the following: a high-quality veal bone supplement that is free of toxic chemicals and metals; a nutritional connective tissue support; a full spectrum amino acid; a multiple mineral support; and special nutrients for ligament function and repair. If inflammation is present in a muscle or joint, you can also utilize proteolytic enzymes between meals, as a safe anti-inflammatory agent, and an essential fatty acid supplement. All sources for nutritional supplements are listed in appendix A.

Joints

In my clinical experience I have found that structural alignment is perhaps the most important factor in maintaining healthy joints. When misalignment occurs in a joint, it is just a matter of time before the joint begins to degenerate and wear out.

Degeneration in a joint occurs when a joint in a misaligned state is unable to properly handle the structural forces that bear upon it. Degeneration occurs naturally when the body alters a joint to become more effectively aligned with abnormal weight-bearing stress patterns, utilizing the piezo-electric effect.

The second most important factor in maintaining healthy joints is the nutritional component, which is the same for connective tissue and joints listed in health tip #15.

Feet and Ankles

Let's take a look at the joints of our extremities and employ some simple methods that will improve their function. We can start with the foundation for the entire structural system of the body, our feet. The structural integrity of our feet is a vital part of our overall health. Our feet are the foundation for the entire body, and they are related to our "under-standing."

The foot is an engineering marvel. Each foot has twenty-six bones that are designed to function like a suspension bridge, and they fit together like a puzzle ring. The heel bone is the largest of these bones and composes the rear portion of the ankle joint, which supports 25 percent of the body's weight on each side. The ball of the foot is the toe side of the suspension bridge, and it bears the other 25 percent of body weight for each leg.

There are actually three arches in the foot that include numerous ligaments to hold the bones of the foot together. The fact that there are so many different components to the function of the foot is the very thing that allows it to be so flexible. Hundreds of ligaments combine functions to support the bones and joints of our feet.

The arches of the foot can support up to 5,000 pounds per square inch of pressure—which is the amount of weight that can come to bear on the foot when running—as these arches also act as shock absorbers for the body. When the arches fall, the entire structure of the body can become unstable, causing a wide variety of structural problems. In the course of a normal lifetime, the average foot travels over 90,000 miles, or three-and-a-half times around the earth. Now that's a long walk!

Healthy, functioning feet are one of the most important factors in maintaining structural health. In my clinical experience, I have found that a majority of people, especially those with chronic health problems, have foot instability problems. If the arches of the feet have collapsed or fallen, other areas of the body will soon follow suit.

HEALTH TIP #16: Support Your Feet

■ Orthotics

The need for arch support is usually obvious, as we often become tired on our feet, constantly lean on structures like walls or chairs, shift our weight from one leg to the other, or frequently need to sit down to take the weight off our feet.

Utilizing orthotics may be as simple as going to your local shoe store to get sized for the right generic foot supports, or as complicated as being casted for orthotics by a chiropractor or podiatrist. When they are necessary, and that may involve 50 percent of the population, orthotics make a huge difference in maintaining structural stability for the entire body. Appendix A contains a list of choices for effective, inexpensive orthotics that can be purchased at your local shoe store. Expensive orthotics are not necessarily better.

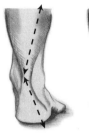 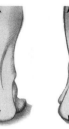

Pronated   Neutral   Supinated

Fig. 5.8: Pronation, Supination, and Normal Foot

An even better solution to foot pronation problems is to strengthen the function of weakened muscles of the foot using specific exercises and the art of applied kinesiology (AK). A doctor of chiropractic trained in AK procedures is usually able to find the cause of weakened foot stability muscles and correct them. When foot stability is restored, the arches commonly return and orthotics may not be necessary at all. Look to appendix A for the contacts for applied kinesiology practitioners.

■ The Three-Way Foot and Ankle Exercise

The Three-Way Foot and Ankle Exercise is an excellent foot, ankle, and knee strengthener, and entails the use of a theraciser (a simple device with a rubber tube and velcro attachment straps). The theraciser greatly assists in the performance of exercises to improve the strength and stability of the foot and ankles. Stretchable rubber tubing can also be used.

If foot, ankle, or knee instability is a problem, this is the exercise for you. Attach one end of the theraciser around the leg of a chair, railing, or stable anchor, and

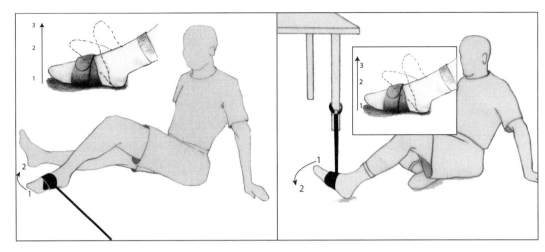

Fig. 5.9: Three-Way Foot and Ankle Exercise #1

Fig. 5.10: Three-Way Foot and Ankle Exercise #2

the other end securely around your foot and ankle. This allows you to use the resistance of the rubber tube to strengthen the full range of motion of your foot and ankle. Move your body as illustrated to allow you to exercise in all three directions. Anchor your heel and allow your foot to travel along its full range of motion at three levels: extension (close to the floor), midrange, and elevated (in the foot flexion position). Keep your heel anchored on the floor throughout the exercise and maintain the tension on the theraciser tube. Ten to twenty repetitions in each position is sufficient. This is a great exercise for regaining foot and ankle stability, reducing knee pain, and helping to restore the integrity of the arches of the feet. See appendix A for theraciser information.

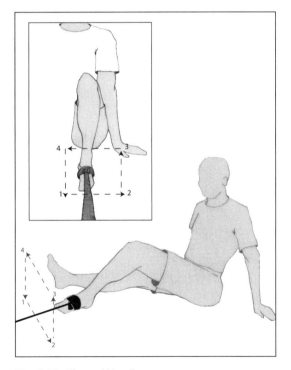

Fig. 5.11: Three-Way Foot and Ankle Exercise #3

Neurolymphatic Reflex Points

Rub the points located in the pubic area (associated with the pelvis) in a clockwise direction twice daily for 15–30 seconds, until tenderness is gone. The Neurolymphatic Reflex Chart is located on page 131.

Knees

The two lower leg bones that connect the ankle joint to the knee joints are the tibia and the fibula. The tibia is the larger, stronger, more weight-bearing bone; the fibula, which is the slenderest, longest bone in the body, is designed less for weight-bearing and more for stabilizing the movement of the knee.

The knee joint is extremely complex because of its unique combination of motion and weight-bearing abilities. The knee flexes, extends, and rotates around a moving axis of motion. This is unusual for a joint, as most axes of movement in the body are fixed. This unique combination gives the knee increased flexibility for added joint motion, but affords less stability.

The knee is surrounded by ligaments that hold the joint together and limit its range of motion. Quick movements place a tremendous amount of stress on these ligaments, which are famous for tearing. The tearing of the anterior cruciate and other ligaments can be caused by muscles that are in a weakened state before the knee injury, which cannot support the stress of complex movement. This weakness is often the result of the organ-muscle relationship, which I described earlier. The muscles of the knee are especially associated with weak adrenal glands and intestinal problems. Ligament tearing also occurs due to the amount of force involved in contact sports such as football or basketball. Even in these cases, a weakness in the muscles often precedes an injury.

The meniscus of the knee is a unique structure that consists of two cartilage pads, shaped like half-moons, that lie between the tibia of the lower leg and the femur of the upper leg. These pads expand the moving surface of the joint and help to keep the head of the femur in the right place, and the cartilage pad acts as a shock absorber to protect the end of both bones. The kneecap is a bone that simply protects the front of the joint from injury.

HEALTH TIP #17: Knee-Strengthening Exercises

To strengthen your thighs and hamstrings, utilize the Alignment Series, Flexibility Exercises, Two Foot Stretches, Foot Stability Exercise, and Three-Way Foot and Ankle Exercise, along with the general strengthening exercises provided in chapter 4. Exercises such as bicycling, swimming, walking, and doing active-stretch yoga are also beneficial. Evaluate the function of your adrenal glands and intestines by utilizing the information provided by your signs and symptoms as a key to understanding what your body is trying to tell you.

▦ Stabilize Knee Function

A Cho-Pat acts as an external ligament to stabilize a knee joint whose ligaments have been overstretched. Use it when knee pain exists or when playing sports or other physical activities. The Cho-Pat knee support is small yet strong, and unlike most knee braces, it does not interfere with the muscle function of the lower leg. Information on Cho-Pat knee supports is included in appendix A.

▦ Neurolymphatic Reflex Points

Rub the tender points associated with the adrenal glands and the large and small intestines. Rub in a clockwise direction twice daily for 15–30 seconds, and continue daily until tenderness is gone. The Neurolymphatic Reflex Chart is located on page 131.

Hips

The hip joint is formed by the union of three different bones that naturally fuse together to form the hipbone and hip socket. This natural process of fusion permits structural individuality to occur and allows the joint to conform perfectly to match the ball of the femur.

The right and left hipbones join the sacrum to form the pelvis, or pelvic girdle. The pelvis resembles a basin or bowl that contains and protects a variety of organs, such as the bladder, colon, rectum, uterus, and vagina.

The hip joint, like the knee joint, is surrounded by fibrocartilage and ligaments. These ligaments help to keep the movement of the joint in check and to protect the hip socket. A tough ligamentous capsule surrounds and protects the hip joint.

HEALTH TIP #18: Hip Exercises

▓ The Hip Roller

For this exercise, lie on your side on a 3- or 6-inch foam roller to stimulate the tensor fascia lata muscle along the iliotibial band (ITB). The iliotibial band runs from the hip to the knee, and it is located down the side of the leg along the seam of your pants. The amount of pressure one uses on the roller can be regulated by assuming more or less of your weight with your hands and feet, as illustrated.

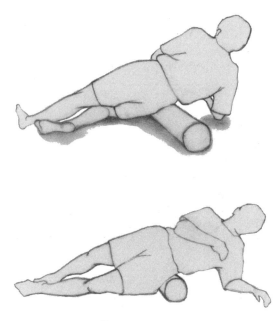

Fig. 5.12: Hip Roller

Slowly move the roller up and down your side from the hip joint to the knee. Limit the amount of time spent on the ITB to a minute or less. Make sure to minimize the amount of pressure applied to the joints themselves. This exercise provides deep massage for the hip joint and its associated muscles; stimulation and strengthening for the muscles that support the hip socket and laterally stabilize the knee; gentle alignment of the femur inside the hip joint; and stimulation of the neurolymphatic reflex points located along the length of the ITB. If the roller is painful on the hip or ITB, take more of your weight off the roller. See additional information in appendix A for the sources and use of foam roller exercises.

Other things you can do for your hips:

- Utilize the Hip Elevator, the Alignment Series, the Yoga Psoas Stretch, and all three versions of the Squat as presented in chapter 4.

- Include nutritional support for connective tissue, especially veal bone and specific joint support formulas located in appendix A.
- Rub the neurolymphatic reflex points to aid the large and small intestines and support hip stabilizer muscles. The Neurolymphatic Reflex Chart is located on page 131.

Shoulders

The shoulder is actually composed of five different joints. As with the knee, the shoulder sacrifices stability for its wide range and complexity of movement. The shoulder has numerous structural supports that provide stability throughout its range of motion, which include the ribs, the clavicle or collar bone, the scapula or wing bone, and the humerus or upper arm bone. Any misalignment of these structures will significantly compromise shoulder function. The Shoulder Alignment Exercise offered here will help to keep these structures aligned.

Both shoulders come together to form the shoulder girdle, which functions as one stabilized unit held together by countless ligaments and supported by scores of muscles. The ligaments limit the amount of movement in the shoulder, while the muscles help to maintain the strength and integrity of the joint. If you hang by your hands from an overhead bar, you can get a sense of how much the shoulder joint can actually expand, which makes the strength of the shoulder muscles essential for normal shoulder function to occur.

If muscle weakness is present in the shoulder, ligament damage can easily occur, as the stress and strain of normal shoulder activity weighs heavily on its ligaments and tendons. In this weakened state, our Innate Body Wisdom begins to restrict movement in the shoulder in order to protect the joint from further damage.

The muscles that stabilize the shoulder attach around a 360-degree arc of motion, which also indicates how the shoulder should be exercised. The equal tension afforded by this circle of muscles helps to keep the shoulder joint in place. If any of these muscles are in a weakened state, it increases the stress placed upon the others.

The level of structural balance present in the shoulder often reflects the condition in other structural areas of the body, namely the pelvis, feet, neck, and midback. The muscle-organ relationship also comes into play in the shoulder, and includes primary components of the digestive system, namely the liver, gallbladder, lungs, and stomach. A weakness in any of these organs will often show up as tenderness, pain, or dysfunction in the shoulder joint.

The shoulder also contains bursa, which are fluid-filled sacks that cushion the bones during movement. When shoulder motion is altered, inflammation of the bursa can easily occur and cause a wide variety of symptoms, including bursitis. These symptoms can be remedied by reestablishing the normal structural balance in the shoulder joint and introducing a natural anti-inflammatory agent.

Like all joints, the shoulder has a joint capsule (composed of ligaments) that completely surrounds the shoulder joint. Normally, the joint capsule is loose and relaxed to permit a generous amount of joint movement.

HEALTH TIP #19: Exercise and Align the Shoulders for Optimal Function

Shoulder circles are accomplished with extended arms moving slowly in concentric circles, starting with the smallest possible circle and ending with the largest possible circle.

All movement is around the 360-degree cone of motion for the shoulder. Repeat each circle several times both clockwise and counterclockwise. A small one- or two-pound weight may be added when this exercise becomes too easy.

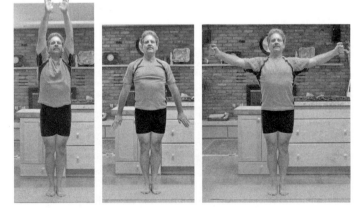

Fig. 5.13: Shoulder Circles

Shoulder alignment is accomplished by gently assuming a prayer position, with your palms facing together behind your back.

Initially the tips of the fingers may be the only part of your hands that touch. In due time, however, the palms will slowly come together in the area between the shoulder blades. Gently performing this exercise in the shower with soapy hands can make it a lot easier.

The following simple stretch for aligning the humerus helps the upper end of the humeral joint. This joint often becomes misaligned when we lie in bed on the side of shoulder pain.

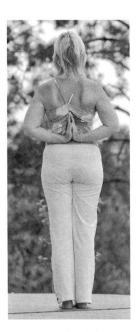

Fig. 5.14: Shoulder alignment, Hands in Prayer

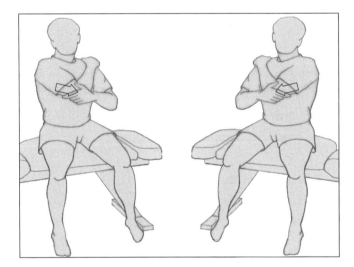

Fig. 5.15: Humerus Alignment

In the sitting position, gently stretch the shoulder joint by pulling the elbow toward the opposite side of the body, as illustrated above. Stretch both shoulder joints, and hold the stretch for 10–15 seconds each.

Use the Shoulder Stretch Exercise if the Shoulder Alignment Exercise is impossible. This indicates that shoulder function is significantly impaired, and you should perform the stretch to limber up your shoulders.

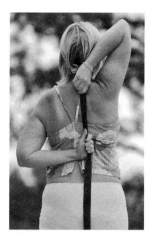

Fig. 5.16: Shoulder
Stretch with Strap

Find a hand towel, belt, or strap, and lay it over your shoulder. Reaching behind your back, grab the top of the towel with one hand. Next, grab the bottom of the towel with your other hand, reaching across your lower back. Slowly inch your hands together. At some point, your hands may even touch each other, and the Shoulder Alignment Exercise can be practiced.

Rub tender neurolymphatic points for the liver, gallbladder, stomach, and lungs, as indicated on the Neurolymphatic Chart on page 131.

Add the anti-inflammatory action of omega-3 oils, ice, and fish and flaxseed oils to safely reduce inflammation. Four grams of fish oil and flaxseed oil daily will help to reduce inflammation without the significant side effects of anti-inflammatory drugs. Sources for mercury-free fish oils and flaxseed oils extracted from whole food sources are listed in appendix A. Icing the shoulder for 20 minutes, one to three times per day, is also useful in reducing inflammation.

Anti-inflammatory enzymes taken between meals, two hours before or after a meal, dramatically improve the body's anti-inflammatory capabilities. Protocols for taking enzymes, and their sources, are listed in appendix A.

Persistent shoulder pain should be addressed. A chiropractor specializing in extremity adjusting and/or applied kinesiology is by far your best bet.

Elbows

It is interesting to note the parallels between the extremity joints in the body. The elbow and the knee joint are both hinge-type joints; the shoulder and the hip are both ball-and-socket joints; and the hands and the feet each contain multiple bones and joints working together. Except for the adaptive changes that have occurred due to weight-bearing needs, these related joints are near mirror images of each other.

This is especially true of the elbow and knee, both of which contain a combination of three joints in one. The knee is composed of the larger weight-bearing tibia and slender fibula bone; the larger radius bone and slender ulna constitute the bones of the elbow.

The elbow is especially important because it rotates the hand. The ulna bone is on the little-finger side of the forearm, and it functions to stabilize the joint. The radius bone on the thumb side of the forearm handles the weight-bearing issues.

These two bones, the radius and the ulna, are held together by ligaments, tendons, and muscles that help maintain the proper alignment between the bones so they can move together in harmony. The elbow joint flexes, extends, and rotates all at the same time, which can be very complex when an elbow joint becomes misaligned.

The various ligaments of the elbow joint can become stressed by a variety of overuse injuries, such as using a hammer, playing racquet sports, doing computer work, or performing other work-related movements that cause misalignment and inflammation of the elbow joint and wrist.

HEALTH TIP #20: Elbow Exercises

1. Use the Shoulder Alignment exercise to align the elbows. The Hands in Prayer Exercise provides an excellent alignment tool for both elbows and shoulders.
2. The Taping Method listed below in health tip #21 is also great for aligning the elbow joint. Occasionally, when very chronic elbow problems are present, a traditional velcro forearm brace is also needed for a short period of time, accompanied by immobilization. The forearm brace is sometimes necessary during lifting, playing racket sports, or performing other activities that create a great deal of torque on the elbow joint. In chronic cases, alignment is strongly recommended by a doctor of chiropractic. In cases of chronic inflammation, ice can also be used for a period of 20 minutes and is helpful up to three times a day. The use of the anti-inflammatory nutritional protocol and enzyme nutrition listed in this chapter is also recommended.
3. Rub the neurolymphatic reflex points associated with the stomach and pancreas as indicated on page 131.

Wrists and Hands

You may have noticed the amazing similarities between your hands and feet, and between the bones of the lower leg and forearm. Although each hand has one more bone than in each foot, the rest of the bones are almost identical.

There are a series of eight cubical-shaped carpal bones in each hand that transfer forces between the lower arm and the metacarpals. There are seven tarsal bones in the foot that perform the same function in the lower leg. The hand has five metacarpal bones, and the foot has five metatarsal bones. The hand and the foot both have fourteen phalanges, the anatomical name for fingers and toes.

Of course, there are major differences between the functions of our hands and feet, despite the fact that there are people who can write with their feet or walk on their hands. The tarsal bones in the foot bear much more weight and are larger and stronger than those in the hands. On the other hand, the movement of the fingers is much more delicate and precise than the movement of toes could ever be.

In general, the hands are designed for more precision movements, which is evidenced by the amount of our brain dedicated specifically to our thumbs. Both the hands and the feet are yet another example of how the need for function determines how our Inner Intelligence creates and adapts our structure.

HEALTH TIP #21: Stabilize the Function of Both the Wrist and Hand

In the same way a Cho-Pat used below the kneecap can stabilize it, a thin piece of non-stretchy athletic tape or a thin watchband can be used around the wrist to stabilize the function of both the wrist and the elbow. When problems with the wrist or elbow exist, place a thin piece of tape snugly around the wrist as indicated in the illustration. Make sure the tape is not tight. There should be no pain or swelling after the tape is applied.

The tape is placed around the wrist on the finger side of the ulna bone as illustrated. If possible, keep the tape in place for 2–3 days. Ice can also be applied to the wrist for 20 minutes, up to three times a day when necessary. Taping the wrist in this way has helped thousands of my patients to overcome wrist and elbow problems. If wrist problems exist, it is a good idea to retape the wrist before lifting heaving items or playing sports.

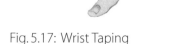

Fig. 5.17: Wrist Taping

Support the elbow and wrist nutritionally with a veal bone supplement and total joint support supplements, as listed in appendix A.

Conclusion

My intent in this first section has been to introduce practical ways to align your structural system and to help you create your own structural health care program. Ultimately, your program will also need to include the assistance of a qualified structural health practitioner who understands the structural integrity of the body and is able to correct your structural imbalances. I feel that there is no other health practitioner that is as well suited in this regard as a doctor of chiropractic. The process of finding the right chiropractor for you may be as simple as getting a referral from a friend, or trying the chiropractors in your immediate area. I have included a short list of chiropractic referral organizations in appendix A for chapter 3 that will help you find your way.

The exercises presented in this section will help you attain and maintain structural balance and will lead the way toward multidimensional wellness. In addition to the exercises listed, general fitness exercises are also recommended to increase your strength and stamina. These exercises include walking, yoga, Pilates, swimming, bicycling, cross-country skiing, and, if your feet are structurally sound, running.

People seem to beat themselves up in the name of fitness. If you have the right information, and know how to implement the right strategies for your particular body type, there is no need for painful experiences to occur. Fitness exercises, if done correctly, should benefit your entire multidimensional self without creating trauma or pain. As a matter of fact, pain is feedback from your body that you have gone too far.

Since fitness is not within the scope of this book, I want to mention several books that more than adequately address the subject. A list of these books is contained in the bibliography.

The alignments and exercises that I have chosen to share are those that have been successful for my patients and for me. Hopefully, the structural section of this book will provide you with the awareness and the tools to balance your structural system and to maintain a nerve system that is free from interference.

The important part of any structural practice is to bring these practices into your daily life and to make them your own. It is only then that they will have power for you. If you make these principles and practices an integral part of your health program, they will not only change the structure and function of your nerve system, but they will effectively work to change your life.

When you become aware of exactly what your Inner Intelligence is telling you, and implement the necessary changes, beneficial results will begin to show up in every realm of your life experience. This is true of your structural balance, your exercise program, your state of mind, your feeling realm, and the spirit that you embrace.

Every lasting change in the body begins and ends with your awareness. When you are aligned with your Inner Intelligence, you are aligned with the awesome power of Nature. And when you are aligned with the power of Nature, there is nothing that is beyond your reach.

Chapter 6

The Endocrine System

THE ENDOCRINE SYSTEM is the key to the biochemical component of health in the same way that the nerve system is the key to the structural component. In reality, the functions of these two systems are so interrelated that they can essentially be referred to as one system: the neuroendocrine system.

The nerve system exerts lightening quick electrical impulses throughout the body, while the endocrine system quickly communicates with neurochemical hormones. Both forms of communication can control and coordinate millions of functions in the body every second.

The manufacture of hormones by the endocrine system allows it to regulate the metabolic function of every system, organ, tissue, and cell in the body. Essentially, these hormones are chemical messengers that allow the Intelligence of the body to create a balanced internal environment.

The endocrine system is so important to the core function of our body that any malfunction can cause myriad signs and symptoms in a variety of organs and systems. Check out the wide variety of symptoms in the implications section associated with each endocrine organ.

Did you ever notice when listening to an orchestra, especially a great one, how each instrument blends so well with the others, creating a sound that is exponentially greater than any one instrument can produce by itself? This provides a perfect analogy for the endocrine system. It is composed of a wide variety of instruments that contribute to the awesome symphony in the human body. And the whole truly is greater than the sum of its parts. At the same time, if an instrument/hormone is out of tune, it can easily be heard above the rest of the orchestra, and the once beautifully blended music becomes marred. It is important to see each component as it relates to the whole system. But if the endocrine system is the orchestra, who is the maestro or conductor?

It's a good question. Before I answer, I'd like to introduce the endocrine orchestra. Review the accompanying illustration, and let's take it from the top.

The instruments with the highest pitch are the pineal gland, the pituitary gland, and the thyroid gland. The thymus gland, centrally located at the heart of the endocrine system, is in the midrange, while the pancreas, adrenal glands, and the sex glands—called the gonads (ovaries in women, and the testicles in men)—round out the lower ranges.

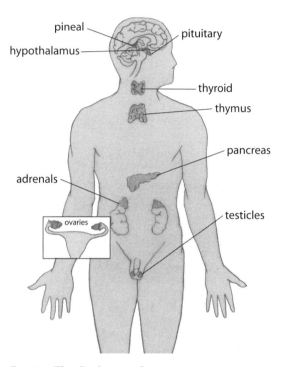

Fig. 6.1: The Endocrine System

When you come to chapter 12 and explore the emotional component of health, you will see how each endocrine gland does, in fact, correspond to certain tonal frequencies and emotions. Specific musical tones will not only strengthen an endocrine gland but can help clear out stuck emotions. You can learn to use sound as a way of clearing negative emotions associated with the endocrine system. This is a very powerful tool for healing.

Each endocrine gland has a huge range of influence within the body due to the action of powerful hormones that circulate the bloodstream. Much of the power and energy generated by the human body is created in the endocrine system, which is why I refer to it here as the power drive system. Basically, the endocrine system transforms our subtle energy fields into seven major power centers. In my experience, the endocrine system represents the magnetic, feeling, feminine, right-brained aspect of life in the human body.

Maestro, Please

There are actually a few different conductors in our endocrine system orchestra. The pituitary gland is called the master gland because it directs the actions of the endocrine glands that are below it. In most cases, the pituitary receives its instructions from the hypothalamus in the brain, which in turn receives its instructions from the pineal gland. Ultimately, the hypothalamus, pituitary, and pineal glands receive instructions from the Internal Intelligence of the body. So, the grande maestro of the endocrine system orchestra is in fact our own Inner Intelligence.

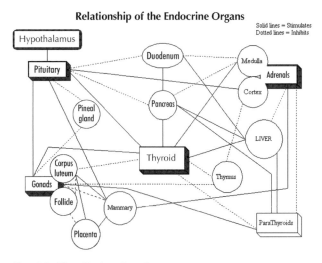

The pineal, hypothalamus, and pituitary glands respond to higher levels of vibration in the body. In our endocrine system–orchestra analogy, these organs would compose the soprano section. The pineal gland is also capable of effecting important

Fig. 6.2: The Endocrine System

brain structures, as it interconnects with the function of the nerve system. Like so many areas of the body, the endocrine system is such a complex system that much of its action remains a mystery. Included here is one of my favorite illustrations of the endocrine system, created by the famous endocrinologist Dr. Henry Harrower. For me, this illustration provides a high wow factor.

Hormones

What we do know about the endocrine system is that its glands secrete a wide variety of hormones that travel rapidly through the bloodstream, and influence target organs throughout the body, which in turn effect all of our forty quadrillion cells.

Biochemically, hormones are composed of a combination of proteins and steroids, which become extremely important when a person is nutritionally deficient and unable to make hormones that function properly. When deficiencies of protein or essential fats occur, the chemical message that hormones normally carry to target organs cannot be delivered.

The common result is that the Intelligence of the body is unable to maintain a balanced internal environment, which produces a cacophony of biochemical imbalances that eventually lead to dis-ease.

A target organ is an organ or group of cells that respond to the instructions of circulating hormones. Each hormone carries a specific message that only certain target organs can receive. When these hormones successfully reach their destination, a chemical message is also sent by the target organ, letting the body know that the message has been received.

This process is similar to what happens when we send a facsimile. When the chemical message from an endocrine organ has been successfully received, a return message is immediately sent back by the target organ indicating that the transaction is complete. When our Inner Intelligence receives the message from the target organ, it stops sending the chemical message. This process illustrates communication at its finest, but can provide an opportunity for chemical communication to go astray. If nutritional deficiencies exist, a part of this important chemical conversation never occurs.

The Pineal Gland

Below is an illustration of the pineal gland and its location in the center of the brain. It is interesting to note that the pineal gland is actually the remnant of a third eye that appears early in the developing fetus. Confirming what mystics have been saying for centuries, the third eye is responsible for our inner sight (insight) and directly connects us to our spiritual self.

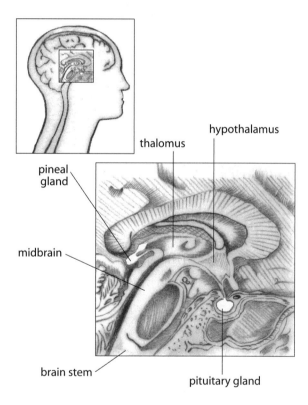

Fig. 6.3: Pineal, Pituitary, and Hypothalamus Glands

The pineal gland functions as an integral part of both the nerve and endocrine systems, and somehow translates subtle energy fields of light into both electrical and biochemical signals. Truthfully, what we know about this amazing endocrine organ could be put on a postage stamp.

Clinically, each endocrine organ has a very specific nutrient that makes it work. Unbelievably, the specific nutrient for the pineal gland is light. That's right: In order to function normally, the pineal needs to be exposed to the entire spectrum of light. It is activated by light, transmits light, translates light, responds to the quality of light, and this mysterious organ may even magnify the effects of light for the rest of the body.

The pineal gland also regulates the hypothalamus, and it influences the thyroid, thymus, pancreas, adrenals, and sex glands. The pineal gland secretes the hormone melatonin, which it produces in total darkness and which relates to the rhythms of our inner biological clock.

Scientifically, melatonin has been found to regulate seasonal cycles, sleep cycles, daily body rhythms, the day and night cycles in the body, and countless brain functions. Melatonin increases the effectiveness of the immune system by suppressing the adrenal hormone cortisol, and is a powerful antioxidant that has the ability to fight free radical damage, which is a primary factor in aging. Melatonin also acts as an antistress agent.

Melatonin is a derivative of the nerve transmitter serotonin and is derived from the amino acid tryptophan. The levels of serotonin in the brain are known to effect mood swings, emotional health, and overall behavior. Low serotonin levels are directly associated with depression.

Research has shown that the pineal gland in birds and other animals contain magnetic material at the heart of their navigational system. Current research demonstrates that this may be true for human beings as well. It appears that the pineal gland responds to magnetism as well as to light.

In recent years, it has also been determined that the pineal gland becomes disturbed by abnormal electromagnetic field radiation, or EMFs. Abnormal levels of EMFs can be emitted from overhead power lines, electrical wiring in our homes, X-rays, fluorescent lights, electrical appliances, telephones, computers, cellular phones, microwaves, televisions, automobiles, airplanes, clock radios, and the list goes on and on.

The electromagnetic disturbances produced by the huge number of EMF devices in our culture not only effect the production of melatonin by the pineal gland but also the overall health and well-being of the human organism. After all, at our core, human beings are electromagnetic in nature, and if that energy flow is disturbed, the health of the entire organism can be jeopardized.

The pineal gland can provide a direct connection to Spirit for human beings. When the pineal is healthy, active, and alive, we become sensitive to the finer frequencies of light, and we become aware of the more subtle levels of our human experience. If the pineal is impaired, the magical music of Spirit recedes into the background, and the possibility of multidimensional wholeness becomes a distant reality.

Implications of pineal gland dysfunction include sleep disorders, such as seasonal affective disorder (SAD), depression, a host of emotional disorders, disturbances in body temperature, jet lag, problems in the reproductive system, premature aging, and the possible proliferation of cancer cells.

HEALTH TIP #1: Enhance the Functioning of Your Pineal Gland

1. Enhance the function of your pineal gland by keeping all electrical devices at least six feet away from the head of your bed—this includes clock radios and TVs. Use an EMF protection screen on your computer. If you are exposed to large amounts of EMFs from computers, cell phones, and electrical lines, wear an EMF protection device or an EMF magnet that can be easily carried in your pocket. Meditation, toning, singing, and vibrational healing have all been shown to be effective in strengthening the extremely sensitive pineal gland.

2. Nutritional support for the pineal gland includes the amino acid tryptophan, folic acid, vitamin C, vitamin A, zinc, pineal glandular extracts, and vision, color, and light therapy. See appendix A for a list of sources to maintain a healthy functioning pineal gland, and see chapter 13 for the positive attitudes, emotions, colors, and sounds that support pineal function.

The Hypothalamus and the Pituitary Gland

The pituitary has been called the master gland because of the level of control it exerts over the rest of the endocrine system. The pituitary gland has been called the workhorse of the endocrine system, as it reacts to the feedback it receives from the body and sends instructions to other endocrine glands to produce balancing hormones.

The pituitary gland is directly below and connected to the hypothalamus as shown in figure 6.3 on page 150. The pituitary gland is nestled in the small saddle of the sphenoid bone, and if you gently push your tongue up into the soft part of your palate, you will be pushing on the underside of your pituitary gland.

Because the pituitary sits within a cranial bone, it is intimately connected and adversely affected by cranial misalignments. The sphenoid bone lies directly behind the eyes and includes the sensitive temple area slightly above and in front of both ears.

The pituitary gland has two distinct parts, the anterior and posterior pituitary. The anterior pituitary produces six hormones: one that stimulates growth throughout the body; two that stimulate the sex glands; one that stimulates milk production in a mother soon after birth: one that stimulates the thyroid; and one that stimulates the adrenal glands.

The posterior pituitary secretes two hormones: one that increases water absorption by the kidneys and another that stimulates the contraction of the uterus during childbirth. The posterior pituitary is composed solely of nerve tissue and is functionally a part of the nerve system.

The hypothalamus has the ability to access both the nerve and the endocrine systems, and is a major player in the communication crossover between the two. The hypothalamus accesses the nerve system through the automatic or autonomic nerve system, which includes both the sympathetic and parasympathetic system. See chapter 3 for more details. The hypothalamus has the ability to control heart rate, blood pressure, digestion, elimination, and a multitude of other system and organ functions in the body.

The hypothalamus is directly connected to the endocrine system by the pituitary gland, and actually stimulates the pituitary to secrete a variety of hormones that regulate the thyroid and parathyroid glands, the thymus, pancreas, adrenals, and sex glands. The hypothalamus is also connected to the limbic system, which functions as the center for feelings and emotions in the body.

The pituitary has a vast area of influence in the body and can ultimately be the cause of any imbalance in the endocrine glands it influences. Common implications of pituitary involvement are growth-related problems (often initiated by protein deficiency); weight problems, such as obesity; diabetes and other blood sugar–related problems; carbohydrate intolerance; liver-related problems, water retention, and problems with circulation.

HEALTH TIP #2: Enhance the Functioning of Your Pituitary Gland

▓ Utilize Cranial Alignments

The sphenoid bone is really the temple of the pituitary gland. If your temples or the roof of your mouth become extremely sensitive to the touch, or you experience headaches in these sensitive areas, a misaligned sphenoid bone may be the cause of your problems. If tenderness exists in any of these areas, contact a cranial sacral specialist and use the cranial balls as indicated in chapter 3.

▓ The Pituitary Tap

The pituitary lies right between your eyes, directly behind a small bump called the glabella (illustration). Gently tap the glabella about 20 times, several times each day, to help stimulate pituitary function.

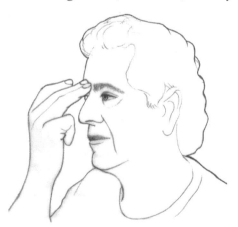

Other strategies for enhancing the functioning of the pituitary gland:

■ Utilize the energy exercises presented in chapter 4, especially the variation of the Squat called the Youthful Pose, which directly stimulates the pituitary gland. All endocrine organs are also supported by the Slant Board Exercise described in chapter 1.

Fig. 6.4: Glabella/Pituitary Tap

■ Nutritional support for the pituitary gland includes the supplemental use of manganese and magnesium, vitamin-E complex, fenugreek tea, and pituitary extracts. If you are a pituitary type, as described in chapter 7, follow the pituitary diet. Sources for all nutritional products are listed in appendix A.

The Thyroid Gland

The thyroid gland is a butterfly-shaped organ found in the front portion of the neck, and regulates the body's growth and metabolism. In our powerful endocrine orchestra, the thyroid gland would be considered the alto section.

The word "thyroid" means "door," and was coined by the Greek physician Galen due to its shape. The thyroid is certainly the door to understanding growth and metabolism in the body.

Metabolism in the body is considered the sum total of all the biochemical processes of the body that create energy to sustain growth, development, and repair. Metabolism includes anabolism, which is the building up or growth part of the process, and catabolism, which is the process of breaking down. Both building up and breaking down are essential parts of all processes in the body.

The thyroid regulates the amount of energy used by the body, determines the rate of growth and repair, heightens our mental processes, supports the function of other endocrine glands, helps to govern the amount of protein the body produces, assists in many functions of nerves and muscles, regulates calcium metabolism, determines the amount of oxygen used by our cells, regulates the growth and repair of our skin and hair, and governs many aspects of our reproductive function.

The thyroid has so much influence in the body that a disturbance in thyroid function can result in a wide range of symptoms and functional problems, including major emotional upsets. When

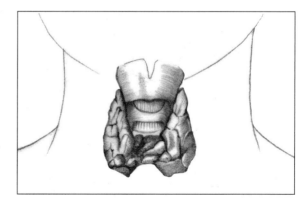

Fig. 6.5: The Thyroid Gland

fits of crying erupt for no apparent reason, think thyroid. If nightmares persist, especially in children, the thyroid could be your main suspect.

As is the case for every organ in the body, each endocrine gland has very specific nutritional requirements in the form of minerals, vitamins, and amino acids. In the case of the thyroid gland, the mineral iodine is the undisputed king. Iodine is absolutely essential for the thyroid to manufacture its main hormone, thyroxin. For blood test enthusiasts, thyroxin is also referred to as T4. Its cousin, which is a more concentrated form of thyroxin, is referred to as T3.

The thyroid gland, which has one of the richest blood supplies in the body, facilitates the absorption of iodine from the blood. The thyroid makes two forms of thyroxin and stores them for up to eight days, or until instructions are received from the pituitary to release thyroxin into the bloodstream.

Elemental iodine, the amino acid tyrosine—which is the Greek word for cheese—and large amounts of enzymes are absolutely essential for thyroid hormones to be produced. If any of these key ingredients are missing or in short supply, thyroid hormones become deficient and metabolic function becomes impaired.

Thyroid hormones increase and activate the energy-producing power plants inside our cells called mitochondria. The thyroid helps these little dynamos produce energy. Thyroid hormones also increase enzyme activity in the body, which aids the body in the break down, absorption, and utilization of carbohydrates. When excess carbohydrates are avoided, thyroid hormones assist the body to burn fat.

Because thyroid hormones help build proteins, they are crucial in the growth process of children. And, as thyroid hormones affect our rate of metabolism, they also can cause significant changes in our weight. Too much thyroid function can cause severe weight loss, while too little thyroid function can lead to obesity. If the amount of calcium circulating in the blood is elevated, the thyroid secretes a third hormone, calcitonin, which helps the body deposit more calcium in our bones.

There are four small glands located on the back of the thyroid called the parathyroid glands. The parathyroids are also part of the endocrine system and produce two hormones that function to balance calcium in the body.

These calcium-regulating hormones function like the (+) male and the (−) female energies we see in so many places throughout the body. An increase in the secretion of one hormone directly increases the amount of circulating calcium in the blood, as well as the amount of calcium absorbed by our bones. An increase in the complementary parathyroid hormone reduces the ability of the body to absorb calcium.

It is interesting to note that vitamin D in the body acts just like parathyroid hormone, increasing the absorption of calcium. Vitamin D is produced when sunlight hits our skin, which is another example of how important sunlight is to a healthy body.

It is also interesting to note that 6 percent of all the blood in the body flows through the bones every minute. At that rate, it takes the body about seventy minutes to adjust the calcium levels in our bones. The amazing speed of this calcium exchange is made possible by the huge surface area of bone crystals in the body. If laid side by side, our bone crystals would more than cover thirty acres!

An underactive or hypothyroid condition causes a slowing down of the body's metabolism and can lead to conditions such as excessive weight gain or obesity, difficulty digesting fats, lowered body temperature, cold hands and feet, an overall lack of energy, fatigue, confusion, memory loss, muscle weakness, a variety of skin conditions, a reduction in circulating blood, excessive hair loss, a thick and swollen tongue, brittle nails, emotional upset, and a sluggish metabolism.

An overactive or hyperactive thyroid causes a speeding up of the metabolism and can lead to conditions such as excitability, anxiety, nervous tension, irritability, premature aging, rapid respiration, fine muscle tremors, heart palpitations, difficulty sleeping, hypersensitivity, exhaustion, excessive hunger, rapid depletion of essential fatty acids, elevated body temperature, and symptoms that relate to wearing out the body due to the excessive speed at which the metabolism is working. A hyperactive thyroid can increase the metabolic rate by over 100 percent.

The associated organs for the thyroid gland are the parathyroid glands. These glands help to regulate and balance calcium and phosphorus in the body. Too little parathyroid activity creates the symptoms of calcium deficiency associated with muscle tetany, irritability of the nerve system, hair loss, and defects in bones, hair, skin, and teeth.

Excessive parathyroid hormone production causes excess calcium to be deposited in the kidneys, bladder, and the intestines, resulting in conditions such as kidney and bladder stones, spurs, and numerous symptoms of calcium deficiency in the tissues of the body, including osteoporosis. The teres minor muscle is directly associated with the function of the thyroid gland.

HEALTH TIP #3: Enhance the Functioning of Your Thyroid Gland

1. Monitor thyroid/endocrine function by evaluating the body's resting temperature. This can be easily accomplished by taking your basal temperature. A basal temperature reading is taken under the armpit first thing in the morning before rising. This measures your resting temperature before you get going. A basal temperature chart with more detailed instructions is supplied in appendix B.

   When thyroid function and metabolism are elevated, an elevated basal temperature usually accompanies this. When thyroid function is depressed, the basal temperature will be lower than normal. Although other endocrine problems can cause temperature changes, the thyroid is at the top of the list. Changes in basal temperature indicate endocrine imbalance.

   The normal basal axillary temperature is between 97.8 and 98.2. The Basal Temperature Chart, along with a blood test evaluating your T3 and T4 levels, will give a good indication of your thyroid function. Muscle testing, performed by a doctor of chiropractic trained in applied kinesiology, can also be a huge help in locating and correcting functional thyroid problems before they turn into major health concerns.

2. Thyroxin production is dependent on sufficient amounts of protein, healthy dietary fats, and natural carbohydrates in the diet. When iodine is deficient in the diet, the thyroid is unable to produce its powerful hormones. This often results in a metallic taste in the mouth and, in severe cases, a swelling of the thyroid gland called a goiter. Iodine deficiencies are more common inland, as iodine is present in fish, solar-dried sea salt, and seaweed or kelp. The RDA for iodine is 0.1 milligrams per day. The best sources of iodine are dulse, kelp, and sea conch. On the contrary, iodized salt is not a good source of iodine for the body to assimilate.

   Caution must be used when taking iodine supplements, as too much iodine has the same inhibiting effect on the thyroid as an iodine deficiency. It is important to muscle test your need for iodine either on your own, as indicated in chapter 11, or by a chiropractic health professional. Using seaweed, algae, dulse, or kelp are much safer iodine sources for the body.

Other minerals that aid thyroid function are manganese, zinc, and iron. Caution must be used when taking zinc or iron supplements, as too much of these minerals can reduce the amount of iodine utilized by the thyroid. A high-quality solar-dried sea salt from a health food store is an excellent source of thyroid-related minerals.

Vitamins that are associated with the thyroid gland are A, B complex (especially folic acid and B12), vitamin C, and vitamin F (essential fatty acids). Make sure that any fish oil supplements have been evaluated for their mercury content. The amino acid tyrosine is also important to thyroid function. Sources for all nutritional products and thyroid formulas are listed in appendix A.

3. Stimulate the neurolymphatic strengthening points associated with the thyroid for 15–30 seconds, 2–3 times each day, to improve the lymphatic drainage related to the thyroid gland. To support thyroid gland function, use the related thyroid points on the Neurolymphatic Reflex Chart, located on page 131 in chapter 5.

4. The accompanying chart of neurovascular holding points can be used to enhance the blood supply to the thyroid gland. Lightly touch and hold related points for 30 seconds, or until a steady pulse is felt under the fingertips. Neurovascular holding points can be used for any organ or endocrine gland.

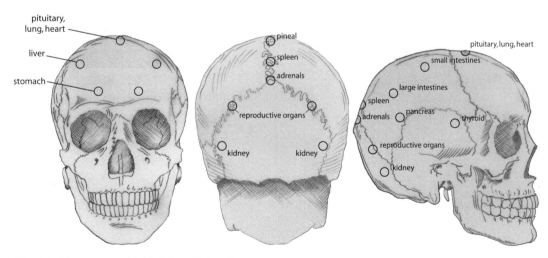

Fig. 6.6: Neurovascular Holding Point Chart

5. Eating fresh ocean fish and dried seaweed that have been monitored for their mercury content is also great for the thyroid. Utilizing dulse and kelp regularly as seasonings is an easy way to support thyroid function. When thyroid problems are suspected, it would be best to eliminate coffee and refined carbohydrates from your diet. Other foods that overstimulate the thyroid are sweets, chocolate, fruit juices, and alcohol.

6. The Thyroid Tap is also beneficial. This tapping is accomplished by flexing your head to one side and exposing the thyroid and parathyroid glands on the other, as illustrated in the accompanying diagram. Gently tap the thyroid gland with your fingers while you hum. This exercise helps stimulate the thyroid and parathyroid glands and can be performed, as needed, on both sides of the neck on a daily basis.

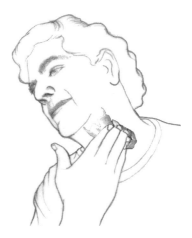

Fig. 6.7: The Thyroid Tap

The Thymus Gland

The next player in our power-packed endocrine system orchestra also directs an incredible amount of activity all on its own. Shaped like a small pyramid, the mysterious thymus gland lies at the heart of the endocrine system. Although the thymus receives instructions from the soprano section, it is considered the director of activity for the entire immune system. Consider it the tenor in our endocrine orchestra. The thymus gland also offers endocrine system control over the cardiovascular and respiratory systems.

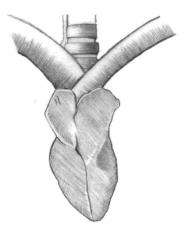

Fig. 6.8: The Thymus Gland

Until the early 1950s, the thymus gland was thought to be just another useless organ, like the tonsils, appendix, and adenoids, until doctors started removing it. The thymus glands of young children were removed for heart surgeries because they were in the way! Unfortunately, without their essential thymus glands, these infants and young children soon experienced complete immune system failure.

It is interesting to note that all of these so-called useless organs are now considered to be an integral part of the lymphatic system, which creates much of our natural immunity. Far from useless, the entire system managed by the thymus gland has been extremely misunderstood.

The thymus gland actually seeds a variety of lymphatic organs throughout the body with immune-producing cells. For this reason it can be considered the mother of our immune system.

Today, the thymus is generally recognized as the most important player in the function of the immune system. Many authorities still believe the thymus atrophies or shrinks during our adolescent years, but this has been shown to be wrong, as most of the thymus glands that have been examined have mainly been from people who had been sick and died. Examination of thymus glands from healthy individuals has rarely been considered. The thymus glands of Yogis who have died from other causes, for example, have been found to be healthy, alive, and full size.

Generally speaking, the cells of our immune system can be divided into two major types, called T cells and B cells. The "T" stands for thymus-dependent cell, and the "B" stands for bone marrow. These cells are specifically called lymphocytes, which are cells of the immune system that originate in the lymphatic system.

The thymus begins to produce lymphocytes in the womb of the developing fetus. These lymphocytes soon move into the bloodstream and migrate to all the tissues of the lymphatic system: the spleen, tonsils, appendix, adenoids, lymph nodes, and specialized tissues of the small intestine. Lymphocytes migrate into portions of our connective tissue, such as our skin, and into the soft inner portion of our bone marrow. On a cellular level, lymphocytes provide the core of our immunity.

So, the thymus gland sets up our immunity by seeding lymphocytes throughout our immune system, and continues to produce and control these T cell lymphocytes throughout the course of our lives. If the function of the thymus becomes diminished, T cells become reduced in number, depressing the effectiveness of our entire immune system.

The thymus gland produces at least one hormone called thymosin, although the possibility that it produces others still exists, since very little is known about its mechanism of action.

Besides regulating our entire immune system, the thymus has also been found to amplify our immunity by instructing bone marrow cells to turn into lymphocytes as they are needed. The thymus helps to reduces our contact sensitivities with the outside world, enhance our production of antibodies, stimulate the production of interferon, and direct the variety of lymphocytes throughout the immune system. Not bad for a useless organ!

The thymus is also an endless source of DNA, which is used for the formation of new white blood cells. The thymus creates new DNA, the basic structural building block of life, which directly connects the thymus with every cell in the human body.

By their very nature, lymphocytes are biochemically neutral. This fact enables a healthy immune system to be poised and ready to neutralize any and all foreign invaders at the drop of a hat. When uncommitted lymphocytes come in contact with any substance that is considered a foreigner to the body, they totally commit themselves to destroying the invader. Like the ruthless yet effective kamikaze pilots of World War II, these lymphocytes give up their lives to destroy the enemy.

A depressed immune system, however, can mistakenly perceive its own tissues as a foreign invader. In the case of autoimmune disease, the body's own immune system begins attacking itself.

Weakness in the thymus gland is often suspected whenever one's ability to resist disease is diminished or when we experience chronic or recurring infections. This is especially true when illness persists for more than seven days. It takes seven days for the thymus to seed the immune system with new cells and make the specific antibodies necessary to neutralize whatever bacteria or viral invader is present.

Research indicates that a weakened immune system may be the ultimate cause for cancer. This makes sense because a healthy immune system normally eliminates the cancer cells that are frequently produced in the body. The Inner Intelligence of the body recognizes cancer cells as nonself, and quickly eliminates them.

Cancer cells only become a problem when the immune system no longer targets them as nonself and allows them to multiply. Once these tiny cells are allowed to multiply, they can quickly overwhelm any system.

A weakened immune system is unable to conduct the same level of surveillance throughout the body as a vibrantly healthy one can. The immune system will get the main jobs done, but some of the smaller ones seem to slip through the cracks.

Immune system weakness initially shows up as smaller ailments, such as allergies, swollen glands, fatigue, asthma, or skin problems. If these small weaknesses go unchecked, they will eventually drag down the rest of the immune system.

Is a weakened immune system a precursor to cancer? The evidence seems to be leaning in that direction. We know for certain that having a weakened immune system is a bad situation to be in, made worse by the overuse of antibiotics. Although antibiotics can be lifesavers, their abuse has created microbial monsters in the form of more virulent strains of bacteria. Viruses are already immune to antibiotics.

Through the abuse of antibiotics and other wonder drugs, monster bacteria have come back to haunt us more and more each year. Our immune systems are becoming weaker, while bacteria and viruses are becoming stronger.

Right now we are seeing a resurgence of so called "cured" infectious diseases. This is because new resistant strains have developed in every type of bacteria. Even antibiotic manufacturers complain that the continued use of antibacterial cleaning agents is making antibiotic use less effective in the body.

With the strengthening of bacteria and viruses, we all need to have super immune systems. What most of us have now are immune systems that are underfed and overworked.

If we take this threat too lightly—as we have taken the threat to our planet's immune system—it is unlikely we will be able to recover. In my opinion, the key to having a healthy immune system is first and foremost to maintain a healthy thymus gland.

Emotions also play an important role in the function of the thymus gland, as the thymus relates to both the physical and emotional heart. The Greeks referred to the thymus gland as the protector of the heart. Today, research has shown that when negative emotions such as fear, hate, envy, or jealousy take over, our thymus gland and immune system weaken. Conversely, when we embrace positive feelings such as love and joy, the thymus gland strengthens and our entire immune system immediately feels the effects.

When the thymus gland becomes weak, it reduces the ability of the body to resist disease. This reduction in resistance is often the key underlying factor in our inability to sustain health, giving bacteria and virus an entry point into the heart of our defense system. In truth, it is our resistance to disease that plays a much more important role than bacteria or virus ever can in the manifestation of disease.

The thymus also becomes weakened by states of chronic stress, which is evidenced by the intimate relationship between the thymus, the adrenal glands, and the lymphatic system in the stress reaction described by Dr. Hans Selye.

The thymus gland is adversely affected by smoking, overtraining, antibiotic use, pesticides, toxic metals, toxic chemicals, parasites, fungal infections, longstanding bacterial and viral infections, and allergies to foods such as sugar, wheat, and dairy products. Rough skin is also a sign of thymus weakness.

The organs associated with the function of the thymus gland include the heart, lungs, and bronchial tubes, as well as the entire lymphatic system, which includes the spleen, tonsils, adenoids, parotid glands, appendix, part of the small intestine, and a host of lymphatic tissue spread throughout the body. The infraspinatus muscle in the shoulder is directly associated with the thymus gland as well.

HEALTH TIP #4: Enhance the Functioning of Your Thymus Gland

- Tap your thymus gland! Tapping the chest over the thymus gland (see illustration) for 15–20 seconds several times a day helps stimulate a sluggish immune system, especially in children. Humming while tapping adds the dimension of sound to the equation and substantially improves the results.

- Providing nutritional support for the thymus gland includes an aqueous thymus extract, which promotes thymus hormone production; vitamin A, which aids against infection; vitamin C complex, which aids in the healing process; bioflavonoids, and essential fatty acids. Also of importance are the trace minerals copper, selenium, and zinc, and foods containing phosphorus. A multiple vitamin containing a full array of trace minerals is also rec-

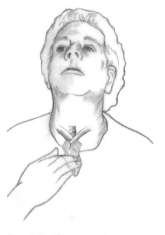

Fig. 6.9: Thymus Tap

ommended to maintain a healthy immune system. Sources for all these nutritional supplements are listed in appendix A.

- Eat fresh fruits and vegetables to support the thymus gland, especially leafy green vegetables, green drinks (see appendix A), and supplementation with a high-quality blue-green algae.

- Limiting coffee intake and refined carbohydrates is also extremely effective. Eating sweetbreads (the thymus glands of beef) or using thymus glandular extracts can help to rebuild a chronically weak thymus gland. As with any red meat, be particularly aware of its source. The best choice is always organically raised beef, free of hormones and antibiotics.

- Stimulate the neurolymphatic strengthening points associated with the thymus gland to improve immune system function. The associated neurovascular holding points for the thymus also help to enhance its blood supply. For best results, hold these points until a synchronized pulse is felt under the fingers on both hands. See the Neurolymphatic Reflex Chart on page 131 in chapter 5, and the Neurovascular Holding Point Chart for the thymus on page 159 earlier in the chapter.

- Thymus function is greatly enhanced by deep breathing, toning, singing, and emotional clearing. The emotional clearing process presented in chapter 12 is highly recommended, especially for those with chronically weakened immune systems.

The Pancreas

The next endocrine organ on the list is actually two organs rolled into one. The endocrine portion of the pancreas secretes hormones directly into the bloodstream to regulate blood sugar in the body, and the digestive portion is an exocrine gland that secretes digestive enzymes into

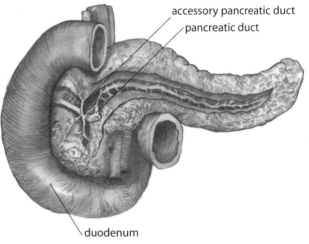

accessory pancreatic duct
pancreatic duct
duodenum

Fig. 6.10: The Pancreas

the upper portion of the small intestine. The digestive portion of the pancreas will be discussed in chapter 7.

The portion of the pancreas that is a part of the endocrine system consists of specialized cells collectively called the islands of Langerhans, named after a seventeenth-century German physician. Only 1.5 million of these islands are scattered throughout the pancreas, producing pancreatic hormones. Although the pancreas secretes a total of four hormones, it is insulin and glucagon, involved in blood sugar metabolism, that interest us the most.

Insulin and glucagon are both major regulators of blood sugar in the body. Insulin stimulates the body to lower our blood sugar level by moving glucose out of the bloodstream and into the cells as a steady source of energy or fuel. Glucagon has the opposite effect: It raises our blood sugar level by releasing stored glucose in our liver and muscle tissue for quick energy. Other regulators of blood sugar are produced by the adrenal glands.

The complementary relationship between insulin and glucagon is another version of the male and female energies working together in the body. Wherever we look in the universe, these complementary energies appear to fit perfectly, except with many human beings it seems. Perhaps these examples of perfect relationships can provide clues about how these energies can work together within ourselves and in our relationship with others.

Blood sugar or glucose is one of the major energy fuels used by the body; it supplies 98 to 100 percent of the brain's energy needs. Glucose, the Greek word for sweet wine, is much different from the refined white sugar that many of us put on our dinner table.

Glucose is a sugar that occurs throughout nature and is easily assimilated by the body. Table sugar, or sucrose, is a combination of glucose and fructose (fruit sugar), and is a refined carbohydrate that is devoid of any of the vitamins, minerals, or nutrients that formally accompanied sugar in its natural state. Refined table sugar, which the average American consumes at a rate of over 125 pounds every year, can cause multiple health problems and create numerous nutritional deficiencies in the body.

Sugar alternatives such as NutraSweet, Sweet'n Low, and aspartame are even more detrimental to your health, as they have been shown to cause over ninety different symptoms. These sweeteners interfere with your body's ability to monitor the calories it has consumed, which leads to overeating. When aspartame is heated to over 86 degrees, it can change chemically and cause a long list of serious side effects.

Honey, on the other hand, has three different types of sugar that are processed at different times in the body. In essence, honey is time-released into the bloodstream, making it much easier for the pancreas to utilize. Unprocessed honey also contains an abundance of natural minerals in proportions the body can easily handle. Other sugars that the body can handle easily include stevia, sorghum, molasses, and date sugar.

Insulin

Whenever any form of refined sugar or refined carbohydrates is introduced, they race into the bloodstream, quickly raising our blood sugar and our energy levels. This rush of sugar stimulates the body to immediately produce insulin in order to move sugar out of the bloodstream and into our tissues and cells. This in turn stimulates our cravings for more refined carbohydrates to increase our energy again, which further stimulates the pancreas to produce more insulin.

Eating refined sugar also prompts the adrenal glands to secrete adrenaline in order to keep blood sugar levels from dropping too low. Adrenaline is a chemical stressor to the body.

Even though refined sugars initially produce a rush of energy, the result in overall lack of energy can easily develop into fatigue, exhaustion, and a general intolerance to refined carbohydrates. Aside from adrenal gland fatigue, an even bigger problem in the overconsumption of refined carbohydrates is that we can burn out the limited number of insulin-producing cells in our pancreas, which is the reason for the epidemic of diabetes that currently plagues our society. Americans today are experiencing a virtual epidemic of diabetes, especially in our Native American populations.

Erratic blood sugar levels are usually the effect whenever we consume a diet high in refined carbohydrates. High-carbohydrate foods include cereals, breads, cakes, and sweets. Unstable blood sugar levels are also produced by foods that contain a high-glycemic index, such as corn, high-fructose corn syrup, rice, and potatoes. Foods with a high-glycemic index quickly elevate blood sugar levels and leave us craving more of the same kind of foods. A chart of high-glycemic foods is presented in chapter 8.

It is also interesting to note that high insulin levels brought on by the overconsumption of high-carbohydrate foods have important implications in the storage of fat in the body. Any excess sugar from high-carbohydrate sources that is not immediately utilized is stored as fat. See a more extensive list in chapter 7, appendix B.

Insulin also acts as a major inhibitor in the break down and utilization of stored fat. In other words, when we eat refined sugars and carbohydrates, we burn glucose for fuel. When we burn glucose for fuel, we stop burning fats and actually increase our fat storage. This is the major reason we get fat when we eat refined foods.

Refined sugars and refined carbohydrates also work to deplete vitamin and mineral stores in the body, create excess fat storage, overtax the pancreas and adrenal glands, and help to increase the level of unhealthy fats circulating in the blood.

When we burn glucose for fuel, we stop burning fats and actually increase our fat storage. This is the major reason we get fat when we eat refined foods.

Glycogen

Another important player in the blood sugar story is glycogen. Glycogen is the form of glucose that is stored in the liver and in our muscles. When blood sugar levels become elevated, the body initially stores the excess glucose as glycogen in our liver and muscles so that the body can access these sugars quickly and easily. When our sugar levels become low the Intelligence of the body calls upon these stored sugars to quickly elevate our blood sugar.

Muscles can also use glycogen directly when they need fast fuel, as it is stored right in the muscle where it is needed the most. If we need to get away fast from a saber-toothed tiger, we have quick access to a limited amount of energy stored inside our muscles that will give us a short burst of speed. Experienced runners usually run at a slower pace, which burns energy from fat, and they save their glycogen for the final kick at the end of the race.

Runners who run too fast for long periods of time burn these stores up quickly, and create a deficiency of muscle glycogen, which leaves them exhausted. When glycogen gets used up, the body starts to break down its own muscle tissue to get the energy from amino acids in our tissues. If this process continues, it can lead to a dangerous condition of muscle wasting.

Glucagon is the pancreatic hormone that releases the glycogen stored in our liver and muscles, raising our blood sugar as the need arises. When we go for long periods of time without eating, high levels of glucagon are found in the blood, which is an attempt by the body to raise our blood sugar. When we start eating again, insulin levels increase, and the glucagon levels decrease in the blood.

When our blood sugar levels are low, we become hungry, and our behavior often becomes altered. When blood sugar becomes excessive, it also adversely affects our behavior. The highs and lows of behavioral changes are manifested in both adults and children in a variety of ways. These symptoms often include attention deficit disorders, depression, high-energy manic episodes, fatigue, irritability, and mood swings that often end in violence. Research has shown that many violent crimes are the direct result of dramatic shifts in blood sugar levels.

The blood sugar and the digestive enzyme portions of the pancreas have two completely different functions, but they are inexorably connected. Overworking the blood sugar portion of the pancreas will negatively affect the quality of our digestion, while digestive excesses will affect the stability of our blood sugar.

Implications of pancreas disorders of the endocrine system include fatigue (temporary or chronic), excessive thirst, energy highs or lows, blurred vision, headaches, nervousness, digestive disturbances, allergies, hypoglycemia, diabetes, erratic behavioral changes and more. The same foods that exhaust the blood sugar portion of the pancreas initially lead to hypoglycemia or low blood sugar. When hypoglycemia exists for a period of time without resolution, hyperglycemia, or high blood sugar, often results in diabetes.

Associated Organs

The pancreas provides the endocrine system connection to the entire digestive and eliminative systems, which directly influences the small intestine, liver, gallbladder, and large intestine. By way of the acupuncture meridians, the pancreas is intimately associated with the spleen; by way of blood sugar, it is directly associated with the adrenal glands. The area surrounding the pancreas is often referred to as the solar plexus and is the solar center for the fire of digestion.

HEALTH TIP #5: Enhance the Functioning of Your Pancreas

If the pancreas could have its way, it would prefer five or so smaller meals evenly spaced throughout the day. The pancreas would also request a relaxed atmosphere in which to dine, with at least 50 percent of its food being raw and mostly organic.

- Try eating five or so smaller meals evenly spaced throughout the day.
- Choose foods that are low on the glycemic index, with 50 percent of your diet coming from raw foods. Eat refined carbohydrates and sugars only occasionally, and little or no caffeine, which adversely affects the pancreas–adrenal connection.
- As frequently as possible, eat in a relaxed atmosphere.
- Provide nutritional support for the pancreas, including low-potency supplementation of zinc, which is one of the main ingredients in insulin; chromium, the glucose-tolerance factor that aids in balancing blood sugar levels; selenium, vitamin A, and essential fatty acids; low-potency vitamin B complex vitamins, all eight essential amino acids, and pancreatic digestive enzymes. Deficiencies of zinc in the soil as well as the absence of B vitamins in our food often create a significant nutritional problem for the pancreas. Sources for nutritional support of the pancreas are located in appendix A.
- Stimulate the neurolymphatic strengthening points and hold the vascular holding points to enhance pancreas function. The strengthening points are located on the Neurolymphatic Reflex Chart on page 131 in chapter 5, and the Neurovascular Holding Point Chart, presented earlier in this chapter, located on page 159.

The Amazing Adrenal Glands

The powerful little adrenal glands are the next members of our endocrine orchestra. The word "ad-renals" indicates their location directly atop the kidneys. The adrenal glands look like little top hats and are the major workhorses of the endocrine system. The adrenals are often called the stress glands of the body due to their involvement in the general adaptation syndrome.

Dr. Hans Selye, who coined the term "stress," observed a triad of findings accompanying an overall pattern of stress in the human body. The three findings in the general adaptation syndrome, or GAS, are the enlargement of the adrenal glands, the shrinking of the thymus and lymph glands, and the appearance of ulcers in the stomach and/or intestines.

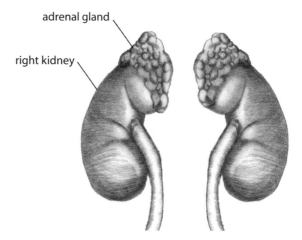

Fig. 6.11: The Adrenal Glands

According to Selye, when these conditions exist, the body is under considerable stress.

The GAS has three stages. Stage one is called the alarm reaction. In this stage the adrenal glands respond to stress by producing an abundance of adrenal hormones. In stage one, the adrenals are working overtime.

Stage two is called the resistance stage. When we hit this stage the body has already been under stress for a period of time, and the adrenals try to adapt to the increased level of stress. They do so by enlarging in size to handle the workload. In this stage the adrenals cannot keep up with the body's demand for their wide variety of antistress hormones.

The third stage of the GAS is the exhaustion phase. In this dangerous phase a person loses his/her ability to cope with stress on all levels of human function. In stage three a person literally runs out of gas and is unable to effectively cope with the stress of their lives. Many of the autoimmune-system diseases experienced today, including rheumatoid arthritis, Crohn's disease, chronic fatigue syndrome, and lupus, involve exhausted adrenal glands.

Stress, as we already know, can exist on all levels of our experience: the structural, biochemical, mental, emotional, and the spiritual. To that we can add something called thermal stress. Thermal stress can occur when we get a chill from a cold draft or air-conditioning, or when we become overheated. When stress levels are already high, thermal stress is enough to be the straw that breaks the camel's back, causing the body to break down into a state of dis-ease.

The adrenal glands are important players for both the endocrine system and overall biochemical balance in the body. In times of stress, the adrenals act as the backup system for the entire endocrine system. Unfortunately, adrenal fatigue is one of the most frequent findings in chiropractic offices across the country because we live such stressful lives. As the pace of our lives increases, the adrenals just get more and more overworked.

Many of us live in a constant state of stress and overdrive—in our jobs, homes, and relationships. Even our exercise patterns frequently create stress and overstimulate our already fatigued adrenal glands. When our backup system wears out, we are setting ourselves up for big health problems in our immediate future.

Each adrenal gland is actually two different organs rolled into one. The adrenal cortex is the outer portion of the gland, and the adrenal medulla is the inner portion. The two are in such close proximity so that their hormones can be utilized together to create biochemical balance.

These little one-inch glands weigh about 16/100^{ths} of an ounce, and manufacture somewhere in the neighborhood of sixty different hormones!

Adrenal hormones exist in three distinct groupings. Let's take a look at a few hormones in each group.

The Adrenal Cortex, Corticosteroids, and Cortisol

The adrenal cortex makes steroid hormones. Steroids are chemicals the body makes that are derived from cholesterol. Steroids are made by the adrenals, the ovaries, and the testicles. Amazingly enough, the adrenal cortex is capable of making all the steroid hormones that are made in the body, including estrogen, progesterone, and testosterone in both the male and female. This is especially significant later in life when the ovaries and testes normally make less of their powerful hormones and healthy adrenals glands come in handy, helping to insure smooth transitions into menopause and later life-stages. When the adrenals are healthy, these transitions are usually smooth. When the adrenal glands are stressed, overworked, and fatigued, these transitions can become a nightmare.

The three groups of adrenal cortex hormones called corticosteroids are mineral balancers, blood sugar regulators, and the male and female hormones.

The mineral balancers get their name because they effect the balance of minerals, or electrolytes, in the body, primarily sodium, potassium, and chlorides. The mineral balancers are also responsible for the balance of salt and water in the body, and are instrumental in balancing the body's pH. The main hormone in this group is aldosterone, which is responsible for 95 percent of the activity in this first group of hormones. The concentrations of minerals in the blood, monitored by the pineal gland, are vitally important to the body. A loss of function in these mineral-balancing hormones would be fatal in less than a week.

The second group of hormones of the adrenal cortex helps us balance blood sugar levels in the body. The primary hormone for the regulation of blood sugar by the adrenals is cortisol.

The blood sugar–balancing hormones of the adrenals are controlled by a negative feedback system in which the body discerns the circulating level of hormones in the blood. When the levels are low, it stimulates the pituitary to secrete hormones to stimulate the adrenal cortex to make more cortisol hormone.

The function of cortisol is a little different from the function of the pancreatic hormones we looked at earlier, as the primary source of glucose comes from breaking down proteins and fats. The action of cortisol on the liver can increase blood sugar levels as much as 10 times.

Cortisol functions to control our reaction to stress and trauma, helps to control our blood pressure, and has an anti-inflammatory effect on our tissues. High levels of cortisol in the blood are an indication of a body that may be in trouble and is in the process of breaking down.

The Adrenal Medulla

The adrenal medulla is the inner portion of the adrenal glands that lie closest to the kidney. This portion of the adrenal glands is actually composed of nerve tissue and associated with the sympathetic nerve system.

The hormones of the medulla are actually produced by nerve endings that are stimulated by the nerve system. These famous hormones have been called the fight-or-flight hormones. There are two of them, and the first is epinephrine, more commonly known as adrenaline. You probably know about the "adrenaline rush" that precipitates an emergency situation where quick action is required, and this little hormone can muster the strength of a giant. Under the influence of adrenaline, people have been known to pick up cars in order to get someone out from underneath. The function of adrenaline, although short-lived, gives us the strength to stay and fight, or to turn and run away with great speed.

Athletes and extreme sports competitors love the feeling that adrenaline brings when it is produced by the body in times of danger. Athletes and others often create extreme or dangerous situations, like bungee jumping or parachuting, in order to produce more adrenaline and the powerful feelings that go along with it. Unfortunately, the body gets accustomed to these pseudo-emergency situations, and more and more dangerous events are necessary to recreate the adrenaline high. As I mentioned earlier in the chapter, adrenaline acts as a major stressor to the body.

People can become stuck in a state of emergency where the adrenals continually produce adrenaline hormone in response to their daily life situations. This experience may be stimulated by work-related deadlines, pressure to perform, or the stress and tension of constant self-imposed demands to get something done in a rush. The overproduction of adrenaline drives our adrenals past the point of normal function, and they are unable to perform their normal tasks.

Extremes in exercise can also be added to the long list of adrenal overstimulation. This rush condition ages the body rapidly and creates many areas of breakdown because our fight-or-flight mechanism is only designed to be used occasionally, when real life-threatening situations exist.

The other hormone produced by the adrenal medulla is norepinepherine. The action of epinephrine/adrenaline and norepinepherine are very similar. Adrenaline is secreted by the medulla 80 percent of the time, and is stronger and more forceful, while norepinepherine is less stimulating and less powerful. It is thought that epinephrine is released when a known stressor is present, and norepinepherine is released in the presence of an unexpected stressor. Both hormones are produced in response to fear and are chemically based on the amino acid tyrosine.

Adrenaline stimulates the heart, nerve system, endocrine glands and kidneys, elevates the blood sugar and blood pressure, and increases the need for essential amino acids used for fuel. Both hormones increase our blood pressure and constrict the blood to our vital organs and skin, diverting blood flow to our muscles, liver, and brain for a quick getaway.

The prolonged effects of these hormones on the body can be a reduction in our metabolic rate, restlessness, anxiety, fear, depression, fatigue, fast heart rate, increased sweat gland activity, slow and ineffective digestion, blood sugar changes, and chronic high blood pressure.

Throughout our entire lifetime, the adrenals only produce about one teaspoon of adrenaline, which indicates how powerful these adrenal-based hormones really are, and how sensitive we are to them.

Evaluation of your multidimensional stress levels provides the keys to owning healthy-functioning adrenal glands. Become aware of the signs and symptoms of adrenal fatigue before emergency procedures become necessary.

Small changes in lifestyle go a long way in rejuvenating these baritones of the endocrine orchestra. It is certainly worthwhile to spend the time it takes to keep these little gems healthy and happy.

Implications

Stress-related illness cuts a wide swath through the field of sickness and disease. Whenever a stress-related problem is present, you will most likely find these little powerhouses right in the middle of the problem.

The list of adrenal-related problems is long and involves multiple body systems. They include blood sugar problems, fatigue, mood swings, insomnia, chronic infections, allergies, symptoms of arthritis, reoccurring inflammatory conditions, swelling of extremities, foot problems, sacroiliac joint involvement, lower back pain, numerous reproductive system problems, midback pain, headaches, knee problems, hip pain, depression, mood swings, emotional disturbances, and learning disabilities.

If adrenal function is impaired, the resulting mineral or electrolyte imbalance can result in additional symptoms, including muscle twitches, heart palpitation or arrhythmia, abnormal sensitivity to light, and swelling or edema in the extremities.

Associated Organs

The adrenals are intimately associated with the pineal gland, hypothalamus, pituitary, thyroid, thymus, pancreas, kidneys, and the sex glands. Hormones from the pituitary gland directly control both portions of the adrenals.

The muscles associated with the adrenal glands include the sartorius, gracilis, posterior tibialis, soleus, and gastrocnemius. Continued weakness in any of these muscles indicates the presence of adrenal fatigue.

HEALTH TIP #6: Enhance the Functioning of Your Adrenals

- There are several important indicators of adrenal gland dysfunction that are relatively easy to evaluate. The first is a blood pressure test called Ragland's sign. The test is performed by taking your blood pressure while lying down or sitting, and recording the readings. The readings are taken again immediately upon standing. When healthy adrenal glands are present, the blood pressure readings should rise by at least eight points. If blood pressure doesn't rise, or is lowered, adrenal fatigue is usually present. Generally, low blood pressure is a sign of adrenal fatigue.

- Another indicator of normal adrenal function is the pupillary light reflex. Shining a light into the eye normally produces a constriction of the pupil. If the adrenals are healthy, the pupil will stay constricted for 30 seconds even with a steady light. If adrenal fatigue is present, the pupil will alternately dilate and constrict (pulse) throughout the 30-second period, which is a sign of adrenal fatigue.

- Overworked, fatigued, or exhausted adrenals call for changes in lifestyle. Reducing stress on all levels of your experience is an important part of the solution. Constantly running around, being perpetually busy, always on the go, and constantly talking on the phone set us up for adrenal exhaustion. The warning signs are usually present before symptoms of dis-ease ever arise. If your lifestyle is stuck in rush mode, adrenal fatigue is not far away. Take the hint before it's too late for the adrenals to regain their strength.

- The anti-inflammatory mechanism of the body is also regulated by adrenal hormones. The mineral-balancing hormones are pro-inflammatory hormones, while the blood sugar hormones are anti-inflammatory in nature. When healthy adrenal glands are present, a balance naturally occurs between the two. It is important to remember that inflammation is always the first stage of healing, so trying to eliminate inflammation with anti-inflammatory drugs is not usually the best answer; in fact, it often adds to the problem. If aspirin and NSAIDS (non steroidal anti-inflammatory drugs) temporarily relieve your condition, this really indicates a need for more essential fatty acid nutrition. Chronic inflammatory conditions, such as arthritis, joint problems, and allergies, are a further indicator of adrenal fatigue and exhaustion. To aid anti-inflammatory nutrition anywhere in the body, include the following: essential fatty acids in fish and flaxseed oils; bromeline and other digestive enzymes taken between meals; the herbs turmeric, horsetail, and rosemary; and vitamin C complex that includes bioflavonoids. You should also use cold packs and avoid heat. See appendix A for sources of anti-inflammatory nutritional formulas.

■ The alignments and exercises offered in chapter 4 are a big help in establishing normal adrenal gland function, as is the Slant Board Exercise offered in chapter 3. Spinal adjustments administered by a chiropractor can also be an extremely useful part of your efforts at re-establishing normal adrenal gland function.

■ Nutritional support for the adrenal glands include the following: adrenal glandular extracts, potassium, organic copper, selenium, vitamin C, vitamin G, niacinamide, vitamin B6, pantothenic acid, licorice root, the amino acid tyrosine, and a mercury-free source of essential fatty acids. Sources for all nutritional supports for the adrenal glands are listed in appendix A.

■ Following the Adrenal Diet outlined in chapter 7, especially for adrenal body types, is also extremely effective. Avoid refined carbohydrates, caffeine, and substances that overstimulate the adrenals, including includes salt, red meat, fried or greasy foods, sugar, marijuana, and alcohol.

■ A splash of cold water at the end of your shower in the morning will be a much better boost to your adrenal glands than another cup of coffee.

■ Stimulating the neurolymphatic strengthening points and the vascular holding points will benefit the function of the adrenal glands. Neurolymphatic reflex points are located on page 131 in chapter 5, and neurovascular holding points are located on page 159 earlier in this chapter.

The Ovaries and Testes

The baseline of the endocrine orchestra is filled out by the gonads, which include the ovaries in the female, and the testicles in the male.

"Ovary" is derived from the Latin word meaning "egg." The ovaries are the paired female reproductive organs that produce both eggs and hormones. At birth, the ovaries contain over of 500,000 immature egg cells. This number is reduced to around 34,000 during adolescence. During the childbearing ages of thirteen and

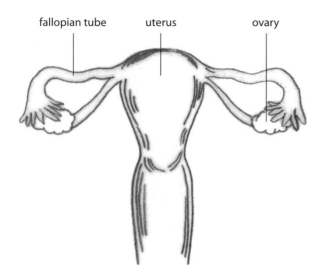

fallopian tube   uterus   ovary

Fig. 6.12: The Ovaries and Fallopian Tubes

fifty, a woman will bring some four hundred eggs to maturity.

Every four weeks one egg matures and is released from one alternating ovary, and enters the narrow fallopian tube. Each ovary has a fallopian tube that opens into the uterus, which is the most powerful muscle in the human body.

If this egg is fertilized by the male sperm cell, it travels to the uterus and attaches itself to the wall of the uterus. The uterus becomes home to the developing fetus, where the amazing miracle of life begins to unfold. If the egg is not fertilized by sperm cell, it passes out of the body during the process of menstruation. This monthly cycle in the female reproductive system is primarily controlled by the hormones of the anterior pituitary gland.

The ovaries produce two endocrine hormones, estrogen and progesterone. In the twenty-eight day moon cycle of a woman, estrogen is dominant for the first fourteen days until ovulation occurs, when progesterone becomes dominant and estrogen wanes.

Estrogen

At least six different forms of estrogen have been isolated in the female. Although estrogen is primarily secreted by the female ovaries, small quantities are also produced by the adrenal glands in both the male and female, and in the placenta, which is the lifeline for a developing fetus. The placenta can produce up to 300 times the amount of estrogen produced by the ovaries.

Only three types of estrogen are produced in significant amounts by the ovaries. These are estradiol—the most potent form of estrogen—estrone, and estriol. Estradiol is twelve times stronger than estrone and eighty times stronger than estriol.

Estrogen has a wide range of effects on the female body.

1. Estrogen acts as a potent steroid that promotes growth and development in the egg follicle, fetus, and other cells of the body.

2. It helps to control the thickness of the mucous secretions in the vagina, which assist the transport of sperm cells to the uterus.

3. Estrogen aids in the development of a thick muscular wall in the fallopian tubes, which assists the egg to move into the uterus as the muscles contract.

4. It helps in the development of a rich lining in the uterus, into which the fertilized egg attaches itself.

5. Estrogen increases fat deposits in the mammary glands.

6. Estrogen develops a duct system for milk production for the newborn infant.

7. Estrogen also directs the pituitary gland to secrete hormones that assist in the maturation process of fetal development.

It is interesting to note that men and women have exactly the same basic breast tissue, especially in the first two decades of life. Under the influence of the right hormones, the male breast can develop sufficiently to produce milk. Presently, there are tribes in Africa in which the male actually takes over the breast-feeding activities!

I would like to emphasize the benefits of breast-feeding. Whenever it is physically possible, breast-feeding should be utilized, as it provides instant immunity for the newborn. Today, colostrum is available in many health food stores and is used to rehabilitate a devitalized adult immune system. This amazing immune-system activator makes all the difference in a newborn immune system and supports immune-system function for a lifetime. In mother's milk, especially in the first few weeks, colostrum is the most important ingredient.

Infant formulas, especially made with soy, do not contain anything close to the nutrients contained in mother's milk and are among the unhealthiest supplements known to man. Infant formulas not only use synthetic vitamins and minerals, which are difficult for the body to utilize, but they contain additives, pesticides, hormones, and harmful chemicals that can cause allergies and allergic reactions in newborns. Natural formulation is beginning to be available, and it is also possible to make your own. For additional ideas, see the Weaning Formula in chapter 9, appendix B.

The liver also plays an integral part in the metabolism of circulating estrogens. The liver helps to deactivate the potency of estrogen in the body by breaking it down into weak forms of estrogen that are easily eliminated from the body in the bile from the liver. If liver activity is abnormal, the levels of circulating estrogen will be abnormally high, causing all sorts of physical, mental, and emotional problems. This fact makes it vitally important to evaluate liver function in all associated female hormone-related problems.

Traces of estrogen are present in the male body, too, especially during puberty and old age. As men age, less male hormones and more estrogen are produced. Interestingly enough, the female hormone estrogen is the main biochemical reason that a man mellows with age.

Progesterone

Progesterone is the complementary hormone to estrogen in the female reproductive system, with the primary responsibility of preparing the lining of the uterus for the implantation of a fertilized egg. Progesterone is secreted more prominently during the second half of the female cycle, just prior to the release of the egg, which is called ovulation.

Progesterone, which means "to prepare for growth," also helps to release the egg from the ovaries. Once an egg is fertilized by sperm cells, progesterone keeps the ovaries from releasing more eggs.

Progesterone also relaxes the muscular contractions stimulated by estrogen in the uterus and fallopian tubes. This helps the egg to implant into the uterine wall and keeps it from being expelled by uterine contractions.

During pregnancy, progesterone stimulates breast development by preparing them for the production of milk, which is a process initiated by the pituitary gland. During pregnancy, the placenta also secretes up to 10 times the amount of progesterone of a non-pregnant female.

Progesterone also helps to break down protein for the development of the fetus. Our Inner Intelligence always makes sure that the fetus has enough life-building nutrients to develop healthy tissue and always provides nutrients to the fetus first, before the mother.

Testosterone

We conclude our look at the endocrine system with the male hormone testosterone. There are at least two recognized forms of testosterone hormones, called androgens. Androgens are male steroid hormones produced in the testicles and the adrenal glands. The amazing adrenals produce at least five different kinds of androgens.

In addition to testosterone, the testes of the male also produce small amounts of estrogen. What this estrogen does, and where in the testicle it is produced, remains unknown.

The regulation of testosterone is dependent on a hormone secreted by the pituitary gland that in turn depends on the hypothalamus of the brain for its instructions.

Testosterone, which is only active for 15–30 minutes after it is secreted, is responsible for the development of male characteristics in the body, which include a deepening of the voice, an increase in body hair, a form of teenage acne, increased sweating, and a toughening and darkening of the skin. Male baldness seems to occur when too much testosterone is produced.

Testosterone has been called the youth hormone because of its effect on increasing muscular development. Testosterone increases the size and strength of the bones in the body by increasing bone matrix and helping the body retain more calcium salts.

Testosterone increases anabolism, which is the constructive portion of metabolism, by increasing cellular activity by as much as 15 percent. This also helps to build muscle and increase body mass. When testosterone is administered, the number of red blood cells in the body increases by 20 percent, which is why the average male has up to one million more red blood cells per cubic millimeter than a female.

Androgens are the steroid of choice for building power and strength in the body, and athletes have been using androgens in one form or another for years to get a leg up on the competition. Unfortunately, there is no free lunch, and the price paid for this life-threatening advantage is unusually steep.

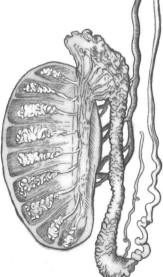

Fig. 6.13: The Testicles

Male Reproduction

Another portion of the testicles do not produce testosterone hormones and contain germ cells that mature into sperm cells or spermatozoa. These cells are surprisingly similar in nature to the ovary cells of the female.

The testicles form in the abdominal cavity and descend into the scrotum during the seventh month of pregnancy. This sac is purposefully located outside of the body in order to provide a lower temperature for the delicate sperm to survive.

A testicle consists of a series of tubules with a central cavity where sperm cells continually mature under the direction of the pituitary gland. From here, mature sperm cells are stored in a two-foot-long tube, called the vas deferens, which lies between the testicles and the prostate. It is in the vas deferens that sperm cells are fed fruit sugar, ascorbic acid, several amino acids, and the B vitamin inositol. When in storage, sperm cells secrete carbon dioxide, which keeps them relatively dormant. Here they can remain fertile for up to fifty-two days.

Another player in the drama of reproduction is the prostate gland. The prostate secretes an extremely alkaline, milky white fluid that is essential for the successful fertilization of an egg. Since vaginal secretions are very acidic, it takes the alkaline secretions of the prostate to balance the pH of the semen in order for it to be effective.

Sperm cells are kept on ice in the vas deferens until just the right moment, when fluid from the seminal vessels (the thick mucus part of the semen) and fluid from the prostate (the thin white alkaline substance) activate the sperm and neutralize the acids of the female.

During ejaculation all three fluids combine via simultaneous contraction of the prostate, the vas deferens, and the seminal vesicles, and some 400 million sperm are activated. They will have twenty-four to seventy-two hours at body temperature to race to their goal of the female egg. Only one of these 400 million sperm will reach the finish line and complete the job.

Implications of female endocrine system imbalance include the following symptoms:

> premenstrual tension
> water retention

swelling of breasts

excessively long or short menstrual cycle

menstrual camps

amenorrhea or absent menses

night sweats

hot flashes

lower back pain

headaches

digestive and elimination system problems

painful menstruation

emotional upset

Too little estrogen can cause diminished menstrual flow problems, while too much estrogen can cause excessive flow problems. Too much progesterone can cause a menses that is too long, while too little progesterone can make the cycle too short in duration. Any of these imbalances can affect the ability of a woman to conceive a child or carry it to full term.

As menses can be seen as an elimination process, abnormal function of the kidney, or the small or large intestines, can cause problems with menstruation.

The liver is another connection with a huge influence on the female cycle. If the large intestine is toxic, the liver also becomes toxic and unable to fully break down and recycle estrogen and progesterone.

In the male, an excess of androgens can create problems with physical and emotional control. Behavioral problems as a result of too much male hormone can create aggressive and violent behavior, which can at times be uncontrollable.

Associated Organs

Organs associated with ovary function are the pituitary, thyroid, adrenal glands, uterus, kidneys, bladder, liver, large intestine, skin, sweat glands, and saliva glands.

The organs associated with the testes are the prostate, kidney, bladder, sweat glands, and saliva glands. The muscles associated with gonadal function are the gluteus maximus, gluteus medius, piriformis, and the adductor muscles.

HEALTH TIP #7: Enhance the Functioning of Your Sexual Organs

Due to the fact that the pelvis is such an integral part of gonadal function, structural alignment of the pelvis and lumbar spine by a doctor of chiropractic is essential for maintaining proper gonadal function.

Taking your basal temperature for a month will evaluate not only the thyroid gland but ovarian function as well. A natural health care practitioner trained in these methods will be able to find nutritional resolutions for thyroid and ovarian imbalances. Muscle-testing procedures performed by an applied kinesiologist can evaluate the function of the ovaries and adrenal glands, and are available through the chiropractic profession. The basic procedure for taking a basal temperature reading is provided in appendix B.

Utilizing the Slant Board Exercise in chapter 2, is extremely beneficial in counteracting the effects of gravity on the uterus. The Squat Series in chapter 4 is especially beneficial.

Stimulating the neurolymphatic strengthening points and the vascular holding points are of great help in supporting gonadal function.

The gonads benefit from the following nutritional substances: essential fatty acids, wheat germ oil, vitamin B, inositol, vitamin D, iodine, zinc, trace minerals, and vitamins A, E, F, and K, as contained in oil-soluble chlorophyll complex.

Substances that adversely affect gonadal function include birth control pills, hormone replacement therapy, hydrogenated fats, denatured fats, and caffeine. Sources of nutritional products for the female and male reproductive system are listed in appendix A.

Today, we ingest unusually high amounts of hormones from our food sources, including poultry, red meats, and especially milk. High amounts of hormones can be a major factor in creating endocrine system imbalances, early sexual development in young adults, and behavioral problems that we encounter in today's world. Eating organic meats and dairy products whenever possible can make a significant difference in the outcome. See chapter 8 for more details on whole food sources.

Following the guideline in the gonadal diet in chapter 7 can be a big help, especially for gonadal body types. The gonads are overstimulated by spices, creamy foods, and red meat.

Conclusion

The endocrine system is an important part of master control for the Intelligence of the body. Working side by side with the nerve system, the endocrine system regulates metabolic function. It oversees a cascade of biochemical actions, the transportation of chemical stimulants, and a host of biological functions that are responsible for the vital health of our cells. And it is the health of our cells that ultimately determines the health of our body.

In order to experience vibrant health biochemically, it is essential for the endocrine system to be functioning at peak performance levels. And, like any orchestra, this requires that each instrument be finely tuned and ready to respond to the master conductor.

The insight and information provided in this chapter will help you better tune your human instrument. Using your signs and symptoms as a guide, you can determine which endocrine organs are most out of tune and how to begin to implement a strategy for change.

The Body Type diet presented in chapter 7 will provide much more insight on how to respond to the specific needs of your endocrine system by creating a diet based on your specific body type. Implementing the Body Type solutions, as well as solutions contained in chapter 8, will help you achieve endocrine system balance.

The methods of testing offered in chapter 9 will allow you to learn more about yourself and your amazing endocrine system, and you will become more specific about the questions you ask. You will realize that all the important information you need about your multidimensional health is being provided for you right now by your Inner Intelligence. You need only continue developing the skills to listen, see, and understand how to translate that information into simple, practical solutions.

The endocrine system is so sensitive that it manifests our feelings and emotions biochemically. This fact, which research has demonstrated over and over again, shows that positive feelings produce beneficial biochemical actions, while negative feelings produce biochemical imbalances. It seems that whatever perception we choose to embrace also becomes our biochemical reality. How we choose to feel about our bodies, ourselves, and the other human beings that populate our world shapes our biochemistry.

Although dietary measures can be a big help in balancing the body, a sick emotional realm can override even the best dietary intentions. This is also true for our structural health, as an unhealthy perspective also has a direct influence on our structural balance.

In reality, our endocrine system is ready to play the type of music we wish to express in our daily lives. If we are a complaining sort, the endocrine system will match our biochemistry to that tonal expression. If we embrace the joy that is available to be expressed in every moment, the endocrine system will match our biochemistry to that.

Ultimately, it is true that we are the composer of our own symphony. We have assembled the greatest musicians of all time, their instruments are tuned and ready, and we have the magic wand of life in our hands. If you listen, you can hear a pin drop. Let the music begin.

Chapter 7

Insightful Nutrition

THROUGHOUT THIS BOOK, you have been reading about our inherent ability to receive valuable information from higher levels of Intelligence. As the faithful servant of this Inner Intelligence, your body transmits a constant flow of information, signs, and symptoms about what is working in your life and what is not working. If you listen for the feedback, recognize how it applies to your life, and make the appropriate changes, your Inner Intelligence will guide you to a life brimming with health and happiness. Your Inner Intelligence will help guide you to discover your ideal diet and assist you in maintaining the highest levels of biochemical balance.

Innately, you may already know what foods your body likes you to eat, and which ones you need to stay away from, by discerning the way you feel following each meal. The idea here is not about eating the foods that you crave, or even your favorite foods, but consuming the foods that increase your overall sense of vitality. To increase the vitality of your body with nutrition, eat more vital foods. For the record, it is often our favorite foods that cause us the biggest problems. This is certainly true in the case of allergies, which are usually caused by the foods we crave the most and eat too often.

The Ideal Diet

In my experience, the ideal diet includes several interconnected components, listed below, which will be discussed in detail in this chapter.

1. Whole foods
2. Body type
3. The key elements of the healthiest diet in the world
4. The principles of food combining
5. pH Balance in the body
6. An awareness of the glycemic index and glycemic load
7. Natural methods of cleansing, detoxification, and elimination

1. Whole Foods

Whole foods form the basis for any healthy diet or eating plan. Whole foods contain food as it was originally designed by nature, including an abundance of vitamins, minerals, and synergistic factors such as enzymes that enable the body to digest them and utilize the benefits. Whole foods also contain a variety of nutrients that have not yet been discovered.

- Eat organically grown whole foods whenever possible. Organic foods eliminate the negative health effects of chemical additives, preservatives, radiation, and pesticides, and deliver the most vital energy possible to the body. Eat raw organic fruits and vegetables on a daily basis, as they still have their enzymes and delicate nutrients intact and provide great fiber. My rule of thumb for a whole foods diet is to eat six vegetables, two fruits, one starch, and one protein per day.

- Eliminate foods containing hydrogenated oils or trans-fats, and vegetable oils that have been denatured by heating during processing. As a rule, the less an oil has been processed, the better quality fat it contains. Hydrogenated oils contain rancid fats that have been disguised by the process of hydrogenation in order to create products with a longer shelf life. Hydrogenated foods include chips, crackers, snack foods, and a host of others. Read labels to avoid this dangerous addition to our food supply.

- Introduce beneficial fats, such as extra virgin olive oil, coconut oil, and cold-pressed vegetable oils from a health food store. These "good" fats are absolutely essential for health, especially the health of your endocrine system. I also recommend taking supplemental omega-3 fish oil (no mercury please), flaxseed oil, and unfiltered omega-6 olive oil on a daily basis.

- When cooking vegetables, steam or stir-fry them with little or no cooking oil if possible. Cooking can turn even the best oil bad. Fried foods provide a direct route to heart disease. Stainless steel cookware seems to be the best. Avoid toxic metal poisoning from aluminum cookware at all costs. See appendix B for the smoke point of many oils.

- Reduce or eliminate refined carbohydrates, which include sugar. Refined carbohydrates usually contain hydrogenated fats, which lead to heart disease, adversely effect blood sugar levels, and deplete the body's stores of minerals and vitamins. Whenever a refined, denatured, or incomplete food is eaten, the body tries to convert it into a whole food by using the vitamins and minerals that it has stored. In this way, refined foods actually magnify nutritional deficiencies, which directly lead to degenerative disease.

- Reduce or eliminate the consumption of caffeine and alcohol, which wear out your body quickly and ultimately lead to ill health and dis-ease.

2. Body Type

Unique factors exist in each human body and comprise your biochemical individuality. Taking these factors into consideration when designing a dietary regime makes the difference between success and failure. I have been especially successful in utilizing the Body Type diet together with body-type-specific exercises with my patients to determine their biochemical individuality.

HEALTH TIP #1: The Body Type Diet

The Body Type diet provides an excellent means of accommodating the vast range of biochemical differences that are present in each human being. I have used it extensively for over twenty years and have found it to be both accurate and effective.

The Body Type diet is based on hereditary factors, and emphasizes the dominance of a particular endocrine organ throughout a person's development. The body type classifications are determined for each person by the dominant action of this specific endocrine organ. This endocrine organ is genetically the source of one's strength and vitality.

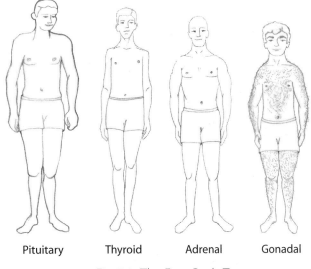

Pituitary   Thyroid   Adrenal   Gonadal

Fig. 7.1: The Four Body Types

The body typing system I use looks at the dominance of a particular endocrine organ. There are four different endocrine body types: pituitary, thyroid, adrenal, and gonadal. This is all about heredity. I'm sure that you can easily recognize hereditary factors that exist in your own family. Some families are tall and thin, while others are shorter and heavier. These family heredity factors can be traced to the dominant function of a particular organ of the endocrine system during development. This dominant organ helps to determine the type of physical development or body type a person has, their specific type of metabolism, food cravings, mental tendencies, and even their emotional makeup.

It is extremely beneficial to know your own body type, as it will aid you throughout your life in maintaining a state of health and well-being. It is especially important not to overwork this dominant endocrine organ, as serious health problems can result when this organ begins to falter. Knowing your body type not only allows you to avoid overstressing this key organ, but it aids in establishing positive habits that help to strengthen it.

You can usually determine people's body type from their physical characteristics: the size and shape of their body, the angle and shape of their rib cage, the size and shape of their head, the shape of their extremities (especially the hands), and the foods they crave. Initially, these foods stimulate and energize a dominant endocrine organ; after several years, however, the organ becomes overstimulated and fatigue begins to set in, which can lead to a host of functional problems throughout the body.

Most of you will be successful in determining your body type from the information listed below. The accompanying illustrations are a big help, especially with weight gain patterns.

■ Weight Gain Patterns

Each of the four body types will gain weight in a specific part of their body that relates directly to their dominant endocrine gland. When the foods and lifestyle that overstimulate that gland are reduced or eliminated, the related weight gain pattern is also reduced.

It is important to note, however, that you can have a weight gain pattern that is different from your body type. Also, a person can have more than one pattern of weight gain.

I have outlined these weight gain patterns and the specific foods that create them. Eliminate the foods that weaken your dominant endocrine organs and create weight gain patterns, and you will strengthen your dominant organ and eliminate the weight. Additional information about weight loss is included in the following profile for each body type.

■ The Pituitary Body Type

Pituitary body types are the tallest of all body types, with large long bones, and a head that often seems too big for their body. Pituitary body types also have large hands with large palms and long tapered fingers, and they are often very creative.

The epitome of the pituitary body type character is Lurch from the old television series *The Addams Family*. Lurch has an exceptionally large forehead ridge over the eyes, enormous hands, and he is exceptionally tall with long extremities. Most basketball players are also pituitary body types. Women with a pituitary body type are physically larger below the waist.

The pituitary gland is stimulated by prolactin in milk, so pituitary types crave milk and dairy products, which can overstimulate and adversely effect pituitary gland function. This is especially evident today, when large amounts of hormones are legally present in milk and dairy products.

Pituitary types don't metabolize simple carbohydrates very effectively. These would include the sugars found in fruit and fruit juices, the lactose present in milk, and the refined sugar and sweeteners found in refined foods. It seems ironic, then, that they tend to crave these carbohydrates.

Pituitary types function best on a high protein (including red meat), low-carbohydrate diet, with little or no dairy products. For this type I usually recommend a high-protein breakfast, a moderate lunch, and a lighter dinner.

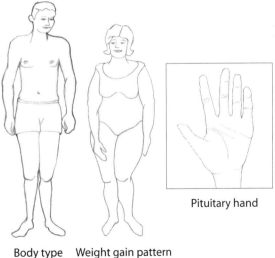

Pituitary hand

Body type   Weight gain pattern

Fig. 7.2: The Pituitary Body Type

Pituitary women usually have symptoms of low estrogen and/or low progesterone.

THE PITUITARY DIET

Abundant amounts of the following:

Ocean fresh seafood, free-range poultry, tofu, raw nuts and seeds, fresh vegetables, water, and herbal teas, especially fenugreek.

Moderate amounts of the following:

Organically raised red meat (beef, lamb, and organ meats), legumes, whole grains, fresh fruits, butter, and vegetable oils.

Avoidance of the following:

All dairy products, sugar, coffee, black tea, fried foods, margarine, Crisco, refined carbohydrates, and fruit juices.

> **Note: Avoidance foods eaten occasionally will cause no real problem to the Pituitary type.**

PITUITARY BODY TYPE WEIGHT GAIN PATTERN

1. Hypo, or sluggish, pituitary weight gain pattern is identified as an overall weight gain of baby-type fat from head to toe, including the arms and hands.
2. Hyper, or elevated, pituitary weight gain pattern tends to concentrate from the waist down.

If you are a P-type trying to lose weight, you should eliminate pituitary-stimulating foods and avoid snacking between meals. Try to leave four or five hours between breakfast and lunch, and five or six hours between lunch and dinner.

■ The Thyroid Body Type

The main characteristic of the Thyroid body type is a long and lean appearance. Whereas pituitary types are usually above six feet tall, thyroid types average from about five feet five to just under six feet. Physically, thyroid types have bones that are long and thin, fine hair, and small white teeth. Their hands are also long but thin, with long, straight fingers and tough nails. Cary Grant could be considered a typical Thyroid body type. T-types are usually nervous and have inconsistent energy patterns.

Since the thyroid gland helps to regulate the speed of our metabolism, thyroid types tend toward elevated metabolism and will crave substances that stimulate the thyroid gland, and elevate their blood sugar and their metabolic rate. These would include sugars, coffee, chocolate, concentrated fruit juices, soft drinks, and alcohol. These substances should be especially avoided by thyroid types.

Thyroid body types can be classic hypoglycemics or people with low blood sugar problems, and they often have a tendency toward depression. They are also prone to arthritis, skin problems, and headaches.

Thyroid types do best on a diet high in protein, high in quality fats, and low in simple refined carbohydrates or sugars. Breakfast is the most important meal for a thyroid type as it helps to stabilize their blood sugar levels. Again, coffee and soft drinks are definitely off limits for a T-type.

If these substances are a part of the T-type's diet, especially in the early part of the day, ingestion will be followed by sharp hills and valleys in both energy levels and temperament. Thyroid types thrive on a high-protein breakfast, lunch, and dinner, divided evenly, with protein at two meals. The best schedule for the Thyroid body type is early to bed and early to rise.

THE THYROID DIET

Abundant amounts of the following:

Eggs, free-range poultry, ocean-fresh seafood, shellfish, tofu, fresh organic vegetables, raw nuts and seeds, water, and raspberry leaf tea.

Moderate amounts of the following:

Red meat and organ meats, legumes, whole grains, butter, vegetable oils, and fruit.

Avoidance of the following:

Coffee and black tea, refined carbohydrates, refined grains, desserts and sugar of all kinds, fried foods, margarine, Crisco, and fruit juices.

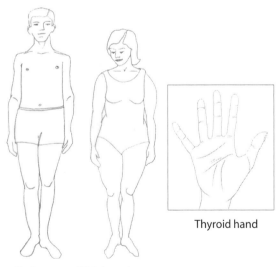

Thyroid hand

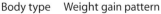

Body type   Weight gain pattern

Fig. 7.3: The Thyroid Body Type

Note: Avoidance foods eaten occasionally will cause no real problems to the Thyroid type.

THYROID BODY TYPE WEIGHT GAIN PATTERN

Soft weight from the elbows to the knees. Most pronounced in the abdomen and hips.

If you are a T-type trying to lose weight, eliminate thyroid-stimulating foods and avoid snacking between meals. Try to leave four or five hours between breakfast and lunch, and five or six hours between lunch and dinner.

■ The Adrenal Body Type

The primary characteristics of the Adrenal body type include a medium height, strong build, triangular face, broad shoulders, and square palms with tubular-shaped fingers. The fingers of the Adrenal type are about the same length as their palms. In general, most men are Adrenal types. The typical Adrenal would be Bruce Willis.

Adrenal types are usually in good health, have strong immune and digestive systems, and are friendly and outgoing. Adrenal types are prone to respiratory problems and allergies, as the thymus and thyroid glands tend to be their weakest organs, and they tend toward high blood pressure and heart problems.

Adrenal types are stimulated by fats and salt. The fats from animal products, especially red meat, overstimulate the adrenals glands. Salty and greasy foods like French fries and chips are also the downfall of the Adrenal type.

Adrenal types should consume a diet high in complex carbohydrates, such as whole grain products, beans and legumes, high in fresh fruits and vegetables, and low in animal fats. Adrenal types thrive on a light breakfast, a medium lunch, and a larger dinner with a small amount of

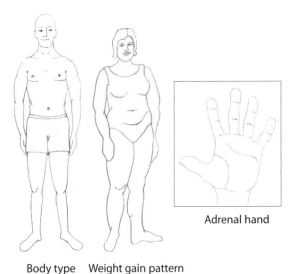

Adrenal hand

Body type   Weight gain pattern

Fig. 7.4: The Adrenal Body Type

protein. Adrenal types also need to drink plenty of pure water. Late to bed and late to rise will make an Adrenal type healthy and wise.

THE ADRENAL DIET

Abundant amounts of the following:

Whole grains, organic vegetables, fruits, legumes, low-fat dairy products, water, and herbal teas, especially parsley.

Moderate amounts of the following:

Ocean-fresh fish, free-range poultry (without the skin), eggs, tofu, coffee or tea, oils, raw nuts and seeds, butter, milk, cheese yogurt, and natural desserts.

Avoidance of the following:

Salt and salty foods, red meat, shellfish, fried foods, margarine or Crisco, sugar and other refined carbohydrates, alcohol, and yellow or aged cheeses.

> **Note: Avoidance foods can be eaten occasionally and cause no real problem for Adrenal types.**

ADRENAL BODY TYPE WEIGHT GAIN PATTERN

Centered around the belly (classic beer/carbohydrate belly).

If you are an A-type trying to lose weight, you should eliminate adrenal-stimulating foods and avoid snacking between meals. Try to leave four or five hours between breakfast and lunch, and five or six hours between lunch and dinner.

■ The Gonadal Body Type

The primary characteristics of the Gonadal body type include shorter height, enhanced sexual development, fine bones, smooth skin, small hands with tapered fingers that are usually shorter than the palms, and thick, coarse hair. Most Gonadal types are women.

The epitome of a Gonadal body type women would be the singer Dolly Parton. Gonadal type males tend to be short and strong with substantial amounts of body hair, often on their backs. Males are usually five feet nine or shorter, and women are usually under five feet three. Gonadal body types are often pear-shaped.

Gonadal types crave rich, creamy, and spicy foods, and red meat, which over-stimulate the gonads (ovaries and testes). This overstimulation eventually fatigues the gonads and results in functional problems in their reproductive system, including symptoms of menopause.

Eliminating spicy and creamy foods from a Gonadal type's diet allows the ovaries or testes to normalize their function and rebuild themselves naturally. Occasionally it is necessary to support these glands nutritionally (see appendix A for details). Gonadal types thrive on a light breakfast, a light lunch, and a larger dinner.

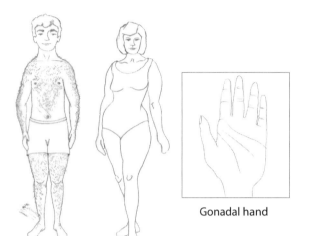

Gonadal hand

Body type   Weight gain pattern

Fig. 7.5: The Gonadal Body Type

THE GONADAL DIET

Abundant amounts of the following:

Fresh vegetables (80 percent cooked), fruits, low-fat dairy products, legumes, whole grains, and red clover tea.

Moderate amounts of the following:

Ocean-fresh fish, free-range poultry, vegetable oils, eggs, raw nuts and seeds, fruit and fruit juices.

Avoidance of the following:

Red meat, spices (Mexican, Italian, Indian, and others), sour cream, cream (especially ice cream), butter, margarine, Crisco, sugar, rich desserts and refined carbohydrates, coffee or tea.

Note: Avoidance foods can be eaten occasionally without any real problems to Gonadal types.

GONADAL BODY TYPE WEIGHT GAIN PATTERN

Larger breasts in both men and women, and dimpled weight gain on hips and thighs (saddle bags).

If you are a G-type trying to lose weight, you should eliminate gonadal stimulating foods and avoid snacking between meals. Try to leave four or five hours between breakfast and lunch, and five or six hours between lunch and dinner.

Exercises to Support Your Body Type

Each of the four body types has an affinity for a particular type of exercise, which includes a combination of cardiovascular, flexibility, and strength-training exercises. Cardiovascular exercises are those that elevate the heart rate for a sustained period of time (20–30 minutes at your ideal exercise heart rate), and include exercises like aerobics, biking, swimming, dance, jogging, fast walking, and cross-country skiing.

Flexibility exercises include yoga postures, active stretching, and range of motion exercises (as indicated in chapters 4 and 5) to improve the flexibility of your neuromusculoskeletal system and enhance your ability to recover from multidimensional stress.

Strength training includes training with free weights or using exercise machines such as Nautilus or Cybex, and exercises that provide resistance training with the use of Therabands or Theraciser. Although each body type benefits from emphasizing one type of exercise, all body types need to include all three types in their exercise program. The dominant exercises for each body type are outlined below.

The Pituitary Body Type: The emphasis for exercising the Pituitary body type is to improve whole body awareness. This is accomplished by avoiding repetitive exercises, such as running and calisthenics, and by integrating the following exercises:

- Strength training 3x week
- Freestyle movement and dance 2–3x week
- Cross Crawl and cross-country skiing–type exercises to improve coordination 3x week
- Tai Chi and Qigong exercises
- Moderate cardiovascular exercise 1–2x week
- Moderate yoga and active stretching to improve flexibility 1–2x week

The Adrenal Body Type: The emphasis for exercising the Adrenal body type is to increase cardiovascular exercise, improve flexibility, avoid heavy weight lifting and contact sports, and to integrate the following types of exercise:

- Racquetball, basketball, bicycling, fast walking, or cross-country skiing to improve cardiovascular health 3x week
- Yoga postures or active stretching to lengthen the body 3x week

- Minimal strength training with low weights and slow repetitions, utilizing the full range of joint motion 2x week
- Core-strengthening exercises

The Thyroid Body Type: The emphasis for exercising the Thyroid body type is to increase strength and endurance, and to avoid exercise with intermittent effort, such as tennis and racquetball. Thyroid body types should especially avoid overtraining, and integrate the following types of exercise:

- Strength training to increase muscle mass, with low weights, low repetitions (10–12), and slow movements through a complete range of motion 3x week
- Slow but steady endurance training 2–3x week
- Swimming, jogging, fast walking, skiing, hiking 2x week
- Yoga exercises and active stretching to maintain flexibility 2x week
- Moderate cardiovascular exercise
- Core-strengthening exercises

The Gonadal Body Type: The emphasis for exercising the Gonadal body type is to integrate the upper and lower portions of the body, and avoid exercises that overdevelop the lower body, such as bicycling, skating, rollerblading, and step aerobics. The following exercises are beneficial for Gonadal body types:

- Strength training for the upper body 3x week
- Strength training for the lower body 2x week
- Movement, dance, cross-country skiing, and fast walking 3x week
- Yoga postures and active stretching for whole body integration 3x week
- Cross Crawl Exercise
- Moderate cardiovascular exercise
- Tai Chi and Qigong exercises
- Core-strengthening exercises

HEALTH TIP #2: The Blood Type Diet

Another diet that includes the aspect of biochemical individuality is the Blood Type diet. Although I personally lean more toward the Body Type diet, the Blood

Type diet has certainly been beneficial for many people. For more information see *Eat Right 4 Your Type* by Peter D'Adamo.

> **A Word or Two for Vegetarians:** Most vegetarians need a comprehensive dietary plan to achieve biochemical balance, and they need to be especially careful to get a complete spectrum of essential amino acids. Being a vegetarian is about much more than simply not eating meat. The dietary suggestions in chapter 7 will support the vegetarian to achieve a vibrant level of health and well-being.

3. The Key Elements of the Healthiest Diet in the World

One of the most promising developments on the nutritional front, as far as I am concerned, is the Mediterranean diet. Of course, this diet isn't new. This is the way the people of the Mediterranean region have been eating (and living) for hundreds, if not thousands, of years. Among people who adhere to this diet and lifestyle, researchers have found substantially reduced rates of heart disease and cancer, and lower death rates in general. That's why it is known as the healthiest diet in the world. What are these people doing that we should know about?

They are eating great quantities of vegetables, a modest portion of meat or fish, fresh fruit for dessert, plenty of extra virgin olive oil, and drinking red wine. And they are taking life slowly, enjoying a siesta at midday, socializing with friends several times a day, eating a late dinner, and dancing until midnight. Sounds pretty healthy to me!

It is relatively simple to eat a Mediterranean diet. Just choose fresh fruits and vegetables—organically grown whenever possible—whole grains, legumes, beans, olives and herbs, limited quantities of meat, dairy, poultry, game and fish, and the magic monounsaturated fat we know as unheated extra virgin olive oil.

You can modify the Mediterranean diet by adding the insight gained from knowing your body type. Reduce your consumption of refined carbohydrates and bad fats, increase the amount of pure water you drink, add the right kind of exercise, and there you have it: a diet even better than the healthiest diet in the world.

HEALTH TIP #3: The Mediterranean Diet Pyramid

You can use the pyramid below to help you evaluate how often to eat which foods on the Mediterranean diet. The pyramid is both simple and self-explanatory. In staying with the principles outlined in this book, it would be good to restrict the consumption of breads, potatoes, pasta, rice, and other grains to just a few times per week.

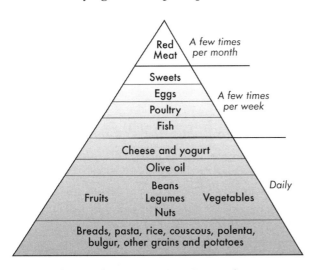

Fig. 7.6: The Mediterranean Diet Pyramid

4. The Principles of Food Combining

Food combining, which I described more fully in the last chapter, can be a powerful tool for alleviating symptoms, especially in the digestive and elimination systems. The principles of food combining include an understanding that we have two distinct digestive systems rolled into one, an acid one and an alkaline one. Our acid digestive system digests fats and proteins, while our alkaline digestive system digests carbohydrates. If we segregate our foods into those simple categories, it will make digestion and elimination much more effective and efficient.

Food combining can be beneficial at any time, but is especially of value as we begin to age and our digestion becomes less effective, or when distress and dis-ease are present in the body. Consult chapter 8 for more guidelines on food combining.

5. pH Balance in the Body

The balance of acid and alkaline levels in our bodies is known as our pH, or potential of hydrogen. Having pH levels in the range in which your body functions most effectively can greatly assist the various functions of the body. As the pH approaches more acidic or alkaline levels, the body becomes less efficient and tends to break down more quickly. That's why I believe it is so important to include a discussion of pH in any discussion of diet.

You can have your pH tested through the saliva, blood, and urine. The pH of the saliva is indicative of the state of alkaline reserves in the body, and constantly changes, especially when we eat. The pH of the urine is more stable than saliva, and usually stays within a small pH range for each person. The pH of the blood is usually extremely stable at 7.4. If blood pH changes more than .5 in either direction, severe health problems can result. Unfortunately, blood pH is difficult to monitor, and we will not consider it in this discussion.

Monitoring your pH levels is a way to help your body maintain the pH range in which it functions most effectively.

HEALTH TIP #4: Testing the pH of Your Saliva

You can monitor your pH by touching pH paper to your tongue first thing in the morning or anytime before a meal. Most experts agree that the ideal pH of saliva is 7.2–7.4, and normal lies in the range of 6.8–7.4. Most pH paper will be calibrated in increments of .5.

HEALTH TIP #5: Testing the pH of Your Urine

Many experts agree that the ideal pH of urine pH is 6.4, and lies in the normal range of 6.3–6.9. A pH of 7.2 is normal for vegetarians. If your urine is outside of these normal ranges, follow the guidelines listed below. If your urine is too acidic, which is usually the case, eating more alkaline-forming foods will help balance your pH and allow your body to function more effectively.

Acid wastes products are the result of normal body functions. These acid waste products lower our pH. When a person eats too many acid-forming foods such as meat, alcohol, or refined carbohydrates, the acid pH is lowered even further, often pushing pH levels out of the desired range and creating additional stress for the body. If your urine pH is too alkaline, which is more rare, eating more acid-forming foods will help balance your pH.

You can also use Nitrozine or pH paper to test the pH of your drinking water. The pH of water should be as close to 7 as possible. Most water sources are acidic (even as low as 5.0), which will increase your acidity, so make sure you are not adding to your acidity by drinking acidic water. See appendix A for methods and products designed to raise the pH of your water.

Balancing Your pH

You may remember from biology class the scale of pH values indicated below. The scale runs from extremely acidic to extremely alkaline. Hydrochloric acid often has a value less than 1, and pancreatic enzymes and bile range from 7.5–8.3.

Fig. 7.7: pH Diagram

Acid						Neutral						Alkaline		
0	1	2	3	4	5	6	7	8	9	10	11	12	13	14

Taking the wide range into consideration, I will use the ideal as a starting point, which means saliva is at 7.4, and urine is at 6.4. Again, these ranges will vary by individual and diet.

The method used to balance pH for both urine and saliva is primarily dietary. If the pH is overly acidic, an alkaline-forming diet is recommended; if the pH tends toward the alkaline range, acid-forming foods will help to balance your biochemistry.

The following are short lists of alkaline- and acid-forming foods. A complete list is included in appendix B under the resources for chapter 5.

Acid-forming foods include alcohol, caffeine, grains, peanuts, sugar, tobacco, and wheat.

Alkaline-forming foods include fruits and vegetables, almonds, avocados, beans, and dried fruit.

Symptoms of excess acidity include fluctuating energy levels, mental fatigue and dullness, depression, headaches, lower back pain, decreased vitality, irritability, and sinus-related problems. Keep in mind that most problems with pH balance occur due to the overconsumption of acid-forming foods. Generally speaking, our environment and lifestyle encourage the condition of excessive acidity in the body.

If you are experiencing excess acidity, add fresh vegetables and fruits to your diet. Both are alkaline forming, easier for the body to digest, make for less stress in the digestive system, and generally account for less wear and tear on the body.

Another way of reducing acidity is through the breath. The body, in its infinite wisdom, innately uses breathing to reduce acidity. Remember, the lungs are the second largest organ of elimination. The technique of integrated breathing presented in chapter 10 will allow your lungs to become more efficient at eliminating toxic waste products and helping balance your pH.

Symptoms of excessive alkalinity include tension, nervousness, muscle tension or spasms, slow recovery from injuries, and traveling muscle pain.

If you are experiencing excess alkalinity, a lack of production of hydrochloric acid in the stomach is the most likely culprit.

HEALTH TIP #6: What to Do About Split pH Readings

If the pH of the your saliva is greater than 7.4 (alkaline) and the pH of urine is less than 6.4 (acid), increase your intake of cereals, breads, and grains. If the pH of saliva is less than 7.4 (acid) and the pH of urine is greater than 6.4 (alkaline), increase the use of high-quality fats, oils (olive, flax, fish, and sesame), and organic dairy products.

HEALTH TIP #7: Colon Cleansing

Colon cleansing, outlined in chapter 8, is also recommended to normalize the internal environment of the colon, along with the addition of probiotics and beneficial yeast cultures, which remove acid waste from the body and are extremely helpful in normalizing pH.

HEALTH TIP #8: pH-normalizing Foot Bath

As part of the cleansing process, the Ion Cleanse footbath is also recommended to normalize pH and assist in removing toxins and toxic metals from the body. The footbath can be used up to twice per week for a period of 10–12 weeks to intensify your cleansing process. After this initial cleansing period, maintenance use is recommended. See appendix A for details on the Ion Cleanse detoxifying footbath.

HEALTH TIP #9: pH-Balancing Complements

When acidity is extremely low for both saliva and urine, pH-balancing nutritional supplements are often recommended. Included in appendix A are several concentrated whole food supplements, a liquid alkaline-balancing formula, and other tools that are excellent for bringing your pH into balance.

6. An Awareness of the Glycemic Index and Glycemic Load

As you discovered in the last chapter, the glycemic index is another important factor in creating the Ideal Diet. The glycemic index is an indicator of the foods that require the most insulin to be produced by the pancreas and the most work by our digestive system. Low-stress foods increase the efficiency of the digestive system, while high-stress foods set up the body for breakdown.

The higher the glycemic index, the more stress is created throughout the body; the lower the glycemic index, the lower the stress levels. Higher stress levels require more adrenaline to be produced by the adrenals glands, while lower stress levels allow the production of endorphins or emotionally beneficial chemicals to be produced. A short list of glycemic food values is listed below, and more extensive resources are listed in appendix B.

When you are considering the glycemic index (GI) of a food, you'll want to also pay attention to its glycemic load (GL), which is a relatively new way to assess the impact of carbohydrate consumption. A GI value tells you only how rapidly a particular carbohydrate turns into sugar, which is essential, but it doesn't tell you how much of that carbohydrate is in a particular serving of food. Both the GI and the GL are important in understanding a food's effect on your blood sugar. A GL of 20 or more is high, and a GL of 10 or less is low. Foods that have a low GL almost always have a low GI.

FIG. 7.8: Glycemic Index and Glycemic Load Table

Foods	Glycemic Index	Carbohydrate per gram	Serving size	Glycemic Load
Dates	103	40	2 oz	42
Cornflakes	81	26	1 cup	21
Jelly Beans	78	28	1 oz	22
Rice cakes	78	21	3 cakes	17
Baked potato	76	30	1 medium	23
Doughnut	76	30	1 medium	17
Soda crackers	74	17	4 crackers	12
White bread	73	14	1 large slice	10
Table sugar	68	10	2 tsp	7
Pancake	67	58	6" diameter	39
White rice	64	36	1 cup	23
Brown rice	55	33	1 cup	18
Spaghetti, white	38	40	1 cup	18
Spaghetti, whole wheat	37	37	1 cup	14
Bread, rye, pumpernickel	41	12	1 large slice	5
Oranges, raw	42	11	1 medium	5
Pears, raw	38	11	1 medium	4
Apples, raw	38	15	1 medium	6
All-Bran cereal	38	23	1 cup	9
Skim milk	32	13	8 fl oz	4
Lentils, dried or boiled	29	25	1 cup	7
Kidney beans	28	25	1 cup	7
Pearled barley	25	42	1 cup	11
Peanuts	14	6	1 oz	1
Cashew nuts	22	6	1 oz	2

7. Natural Methods of Cleansing, Detoxification, and Elimination

Another important part of your ideal diet is the process of tissue cleansing and detoxification.

When animals are sick, they usually abandon their normal diet, and either fast or restrict their diet to green grasses. This innate shift in dietary habits, which only lasts for a short period of time, gives the digestive system a much-needed rest and allows their bodies to heal and detoxify. This amazing healing process, which is considered normal in the world of nature, is something we humans can take advantage of, too.

Fasting and eliminative diets have been used since ancient times to improve physical health, mental well-being, and spiritual insight. In this age of denatured foods and toxic environments, it is especially important to take advantage of the body's ability to do a thorough cleanse. While attending chiropractic school in the early 70s, I spent a considerable amount of time experimenting with fasting and eliminative diets. I would regularly drink only fresh juice for four or five days at a time, and to my surprise I found that instead of becoming weak, mentally slow, and depleted of energy, I was physically energized, light on my feet, and as acute mentally as I have ever been in my life.

This cleansing process gave my digestive system a rest and helped me to rid my body of toxic wastes. The energy my body would normally use for digesting vast quantities of food was used instead to improve my health. Usually after the first day of a cleansing fast, I would find myself with a wonderful, heightened awareness about my body, my surroundings, and my connection to the Source of my life.

In the years that followed, I discovered many different methods of cleansing, ranging from simply adding more fruits and vegetables to my diet, to cleanses that lasted for several weeks.

One cautionary note: I do not recommend juice fasting as an entry point to the cleansing process, as it requires some preparatory work. The first stage of cleansing should be rather gentle, similar to sticking your toe in the pool before diving right in.

It is especially important to give yourself a gentle entry because most of us have large amounts of toxins in our bodies, and trying to cleanse too much too fast can be extremely taxing to the system. A good way to ease into the cleansing process is to create a transition diet. Over the course of a week or several weeks, increase the amount of fruits and vegetables you eat, and reduce the amount of refined carbohydrates. A transition diet will activate the cleansing mechanism in the body and prepare the body for a deeper cleanse. For most people, six vegetables, two fruits, one starch, and one protein per day provides a good transition diet. If you are more familiar with the cleansing process, you can move directly into the first cleanse.

The use of a green food supplement like barley greens, and fresh vegetable juices like carrot or celery juice, taken on a daily basis, will allow for a smooth transition. You can find a listing of some of these fine green products in appendix A.

Whenever you are cleansing, be careful not to drink too much full-strength fruit juice, as it can adversely affect your blood sugar and trigger a cleansing process that is too rapid for your body to handle. A good rule of thumb is to eat fruits and drink diluted fruit juices in the morning, except if you are a thyroid body type, and to eat vegetables and drink fresh vegetable juices in the afternoon and evening. While cleansing, a piece of fruit makes a great evening dessert.

One final note before I introduce the first cleanse: All cleansing diets have an optimum time frame. After you experience the cleansing process a few times, you will begin to discern what type of cleanse your body likes best, when your body wants to do it, and when it is over. Just as an animal stops eating at the appropriate time, your Inner Intelligence will let you know when it is time for a cleanse and when it is time to stop. The Intelligence of the body communicates this when your food doesn't taste that great, when you don't really feel like eating, or when your body doesn't feel that well after meals. Some experts say that cleansing should continue until your tongue is pick and clean; while that's a very good indicator, you don't need to do all your cleansing at once. Use the color of your tongue as a cleanse indicator, and realize that until it is pink, cleansing should still be in your immediate future. This awareness will lead you to find just the right cleanse and its time frame.

My favorite time for a cleanse is in the spring, and it fits right in with spring cleaning; however, summer and fall are also good times for fasts because there is an ample supply of fresh fruits and vegetables, and the weather is conducive. Cleansing in cold weather is usually a bad idea. There are times in winter when your body will want a cleanse, but the spring, summer, and fall are the best seasons to do it. And when you start a cleanse, you want to be committed to following it through.

HEALTH TIP #10: The Seven-Day Detoxification Feast

The Seven-Day Detox Feast is really an excellent cleanse for beginners. Please take note that it is a feast not a fast, which means you will be feasting on fruits and vegetables the entire time. While on the feast, remember to drink your normal ration of water, approximately one half your body weight in ounces every day, as this will aid your body to flush out toxins.

If you begin to feel bad on this cleanse, this is usually an indication that your tissues are especially toxic and need a good, slow cleansing. Return to a transitional diet for a few more weeks, and eat less fruit and more vegetables.

Begin the cleanse the night before by creating a supply of vegetable broth, which you can drink at anytime during the feast.

Broth Recipe

Place about 20 finely cut carrots, with tops if possible, into 2 quarts of water and boil for 15 minutes. Add one bunch of finely cut parsley and a large handful of cut spinach to the pot. Simmer for another 10–15 minutes. For additional flavor, you can add a vegetable seasoning (listed in appendix A). This broth can be taken at any time and will help to raise your blood sugar and flush the body of toxins. The amount of broth you drink can be subtracted from your daily water intake.

Fifteen minutes before breakfast, drink the juice of a medium-sized lemon, freshly squeezed into 8 ounces of hot water. This is a great way to begin your day, even when you are not on the feast. Lemon juice sets up your body for cleansing, helps to normalize your pH, and aids in the digestive process. Rinse out your mouth after taking lemon juice, as it can adversely effect your teeth. If you can feel the effects of the lemon juice on your teeth, gargle with baking soda right afterward.

During the cleanse, use the following breakfast suggestions for each of the seven days.

Fresh juice: Drink at least 8 ounces of fresh-squeezed, organically grown (if possible) orange or grapefruit juice. You may drink more if you desire.

Cottage Cheese: Eat 5 level teaspoons of cottage cheese purchased in a health food store, such as the brand Alta Dena Dairy. Supermarket cottage cheese actually contains plaster of Paris, so don't use that.

Fresh Fruit: Eat at least a half-pound of fresh fruit (you may eat more if you wish). No bananas or avocados please, as bananas are a high-starch fruit, and avocados are too rich in oils for this cleanse.

Herbal Tea: Drink a cup of the herbal tea of your choice, noncaffeinated if possible. Sweeten with a little organically raised honey if you wish. No coffee is allowed during the cleanse.

If you are a heavy coffee drinker, you may suffer from caffeine withdrawal in the form of headaches when you stop drinking coffee. If this is the case, slowly wean yourself off coffee over a 1–2 week period prior to the cleanse.

If you do have a reaction, it indicates that you are most likely addicted to caffeine. If you sense a headache coming on during the weaning process or the cleanse, have a half cup of coffee and it will usually go away. When you have withdrawal headaches, it indicates that a complete three-week break from coffee would improve your physical, mental, and emotional well-being. Three weeks is the amount of time it takes for the body to eliminate addictive substances from the body. If you return to coffee drinking after the three-week hiatus, try drinking it every other day, which will help your body to break the addiction pattern.

During the cleanse, use the following suggestions between breakfast and lunch.

Drink more fruit and vegetable juices, and eat some fresh fruits and vegetables if possible. The more live foods you introduce into your body, the more cleansing you will experience. You can also drink the vital broth at any time. Remember: this is a feast, so eat and drink your fill of acceptable foods.

During the cleanse, use the following suggestions for lunch for each of the seven days.

Vegetable Broth: Drink two cups before your meal.

Salad: Make a chopped salad of fresh raw vegetables. Use a salad dressing of extra virgin olive oil (green in color is best) and lemon juice. Use at least four of the vegetables listed below, and chew your food well.

Dessert: Eat a dessert of fresh fruit with a little honey if desired.

During the cleanse, use the following suggestions for dinner for each of the seven days.

Vegetable Broth: Drink two cups of broth before your meal.

Cooked Vegetables: Select two or three vegetables from the vegetables listed below. Steam them, and drizzle them with extra virgin olive oil. Eat a generous helping.

Dessert: You can make a baked apple or a fresh fruit salad for dessert.

Herbal Tea: Have a cup of noncaffeinated herbal tea with a little honey if desired.

If you are still hungry, eat more fruit, and drink vegetable juice or vital broth an hour or so after eating.

◼ What You Can Expect from the Feast

You may feel some discomfort the first day from having changed your regular dietary habits or from the avoidance of coffee and refined carbohydrates. These substances are addictive, and some people may initially experience symptoms from avoiding them. These symptoms may include headaches, cravings, mood swings, and mental fogginess. The symptoms are short-lived, and usually last for only a day or two. If symptoms do show up, it indicates that you are on the path to your true energy levels. When you introduce this much fresh, live food into your body, your body will be surprised—and happy.

Around the third or fourth day, your kidneys and bowels will begin to move more freely, which is the desired result, as this will aid you in eliminating toxic waste from your body. You may also experience some symptoms of nausea, gas, or a slight (toxic) headache. These are usually indicators that you are having success in your cleansing process, as toxins are now passing out of your body. It also indicates the need to drink more water. Dry skin brushing is a big help at any time during any the cleanse.

As toxins move out of the body they travel through your bloodstream, and it is common to feel them on the way out. After a few cleanses, these simple reactions won't happen much anymore.

At about the fourth or fifth day, you may feel a surge of energy, your complexion may clear up, your eyes often become brighter, and hopefully you will have moments of feeling absolutely wonderful. These are also common side effects of the cleansing process. Be determined to continue the fast for the full seven days. If you feel deprived of your normal foods, think about how many times you have had them before, and how soon you can have them again. Take it from me, breaking your fast for a tempting food is usually a big disappointment.

Acceptable vegetables to eat during your feast include artichokes, asparagus, broccoli, green beans, beets, Brussels sprouts, cabbage, carrots, cauliflower, cucumber, celery, dandelions, endive, eggplant, fresh green peas, green peppers, kale, kohlrabi, lettuce (not iceberg), okra, onions, parsley, parsnips, pumpkin, radishes, rutabagas, spinach, squash, Swiss chard, tomatoes, and turnips.

Transition Diet

When the cleanse is over, your need to eat a transition diet for a few more days so your body won't react adversely. Continue with the lemon juice and the fruits and vegetables, and add small portions of tofu, poultry, and whole grains to the mix. Try to avoid red meat and refined carbohydrates for a little while longer.

This is also a great time to evaluate the foods that you normally eat, and a great time for a dietary change. Ask yourself if you want to reintroduce this food into your clean body, or if you are much better off without it. If you pay attention to your body after you eat, your Inner Intelligence will let you know exactly what it thinks.

HEALTH TIP #11: The Eleven-Day Elimination Diet

I know eleven days seems like a long time, but this is a relatively easy cleanse that can be utilized by most everyone. I have used this cleanse in my practice for over twenty-five years. If you are a beginner, or have chronic symptoms of disease, you may wish to do the seven-day detoxification feast a few times before you try the eleven days. Elderly persons should reduce the number of days to four or five. Listen to the wisdom of your Inner Intelligence, as it will tell you exactly what you need. However, do not listen too much to your babbling mind during the cleanse, especially for the first day or two. Whenever you cleanse anything, the first thing that gets released is dirt and toxins. During the cleanse, your mind and emotions begin to release their own form of toxins, which is absolutely normal. As a matter of fact, cleansing your mind and heart is one of the primary benefits of any cleanse!

The Eleven-Day diet can help as a general cleanser two or three times a year; whenever a cold appears; at a time of crisis; when a fever sets in; when weight reduction is desired; when joints become stiff; when your skin breaks out; or when chronic constipation is present.

▧ Days 1 and 2

Fresh Fruits: For the first few days, only fresh fruits should be eaten. Eat plenty of grapes, melons, tomatoes, pears, peaches, plums, and apricots. Dried fruit may be eaten only if soaked overnight in purified water, which you should also drink. Baked apples can be eaten for dessert.

▧ Days 3, 4, and 5

Juices: Only fresh juices and purified water should be taken into the body for these three consecutive days. Drink one glass of juice every four hours. Utilize fruit juices in the mornings, preferably grapefruit, and vegetable juices in the afternoons. If blood sugar issues concern you, stick primarily to vegetable juices. Days 3, 4, and 5 can be the most difficult part of the cleanse, and certainly the most advantageous. Hang in there with this part of the cleanse, and don't bail out. Once you make it through, you will be glad you did. During these three days of the cleanse you will be battling your mind, and dealing with your desires, as you tap into your addictions on many different levels.

Try to arrange this portion of the cleanse on a weekend, or when your work and play schedule is limited. Periods of rest are absolutely necessary during the entire cleanse, especially during these three days.

▧ Days 6–11

Fruits, Vegetables, and Salads: For these six days, breakfast should consist of citrus fruits, such as grapefruits. Between breakfast and lunch, any kind of fruit may be eaten. Lunch consists of a salad with 3–6 vegetables and two cups of vital broth. If hungry between meals, fresh fruit and/or fruit and vegetable juices may be taken. Dinner should consist of two or three steamed vegetables and two cups of vital broth. Vegetable juice or baked apple may be taken before retiring if desired.

▪ Vital Broth

2 cups carrot tops	2 cups potato
2 cups beet tops	2 quarts purified or distilled water
3 cups celery stalks	Add carrot or onion to flavor if desired
2 cups celery tops	1/2 teaspoon Vegex or Jenson's veggie broth

Chop these finely, slowly bring to a boil, and simmer for approximately 20 minutes. Use only the broth after straining. Keep broth in refrigerator and serve warm. You can also enjoy the vital broth at any time during the transition diet.

After the cleanse is over, be sure to utilize a transition diet for a few days. Avoid protein, and add some rice or another grain to your evening meal. Care must be taken not to binge when the cleanse is completed, as it can negate the beneficial effects of the entire cleanse!

Take slow steps toward your optimal diet, taking care to eliminate some things that you don't want to reintroduce into your diet. Make a conscious choice and follow through with it. In completing this cleanse, you have strengthened your will power and the control over your mind and your desires. Utilize these beneficial changes to the full extent by eliminating unhealthy foods and behaviors.

▪ What You Can Expect from the Cleanse

As with the Seven-Day Feast, you can expect to be hungry for the first day or two. For the next three days you may feel slightly weak and experience some of the toxic symptoms of nausea, gas, and headache created by the elimination of toxins. Make sure that you drink enough water and/or diluted vegetable juice. Going to bed early also helps a lot during the three days of juicing.

Once you reach day five, you are home free, and you may feel a big surge of energy, but be careful not to spend it all. I recommend a hot bath every evening during the cleanse, followed by dry skin brushing, as it aids in elimination and soothes the body and soul. Mild exercise, such as yoga, can be beneficial during the eleven days. The use of colon therapy or home enemas is highly recommended for the first five days. Instructions for taking an enema are located in appendix B.

The benefits of this cleanse are vast, and will improve your ability to digest, absorb, assimilate, and eliminate. The benefits far outweigh the sacrifice. You might remind yourself of that often as you fast.

Once you have completed the diet, you can initiate portions of the diet any time you feel the need. I frequently cleanse for two days on just fruit, or three days on juices, or complete only the last six days of the cleanse. Have fun, and don't give up the ship.

HEALTH TIP #12: My Breakfast Drink

Even though this it not a cleanse, I include a cleansing breakfast drink that I have devised over the years. You can substitute this drink for breakfast unless you have a particularly active lifestyle, in which case you may need additional protein.

The breakfast drink includes a low-potency, full-spectrum, whole foods multiple vitamin and mineral powder; high-quality bonemeal powder for healthy bones, teeth, ligaments and tendons; high-quality mineral whey protein powder; an essential amino acid powder; nutrition for healthy arteries and veins; a source of whole foods B-complex vitamins; vitamin E complex; kefir culture, a great source of pH-balancing chlorophyll; fiber; essential fatty acids, such as flaxseed oil; and fresh fruit. I include all of the fixings here, which you may wish to modify according to your needs.

In a blender, mix the following ingredients:

Fresh fruit—use a banana, frozen fruits, and/or blueberries

Fruit juice—8 ounces of diluted non-citrus juice as a base,
    or purified water

SP Complete—full spectrum multiple vitamin/mineral

Calcifood powder—bonemeal

Capra Mineral Whey—other whey products are much less desirable

Amino Charge—amino acid powder

Lecithin granules—to assist in emulsifying fats

Nutritional yeast—natural source of B vitamins

Unprocessed raw wheat germ—a source of vitamin E complex

Green food supplement—spirulina/Pure Synergy

Flaxseed meal—Bob's is best

Flaxseed oil—Barlean's

Wheat germ oil—helpful when spinal problems return
   (keep refrigerated)

Rice bran syrup—source of B vitamins

Raw almonds—a handful

If you wish, you can vary the amounts of the ingredients to alter taste and consistency. Nutritional yeast and rice bran syrup taste strong, but they are both powerful nutritional supplements loaded with B vitamins. I have found that the addition of a banana greatly improves the taste. I hope that you enjoy this wonderful drink to start your day. Sources for all nutritional products are listed in appendix A.

Conclusion

In this chapter I have provided a variety of tools that will enable you to create vibrant health by balancing your body's biochemistry. This especially comes into play in creating your ideal diet, which is the result of utilizing the wide variety of information offered by your Internal Intelligence.

The first step is to use the information and resources provided in this chapter to establish your body type. Once you do that, a wealth of information will be available to you about your body's specific needs and how to change your weaknesses into strengths. This information, tempered with what you already know about your body, will provide the basis for your ideal diet.

Practice the principles of the Body Type diet until you become familiar with the specifics of your type, including any weight gain patterns that may be present. The insight provided by the Body Type diet will help you to build your health by introducing a lifestyle that increases the vitality of your blood type. See the book list for additional information on Body Typing diets.

The Blood Type diet provides you with additional information on how you can become more specific in refining your diet and your lifestyle. You can use your blood type to gather information about lectins and gain insights as to what your body likes, and how you can provide it.

Use the principles provided by the Mediterranean diet to include the foods that create a healthy cardiovascular system. The Mediterranean diet pyramid provides the guidelines for the creation of the healthiest diet in the world. See the book list for additional resources.

Your job is to learn what your body likes about each of these diets and how you can utilize these factors to create your ideal diet. Fortunately, your Inner Intelligence will give you all the necessary feedback, in the form of signs and symptoms, about what is working and what is not. Remain open and stay in the process long enough for the results to show up. If you constantly evaluate what is working and what is not, on all levels of your experience, you will be successful in creating a new level of vibrant health and multidimensional well-being.

Whenever you stop looking for feedback, you will often become stuck in an old pattern or perspective, and completely miss the changes that are occurring right now. The stress levels in your life are always changing, so why not your health needs? The people who are successful in creating health throughout their lifetime are the people who constantly respond to the changing conditions in their lives.

When you remain in the process of creating health, it allows you to be ready for the unexpected. This perspective not only keeps you from falling into the same old rut, but it will help you to maintain the frame of mind and posture of heart necessary to receive the latest and greatest guidance from your Inner Intelligence. This is true not only for dietary information, but for every level of conscious experience.

You can improve your health even more by implementing the principles of food combining— especially when digestive health problems exist—monitoring your pH, and integrating the basic principles outlined by the glycemic index and glycemic load. All of these factors combine to provide a healthy perspective that will be reflected on all levels of your life experience. The integration of these diets and health-producing practices will expand your ability to create your own health.

The cleansing diets are perhaps the most valuable tools in creating vibrant health. To understand the amazing miracle of tissue cleansing is to be given a precious gift. Ultimately, it is your overall perspective that provides you with the awareness to choose the right health-producing practice. This awareness transfers the vibrant health of your Inner Intelligence to your open heart, through your mind, and into your physical body. Healing naturally occurs as a direct result of the conscious connection with your Inner Healing Presence.

In the wink of an eye, this powerful Healing Presence can easily change your posture of heart, your clarity of mind, and the function your body. All you have to do is to provide the opportunity for healing to occur. When you are willing for healing to occur, and give thanks for your many blessings, this powerful life-changing Presence can accomplish more healing in a moment than some people receive in a lifetime.

Chapter 8

Digestion and Elimination

DIGESTION AND ELIMINATION are two body systems connected by a 40-foot-long digestive tube. The digestive tube has an opening at two ends—the mouth and the anus—and is really considered an outside surface of the body because it is composed of the same type of cells as our skin. It is filled with millions of tiny glands that secrete a wide variety of substances, ranging from extremely powerful acids and digestive enzymes to protective coatings and alkaline reserves. The digestive enzymes are secreted by a quartet of organs, and allow us to digest and assimilate all the major food groups: protein, fats, starches, and carbohydrates.

Digestion begins in the mouth with alkaline saliva, which breaks down starches and carbohydrates found in our food. In fact, 70 percent of the digestion of starches and over 50 percent of digestion of carbohydrates occurs in the mouth. Chewed food proceeds to the acid environment of the stomach, where proteins and fats begin to be digested. Food can remain in the stomach for up to six hours before it moves on to the upper portion of the small intestine. At this stage, the liver and pancreas contribute alkaline digestive juices to the process.

As the food moves down the line, it reaches the middle portion of the small intestine, where nutrients are absorbed by the blood and lymph systems for distribution to the rest of the body. The elimination system begins near the end of the small intestine, and includes the large intestine or colon.

Digestion and elimination are so integrated in the body that they blend together into one functioning unit. For instance, whenever we eat a meal, a reflex is automatically triggered in the large intestine to eliminate the solid remains of our previous meal. The progression of food through the entire digestive and eliminative tube is designed to be a coordinated affair, orchestrated by reflexes from the nerve system to produce continuous movement.

Under normal circumstances, the digestive tube is estimated to hold approximately three meals, which pass out of the body approximately every twenty-four hours. Twenty-four hours is therefore the ideal transit time for a meal from ingestion to elimination.

For most of us, however, this is not the case. Most people who eat three meals a day have only one bowel movement. Some people only experience one bowel movement a week. Whichever the case may be, our digestion and elimination are designed to function together. Eat a meal, eliminate a meal.

An Easy Self-Check of Your Digestive System

You can check your own transit time by eating a meal that contains a serving of red beets. Keep track of when you eat the beets, and notice when beet-red stools show up. The difference in these two times is your transit time. If beet-red stools appear too soon, your digestive system may not have enough time to extract the nutrients from your food. If your transit time is too slow, you may not be able to absorb enough nutrients to keep your body going. This can be a sign that your digestion is inefficient, and you may be absorbing toxic waste material along with your nutrients.

Generally, most people have a slow transit time, which indicates an inefficient digestive system and an overall condition of constipation.

In this chapter, I look at the overall design and function of the digestive system, and how it inherently holds the key to creating your optimal diet. Ultimately, how well your digestive system functions will show you how best to eat. Improve your digestion, and you will absorb your nutrients more effectively, and improve the overall function of your elimination system in the process.

The Mouth

Chewing well is probably one of the easiest and most important things you can do for your digestion. Chewing involves a variety of muscular action in our cheeks and jaw. Even our lips have a purpose in digestion: they keep your food inside your mouth where it belongs.

The tongue is a combination of muscle fibers that wind in three different directions, and it plays an integral part in the digestion of starches. The tongue functions to mix saliva with food, to keep the food mixture in the correct position to be mashed by our teeth, and to push food backward for swallowing. The tongue contains a variety of taste buds that help us evaluate, select, and enjoy a variety of foods.

Who would have thought that when your mother told you to chew your food, she was absolutely right? Maybe she knew that the digestion of starches and carbohydrates is initiated in the mouth, which makes it an absolute necessity to chew your food thoroughly.

Believe it or not, healthy teeth are also a huge component of good digestion, as solid food must be reduced to small particles before it can be digested. Ask anyone with false teeth how important teeth are to digestion. It is amazing to see how each tooth is specifically designed for different stages of eating. Incisors are designed for cutting food, canines for grasping food, and molars for grinding. What wonderful bodies we have.

For many individuals, a lifetime of improper nutrition has lead to unhealthy teeth, which makes normal digestion much more difficult. Gum disease, which is often a sign of protein deficiency in the diet, leads to loosening of the teeth. Dental cavities, a sign of eating too many refined carbohydrates, lead to the loss of healthy teeth. Almost everyone thinks that tooth decay occurs from the outside, when in truth it occurs from the inside. Tooth decay occurs when we ingest foods that are overly refined, processed, and preserved.

Nutrition and Physical Degeneration, an extensive study by Dr. Weston Price on native peoples throughout the world, demonstrates the facts about tooth decay beyond a shadow of a doubt. He discovered that when native peoples ate native foods, tooth decay was rare. As these peoples became "civilized" and their diets changed accordingly, the resulting poor dental health was nothing short of criminal.

Eating refined and denatured foods is a precursor to a mouth full of cavities. Additionally, the ingestion of preservatives, chemicals, and pesticides, which are abundant in both our food and water, is a precursor to the ill health and chronic disease that plague our society today. Healthy teeth mix our food with about 1 1/2 quarts of saliva each day. Saliva enhances our chewing, swallowing, and taste, and it functions to moisten and lubricate our food. Saliva production is frequently initiated by the smell, sight, or the mere thought of food.

Saliva contains ptyalin, an alkaline digestive enzyme and a form of amylase, which digests carbohydrates and starches but has no digestive effect on fats or proteins. This fact indicates the importance of chewing carbohydrates and starches more thoroughly. Saliva production is usually suppressed whenever we become dehydrated, or when we are in a state of emotional stress. In fact, if you experience severe dryness of the mouth and water doesn't seem to quench it, it is often a good sign that you are stressed. If either of these conditions exists, it is usually not a good time to eat.

HEALTH TIP #1: Chew Your Food Thoroughly

Some experts say to chew up to one hundred times per mouthful, which is a little much in my book, but forty or fifty times is certainly in the ballpark. Just for fun, check out how many times you chew before you swallow. Many people swallow their food after only a few chews. Remember, your stomach does not have teeth.

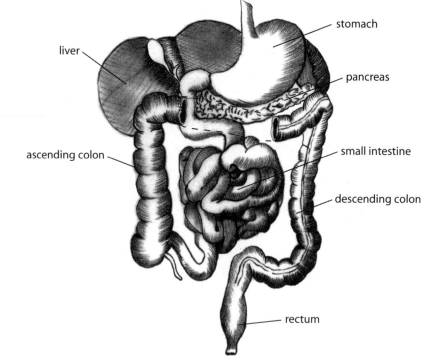

Fig. 8.1: The Digestive Organs

The Esophagus and Stomach

The act of swallowing occurs when the tongue forces the chewed food to the back of the throat, triggering our epiglottis to cover up the airway, which keeps foods and liquids from entering the voice box, the trachea, and the lungs. When we swallow food, it passes into the esophagus, which lies directly behind the air passage to the lungs. When food is swallowed, the muscles of the esophagus initiate a wave of contractions, called peristalsis, that is echoed throughout the entire digestive track. It is this peristaltic wave that pushes the chewed food to the end of the digestive tube.

The cardiac sphincter is the valve between the esophagus and the stomach that helps to keep food in the stomach, much in the same way that the valves of the heart keep blood where it belongs. Sometimes this sphincter becomes weakened, and stomach contents regurgitate back into the esophagus. When this occurs, it often encourages pathogenic bacteria to take up residence in the area surrounding the valve, causing a variety of digestive symptoms, which include stomach irritation.

The stomach is the perfect shape to allow for storage and for mixing of food with our digestive juices. Basically, the stomach is a large muscle with fibers going every which way to help mix the stomach contents with the gastric juices produced by glands in the stomach walls. Stomach contractions are rhythmic and occur most of the time. You may have felt what you call hunger pains, which occur when your blood sugar is low, your stomach is empty, and your body wants more nutrients. These hunger contractions are usually successful in motivating us to get something to eat.

When food is present, glands in the stomach walls produce three kinds of gastric juices, the first of which is hydrochloric acid (HCL). Hydrochloric acid is a strong acid with a pH of less than 1.0. This stuff would burn a hole in your stomach if it weren't for the production of mucus from the stomach walls to protect it. This mucus keeps HCL from digesting the stomach along with our food. HCL also destroys any foreign invaders like bacteria, parasites, and viruses that may be present in our food and drink. When the stomach is healthy, parasites are destroyed in the acid bath of the stomach. It is also HCL that activates the wide array of alkaline digestive enzymes in the body.

The second secretion produced by the stomach is pepsin, which is a digestive enzyme that initiates protein digestion. Pepsin needs an acid medium to become active, so HCL is its perfect complement. If the pH of the stomach reaches 5.0, pepsin stops working and protein digestion stops.

If you drink water or other liquids with your meal, you also dilute your HCL, and your pH becomes raised to the point where pepsin becomes ineffective. At this point, the body tries to make more HCL, which may cause symptoms of acid reflux to occur, especially if the stomach is full. If you take an alkaline antacid at this point, the situation goes from bad to worse. The body keeps making HCL, and we keep trying to douse the fire of digestion with alkaline antacids. Worse still, protein has not been digested properly and may end up putrefying in your intestines. Incomplete protein digestion is noted by putrid smelling gas, which is the end product of poor digestion.

If you want to have good digestion, don't drink when you eat. You can drink fluids half an hour before, or wait until an hour after, without any ill effects.

HEALTH TIP #2: The Trouble with Ice Water

The next time you are offered ice water in a restaurant, turn it down. Water not only dilutes your digestive juices, but ice slows down the biochemical action of digestion. Ice water is the worst possible thing to drink for your digestion. Why they serve it in every restaurant in the U.S. is beyond me.

The stomach also produces a hormone called gastrin, which helps to regulate the amount of HCL that your stomach makes. Hormones require essential fatty acids to work properly, so consuming the right kinds of fats impacts stomach function as well. Too much fat eaten at one time can also cause a problem, delaying the passing of food to the small intestine by up to six hours and creating a major delay in the digestive process.

The stomach juices partially digest fats as well as proteins, which is a big help in determining good food combinations. It's important to remember that digestive juices in the stomach have no effect on breaking down carbohydrates. Carbohydrates are digested by the alkaline juices in the mouth, pancreas, and small intestine.

The nerve system has a big part to play in coordinating all the secretions and contractions of digestion in the stomach. At least three different connections exist in the nerve system for the stomach alone, the most important of which is the vagus nerve, and are intimately connected with our gut feelings. These feelings become evident in phrases such as "I can't stomach this anymore," or "That turns my stomach."

When all the conditions are right, the valve to the small intestine opens and stomach contractions push food through to our amazing small intestine. The emptying of the stomach depends on a variety of factors, including how much protein is in a meal, how much fat you eat, how much liquid you drink, how large a meal you eat, how well your stomach is mixing your food, how much HCL you produce, how long your food has been sitting in your stomach, and how long it has been since you ate your last meal. These factors help determine if there is any room in the upper part of the small intestine to accommodate more food.

HEALTH TIP #3: Eat Small Meals in a Relaxed Atmosphere

- Chew your food well.
- If digestion is sluggish, supplement with digestive enzymes.
- Eat a whole foods diet.
- Don't drink anything during meals.
- Decrease your consumption of sugar and refined carbohydrates.

If you have stomach problems, including if you experience pain or discomfort, gas, burping, acid reflux, or acid indigestion directly after eating or within an hour after eating, your stomach will benefit from eliminating or avoiding fried foods, coffee, black tea, carbonated beverages, strong spices, black and white pepper, chili peppers, vinegar, mustard, tobacco, and alcohol.

To help ease stomach pain, add raw cabbage juice to your diet, which contains vitamin U for ulcers. You can also try raw potato juice, aloe vera juice, flaxseeds, or slippery elm, licorice, and chamomile teas.

Remember the importance of correcting the underlying cause of your problems on the structural, chemical, mental, emotional, and spiritual levels of your life.

The structural component of health related to stomach function centers around the nerves of the sixth thoracic vertebrae, which lies directly between the shoulder blades. Pain in this area is often indicative of stomach and/or gallbladder problems. If stomach or digestive problems exist, this is an important area of the spine to have evaluated for structural misalignments by a doctor of chiropractic.

Acid Reflux and Hiatal Hernia

Acid reflux, which is experienced by millions of people in the U.S., can often be corrected by resolving a hiatal hernia (HH), a condition in which the stomach gets pulled up into the diaphragm. When a hiatal hernia is present, there is just not enough room for the diaphragm to expand fully because the stomach is in the way, and this effects the function of the lungs, the diaphragm, and the stomach. The hiatal hernia has been called "the great mimic," as it mimics a variety of symptoms in the body. These symptoms include a variety of digestive problems, such as regurgitation of stomach contents, chronic belching, symptoms of acid indigestion immediately following a meal, gastritis, difficulty in digesting fats, acid reflux, burning in the sternal area (caused by regurgitation of digestive juices going back through the cardiac sphincter), hiccups, and a variety of esophagus problems, including difficulty in swallowing.

Symptoms involving HH also extend to the respiratory system, and often manifest as a restriction in breathing capacity. The feeling of not being able to take a full breath, or general shortness of breath are often related to this pseudohernia of the diaphragm.

Heart-related problems are frequently mimicked by a hiatal hernia. These include acute signs of angina (heart attack) and other coronary-related pain. If acute heart-related problems are suspected, they should obviously be checked out by a heart specialist.

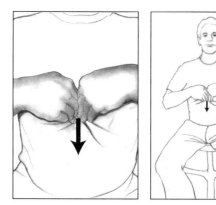

Fig. 8.2: Correction of Hiatal Hernia

But if no severe heart problems are found—which is often the case—chances are that the great mimic is at work.

Symptoms of a hiatal hernia are usually aggravated after eating a large meal, after vomiting, or when lying flat on your back after eating. Persistent symptoms of a hiatal hernia should be checked out by a doctor of chiropractic trained in techniques designed for the correction of a hiatal hernia.

Hiatal hernia can often be addressed successfully through self-care techniques like the one you'll find in health tip #4 below.

HEALTH TIP #4: Correcting a Hiatal Hernia

Applying Direct Pressure

Familiarize yourself with the anatomy surrounding the diaphragm and stomach, as indicated in the accompanying illustration. Locate your sternum. Anatomically, the sternum is likened to a sword. It is very important that you avoid the very tip of the sternum, called the xiphoid process, as it is very delicate. The contact for reducing hiatal hernia is two inches below the tip of the sword.

Sitting back comfortably in a chair, with your feet stretched out in front of you, contact the HH point two inches below the center of the sword tip. Take a deep breath while maintaining contact with the HH point. Press in and down on exhalation, using about 5–10 pounds of pressure. (You can use a bathroom scale to determine how much pressure is equivalent to 5–10 pounds.)

Maintain the contact on both inspiration and exhalation for three consecutive breaths, and then relax and breathe normally

This procedure may be applied 2–3 times a day over the course of several days. Most of the time this self-correction procedure will be successful, but if pain continues after several days, see a chiropractor trained in this applied kinesiology technique for further correction. Stimulating the hiatal hernia reflexes, and the lymphatic drainage points for the diaphragm indicated in the accompanying illustration, can be of great benefit. If these reflexes are tender or painful, it is a good indication that a hiatal hernia and gastric inflammation are present.

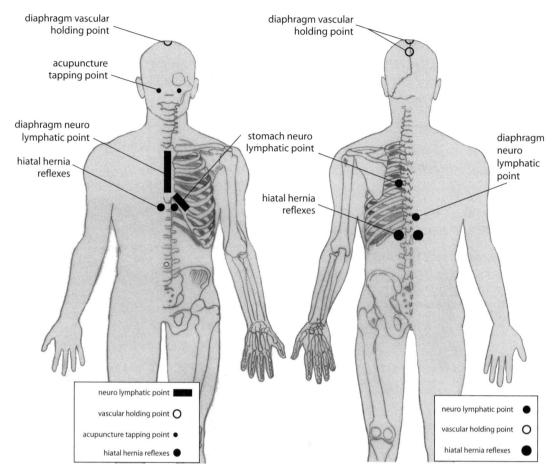

Fig. 8.3: Reflex Point Chart for Hiatal Hernia

■ Reflex Points

The reflex points for hiatal hernia are located about an inch or two below the sword tip on either side of the sternum. Press gently or rub these points, using 5–10 pounds of pressure, to effectively reduce hiatal hernia symptoms. The reflex point on one side is often more tender than the other and indicates the side of the diaphragm that is most involved in the pseudohernia.

Stimulate these points for only 15–30 seconds at a time, as they can get extremely tender, especially the following day. Also, rub the large reflex point for the diaphragm that runs the length of the body. This diaphragm point is often extremely tender when long-standing hiatal hernia problems exist. Use only 2–5 pounds of pressure (or less) on this sensitive diaphragm point. Rub all points as indicated, three or four times per day, until all soreness is eliminated, which in some cases may take up to several weeks. Please pay particular attention to stay away from the tip of the sword.

Remember to always contact your Inner Intelligence before performing any of the procedures offered in this text. Awareness will insure your success, keep you from hurting yourself, tell you when to perform a procedure and when it is complete.

There is also an emotional component connected to a hiatal hernia, as our gut feelings are usually involved whenever our stomach is. I have found that stress and worry are emotional precursors to a hiatal hernia.

Resolving a stressful gut requires a general relaxation about the situations and events in one's life, especially concerning the future. Evaluating one's multidimensional stress load is certainly indicated. Essential solutions also involve a quiet and relaxing atmosphere in which to eat, and taking one's time while eating. Eating small meals is helpful, but until the stomach is pulled down from the diaphragm, symptoms will usually continue. Sources for the nutritional support of inflammatory stomach conditions are listed in appendix A and are important for resolving the cause of hiatal hernia.

The Small Intestine

If you want action, the small intestine is the place. So much happens here that it is hard to keep track of it all, especially in the upper portion, called the duodenum. The duodenum gets its name because of its length, which is twelve fingers' breadth.

The duodenum does a lot of different things at the same time. Your food, called chime at this stage, comes into the small intestine from the stomach as an acid mixture containing partially digested proteins, fats, and carbohydrates. From here, the liver, pancreas, and small intestine take over the digestive process.

The digestive portion of the pancreas contains enzymes that are capable of digesting protein, fats, and carbohydrates. There are actually six different alkaline enzymes secreted by the pancreas for the digestion of protein alone. Pancreatic amylase breaks down starches, sugars, and other carbohydrates, while pancreatic

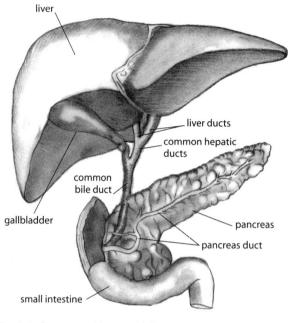

Fig. 8.4: Pancreas, Liver, and Ducts

lipase helps break down fats into fatty acids. "Lipo" means fat, as in liposuction. I mention these enzymes and their actions to assist you in recognizing the role of these digestive enzymes in your nutritional supplements. Cells in the pancreatic ducts are also the source for large amounts of bicarbonate, which have a neutralizing effect on the acid coming into the small intestine from the stomach.

You could say that the pancreas is a big gun in the digestive process. Along with the small intestine, it can handle the digestion all three food groups: proteins, fats, and carbohydrates. As opposed to the acid-producing digestive juices of the stomach, pancreatic enzymes are very alkaline, ranging between 7 and 8 on the pH scale. The pancreas has to work hard to produce enough enzymes to neutralize the acid pH of chime from the stomach, which it secretes directly into the duodenum of the small intestine. The pancreas uses two different passageways to the small intestine, one of which is shared by the liver and gallbladder.

The liver is the largest organ of the digestive system. In truth, the liver is the largest gland in the entire body, and is located on the right side directly under the dome of the diaphragm. Although the liver has between 500 and 1,000 different functions, its digestive contribution is singular: it produces bile.

The sole purpose of bile, and its active ingredient bile salts, is to predigest or emulsify fat that can be digested by the small intestine and absorbed by the lymph system. A continuous trickle of bile is produced by the liver and stored by the gallbladder. The gallbladder is a storage tank for bile, which is squeezed into the small intestine when sensors in the small intestine determine the presence of fat. The higher the fat content in the small intestine, the more bile is released by the gallbladder. Do you see how incredible our digestive process really is? And most of this happens without us even knowing about it.

If someone has their gallbladder removed, the steady drip of bile from the liver goes directly into the small intestine. This small amount of bile is not very effective in emulsifying fats. So while it is true that people can live without a gallbladder, most likely their fat digestion will be inadequate for the rest of their lives. If you have had your gallbladder removed, you should take bile salt supplements, especially when you consume a particularly rich, fatty meal. Sources for bile salt nutrition are listed in appendix A.

Every day, about a quart of bile is produced and stored in the gallbladder, along with a quart of saliva, two quarts of gastric juice, a quart of pancreatic enzymes, and three quarts of secretions from the small intestines. This explains why you need to drink a lot of pure water.

Surprisingly, it's the small intestine itself that completes the digestive process for proteins, fats, and carbohydrates in the body, with millions of tiny glands located throughout its 25-foot-long tube. The small intestine moves the chime along its way using alternate muscle contractions called peristaltic waves, initiated by the nerve system. This peristaltic movement stimulates enzyme production through-out the small intestine. The small intestine completes the digestion of fats into fatty acids, proteins into amino acids, and carbohydrates/starches into three simple sugars: glucose, galactose, and fructose.

The simple end products from the digestion of proteins and carbohydrates are directly absorbed into the bloodstream via the villi of small intestine. Fat, which is also absorbed by the villi in the small intestine, is absorbed directly into the lymph system before it is transferred to the blood directly above the heart. The wrong kind of fats go straight to your heart.

Villi are little outcroppings in the small intestine that increase the body's ability to absorb water and nutrients. Millions of these tiny hair-like structures fill the small intestine, dramatically increasing its surface area by over twenty times. Villi act like little hairs that suck water and nutrients into the blood by way of the small intestine. Of the 10 liters of fluid that are present in the small intestine, $9\frac{1}{2}$ liters are reabsorbed by the villi. As a result, our small intestine has a surface area of over 550 square meters, approximately the size of a tennis court!

Electrolytes are also absorbed by the small intestine. Sodium chloride and other important ions make possible the transport of nutrients and water. These electrolytes create the pumping action that allows for an enormous amount of absorption to occur in the small intestine.

Calcium and other minerals are poorly absorbed in the alkalinity of the small intestine and require the acid medium of the stomach to be absorbed. Loss of stomach acid or periodic ingestion of antacids severely limits the amount of calcium and other minerals that can be absorbed by the body.

Some alkaline antacid products actually tout the fact that they contain calcium, even though their high levels of alkalinity will almost completely block the absorption of calcium by your body.

The structural component for the small intestine is centered around the function of the twelfth thoracic vertebrae. If misalignment occurs in this very vulnerable transition area of the spine, the many functions of the small intestine can be severely altered.

HEALTH TIP #5: Enhance the Functioning of the Small Intestine

- Avoid or eliminate wheat products, dairy products, and other mucus-forming foods that decrease the small intestine's ability to absorb nutrients.
- Supplement your diet with a full array of digestive enzymes.
- Eat a whole foods diet. The addition of fiber and roughage improves the steady movement of the chime through the intestine.
- Be sure to drink enough pure water in your diet.
- Chew your food well.
- Cleansing the liver and gallbladder, as illustrated later in this chapter, is beneficial for both the small and large intestine
- Supplement with acidophilus bifidus bacteria to increase the efficiency of elimination in both the large and small intestine.

A complete list of enzymes and nutritional support products for the intestines are included in appendix A.

The Liver and Gallbladder

Even though we only use about 1/6th of the liver's capacity at one time, it is an organ that needs both our attention and our assistance. As mentioned, the liver produces bile, which helps to emulsify fats and oils in the digestive system and even helps us to absorb calcium. The liver also uses bile as a means to lubricate the intestines, and eliminate toxins and poisons from the body. When too many toxins overload the intestines, it also backs up and affects the liver and gallbladder. Bile becomes thick and toxic to the point where it adversely affects the digestive process and can interfere with many other functions of the liver. The liver itself can become toxic through the use of drugs, medications, alcohol, and from pollution, toxic chemicals, toxic metals, the numerous additives and preservatives in our food and water, and environmental poisons, such as pesticides and herbicides. Toxins usually have a cumulative effect on the liver, and continue to build up over a period of years.

Another function of the liver is to break down and recycle used hormones in the body, and as a result, the liver is a great regulator and balancer for hormone activity. The liver also contributes to the balance our blood sugar levels, the clotting of blood, water retention, fluid balance, and utilization of the oil-soluble vitamins A, D, E, and K. Symptoms of liver and gallbladder problems may include fatigue, loss of appetite, a constant feeling of fullness, digestive problems, a wide variety of skin problems, and constipation. Other indications include sore knees or knees that are slow to heal after an injury; pain in the right scapula, right shoulder or midback areas; pain and tenderness under the right ribs and sternum; intolerance to greasy foods; foul, smelly, or floating stools; hemorrhoids; and the feeling of being overly full after eating.

Because the liver and gallbladder are so important and work so hard to filter out toxins, it becomes important to clean out the filter once in a while. The gallbladder acts as a storage tank for bile, gets congested and toxic, and often contains hundreds of cholesterol-based gallstones.

Cleansing the liver and gallbladder is most effectively accomplished by using the Gallbladder Cleanse and the Liver Flush on two different occasions. The Gallbladder Cleanse and the Liver Flush are best utilized during the spring, summer, or fall seasons, but they can be used sparingly during the winter months, depending on your location and life circumstances. The Gallbladder Cleanse cleans the storage tank and the bile ducts of sludge and gallstones, and it improves drainage of bile and toxic wastes from normal liver activity. The Liver Flush flushes out toxins and stored chemicals, drugs, waste products and stones that build up inside the liver as a result of living and eating on planet Earth in this highly toxic environment. The Gallbladder Cleanse and Liver Flush give our digestive system a well-deserved rest, and can be used on a semi-annual or annual basis.

The structural relationship associated with the liver and gallbladder centers around the fourth and fifth thoracic vertebraes, which is an area located between the shoulder blades. If misalignments occur in this area, it can interfere with any number of liver or gallbladder functions. Any aberration in liver or gallbladder function can effect millions of interdependent functions throughout the body. The Gallbladder Cleanse is not for the faint of heart, but it is safe and highly effective. Swedish bitters are also effective with liver and gallbladder problems.

When cleansing the liver and gallbladder, it is important to begin by opening the bile ducts associated with the gallbladder. For this reason, before starting any cleanse, I usually recommend the Gallbladder Cleanse.

HEALTH TIP #6: The Bile Duct and Gallbladder Cleanse

1. From Monday until noon on Saturday, drink a quart of unfiltered unsweetened apple juice daily and add 40 drops of orthophosphoric acid, as provided in Phosfood Liquid. Use unfiltered apple juice from a health food store to keep chemical additives to a minimum. If blood sugar problems exist, you can skip the apple juice completely, add 40 drops of Phosfood Liquid to a quart of distilled water, add a teaspoon of pectin, and eat an apple a day. Or, add one cup of apple juice to a quart of water and 40 drops of Phosfood. You can do this in addition to your normal, healthy diet, regular supplements, and medication if applicable.

2. Eat a healthy, live food lunch at noon on Saturday.

3. Two to three hours after lunch, take 6–8 capsules of disodium phosphate, or 2 teaspoons of Epsom salts, or flavored magnesium citrate in one ounce of hot water. Drink a small amount of fresh-squeezed citrus juice.

4. Two hours later, repeat step 3 at least one hour before dinner.

5. Saturday's dinner should only consist of citrus or fresh-squeezed citrus juice.

6. At bedtime drink 4 ounces (half a cup) of unrefined, extra virgin, first-pressed olive oil with the juice of half a lemon. Follow this with a small glass of grapefruit juice.

7. Go to bed, lie on your right side with your right knee pulled toward your chest for 30 minutes, which stimulates the gallbladder to empty its contents. Go to sleep.

8. Upon rising, and at least one hour before breakfast, take 6–8 capsules of disodium phosphate again, 2 teaspoons of Epsom salts, or flavored magnesium citrate in two ounce of hot water. You may also drink a small amount of fresh-squeezed citrus juice.

   Sunday is your cleansing day, which is when gallstones usually show up in your stools. Continue with your regular diet, eating primarily fresh fruits and vegetables and drinking plenty of pure water with lemon. You will usually have a loose bowel movement within an hour of step 8, or in some cases it may happen the night before.

9. After this loose bowel movement, check for small floating balls of varying sizes and color. Finding 50–100 gallstones is not unusual.

Be prepared to rest after this procedure, as you will most likely feel tired and weak.

If stones are present, it indicates the need to perform this procedure again in 2–3 months, and again in 6 months, depending on the number of stones produced.

If you experience nausea when taking the olive oil, get up and walk around, prop yourself up with pillows, or do whatever is necessary to prevent vomiting. If you do throw up the mixture (which is rare), this indicates that you should repeat the procedure again at a later date.

Always perform this procedure with the knowledge and aid of your health care provider. Sources for all products are located in appendix A.

HEALTH TIP #7: The Liver Flush

After your gallstones are at a minimum, you may wish to try a different version of liver cleanse called the Purification Diet, or Liver Flush. This is an easier version for cleansing the liver and is a great way to cleanse the liver several times a year. The Liver Flush is my favorite cleanse.

It can be utilized whenever it is needed, or traditionally twice a year. The length of the flush can vary anywhere from one day to two weeks in duration. I initially recommend the Liver Flush to my patients for a period of five consecutive days, but it can also be useful for just a day or two at a time. The Liver Flush will help the liver to eliminate toxins from the body, which will help you improve your level of biochemical balance.

Energy usually remains high on the cleanse as long as you eat enough food. Don't starve yourself, and most likely you will be happy. The Liver Flush will help to normalize weight, and when you are done, it will increase your sensitivity to the dietary needs of your body. The Liver Flush will lubricate the colon, break down old fecal matter in the intestines, cleanse the liver, and eliminate excess mucus throughout the body.

The Liver Flush Drink

In the morning, mix together in a blender the fresh-squeezed juices of several oranges and half a lemon, 1–2 cloves of fresh garlic, and 1–3 ounces of extra virgin olive oil (the dark green color is best). Start with just 2–3 tablespoons of olive oil, and build up to more as you can handle it. Believe it or not, the Liver Flush drink actually tastes good, especially if you use a blender.

A note about garlic: Fresh garlic is by far the best, and crushed prepared garlic is next best. If you just can't stand garlic, kyolic purchased from a health food store has the offensive taste and smell of garlic removed.

Chewing a little parsley or a few seeds from a lemon or an orange will help with the garlic smell. The more effectively you cleanse your body, the less you and your friends will notice the garlic smell and taste!

▓ The Liver Flush Tea

Follow the Liver Flush by drinking a cup or two of Liver Flush Tea made from the following herbs:

>   1 tsp. comfrey
>   1 tsp. fennel
>   1 tsp. licorice
>   2 tsp. flaxseeds
>   1 tsp. fenugreek seeds

Add chamomile if you have an upset stomach.

The hot liquid speeds the oily mixture through the digestive system and prevents nausea. The use of honey in the tea is not recommended. Take the Liver Flush drink first thing in the morning, followed by the tea, and don't eat until noon.

▓ Lunch and Dinner during the Liver Flush

The rest of the day you can eat exotic salads with extra virgin olive oil and lemon juice dressing, and more garlic if you can handle it. Eat a variety of steamed or baked vegetables. Potatoes can be eaten raw or juiced, as cooking turns them into a starch, which is excluded during the cleanse.

Fresh, baked, or dried fruits are also fine, as are avocados, pineapples, and other exotic fruits. Try not to combine sweet fruits like bananas, apples, and pears with acid fruits like citrus or pineapple, as the combination often negates the benefits.

Baked apples or bananas are a great dessert, and cooked squash is a satisfying substitute for starches. Artichokes are good cold and can be cooked ahead of time. A few figs are also an aid in the cleansing process. Making soups using the water from your steamed vegetables is also an excellent idea. Be creative and drink plenty of pure water.

Sprouts and high-protein vegetables are always a great asset to any cleansing program. Considering eating fresh peas, another avocado, wheat grass, and fresh green vegetable juices that are high in chlorophyll.

Foods not permitted during the Liver Flush are alcohol, sugar, grains, legumes (except peas and sprouts), caffeine, and anything containing meat, fish, or eggs. In order for the cleanse to be effective, follow this list as closely as possible.

HEALTH TIP #8: Liver Detox

Eliminate hydrogenated fats, denatured oils, and fried foods from your diet, and limit melted cheese, refined foods, and alcohol. Eat small meals and increase the consumption of B vitamin foods such as brewer's yeast, seeds and nut butters, raw wheat germ, whole grains, beets, beet juice and dilute lemon juice.

The Organ Release Technique for the liver is an excellent way to release liver and gallbladder stress and congestion.

Become aware of the level of tension, stress and/or pain in your abdominal organs by lying on your back and checking them out. Use the organ map on page 250 to find the location of your organs. Pain or tension in any organ indicates the

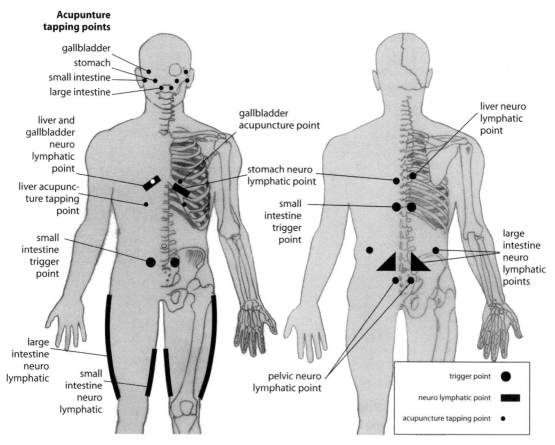

Fig. 8.5: Treatment Point Chart for Digestive Organs

need for this valuable technique, especially in the liver and gallbladder. Use the specific points on the map to help release liver and gallbladder tension. The location of organ release points for the liver, gallbladder and the emotional release point are included toward the end of this chapter.

Stimulate the neurolymphatic points for the liver and gallbladder.

Lightly touch the associated vascular holding points for the liver and gallbladder.

Tap the related B&E point for the gallbladder.

The Pancreas and the Glycemic Index

The pancreas is a workhorse in the digestive system and is responsible for neutralizing our stomach acid. The pancreas manufactures digestive enzymes that are designed to digest proteins, starches/carbohydrates, and fats, and has a big job to do in the body. We can help out our pancreas by giving it a break from difficult to digest refined carbohydrates, such as sugars, soft drinks, starches, breads and cakes, and by eating foods that are low on the glycemic index scale. I have been using the glycemic index for years to indicate high-stress foods. The glycemic index measures the amount of insulin the pancreas produces in response to specific foods and drinks. The lower the glycemic index, the less insulin produced by the pancreas, and the less it has to work.

The pancreas has enough to do without excessively producing insulin. Even though insulin is secreted by the endocrine portion of our pancreas, the gland functions as a whole. Stress one part of the pancreas, and you stress the whole organ. This principle is also evident when the digestive portion becomes overloaded and adversely effects the endocrine portion. I have noted this situation when parasites are present in the intestine. Through sensors in the intestine, the pancreas detects the need for protein digestion, which it will continually try to manufacture in order to digest the parasites. Although this is sometimes effective, it often results in increasing pancreatic stress.

HEALTH TIP #9: Enhance the Functioning of the Pancreas

The glycemic index listed in chapter 7, appendix B, indicates which foods require the most insulin by the pancreas. Foods like bagels, refined sugars, breads, refined cereals, potatoes, and corn top the list. Whole foods, including whole grains, generally have a low glycemic index and allow the pancreas to work less.

It is also important to note that when we eat a food in its whole or natural state, it contains significant amounts of fiber, which lowers the glycemic index of that food. Fats eaten with a meal, in the form of extra virgin olive oil, avocados, and small amounts dairy fat, also lower the glycemic index by increasing digestion time, which gives the pancreas a breather. Refined foods need to be digested quickly and require large amounts of insulin, and quickly raise blood sugar levels.

Make a copy of the glycemic index and Glycemic Load Chart in chapter 7, and put it on your refrigerator. Access to a more complete list of carbohydrate utilization is provided in chapter 7, appendix B.

Nutrition for the Pancreas

It is often helpful to include a digestive enzyme formula with your meals. The most common pancreatic enzymes include protease, amylase, lipase, invertase, lactase, and cellulase. Also of great assistance to pancreatic functioning is proper food combining, reducing the consumption of wheat and dairy products, zinc supplementation, and whole food sources of B-complex vitamins. Balancing blood sugar levels also aids in stabilizing the digestive portion of the pancreas. Do your pancreas a big favor and eliminate soft drinks from your diet, as they are the biggest offender in unhealthy pancreatic functioning. Instead, drink water and lemon, or lemon Recharge juice, which will raise the levels of your electrolytes instead of raising your glycemic index.

It is also important to remember that enzymes found in whole organic foods are used by the body to digest that food.

The structural relationship to the pancreas centers on the seventh thoracic vertebrae, which is located directly between your shoulder blades. Pain between the shoulders can be a result of structural interference to the liver, gallbladder, stomach, and the many important functions of your pancreas.

The Ileocecal Valve

The small intestine and large intestine are connected together by a pouch called the cecum, which is about the size of a tennis ball. The cecum contains the appendix on one end and the ileocecal valve (ICV) on the other. The ICV allows chime to enter into the large intestine and keeps it from returning to the small intestine.

The appendix, like many other areas of the lymph system, has been thought to have no useful function. I was trained, however, to view the appendix as the oil-can of the intestine. When the appendix is removed, constipation is often the consequence. The appendix can become troublesome, especially with today's diet of refined foods and large meals, and it is frequently removed surgically due to irritation or infection. In some states, if a surgeon enters the abdominal cavity for any reason, she must remove the appendix even if it is in perfect health.

An even longer list of digestive troubles points to the ileocecal valve. The ICV normally opens and closes when chime needs to pass from the small intestine to the colon. This valve often gets stuck in the open or closed position, causing myriad symptoms.

ICV problems can arise after periods of unhealthy dietary habits, lifestyle indiscretions, structural misalignments, and emotional imbalances that lead to irritation or hypersensitivity in the walls of the intestines. The intestines become irritated in much the way your skin gets irritated when you use toxic cleaning agents. Bingeing on refined foods, sugar, alcohol or soft drinks irritates the lining of your intestines, and toxic emotions have even more of an irritating effect. When we become irritated about something in our lives, so do our intestines.

Other symptoms of ICV involvement include fever, headaches, dizziness, flu symptoms, nausea, shoulder pain, lower back pain, ringing in the ears, faintness, sinus infection, sudden thirst, and dark circles under the eyes.

ICV problems are often initiated by eating foods that overstimulate the valve. This list includes sugar, caffeine, too much fat, toxic chemicals in foods, food coloring and additives, and phosphates in soft drinks, alcohol, cocoa, and chocolate.

ICV problems can also be initiated by eating too much roughage at one time, including popcorn, chips, nuts, whole grains, large amounts of salad, pickles, tomatoes, and too many raw fruits and vegetables, especially if you are not used to eating them. Other causes of ileocecal valve problems are spicy foods, pepper, chili peppers, and other intense spices. Popcorn is probably the biggest offender in causing ICV problems, as it contains large amounts of indigestible cellulose. Cellulose provides good fiber for the intestines and aids our elimination, but too much of a good thing can also cause a problem. Start slowly with fiber, and build up the amounts you ingest over a period of time. Otherwise, you may trigger your ileocecal valve to get stuck, which will cause you major problems.

The structural relationship to the ileocecal valve centers around the twelfth thoracic vertebrae. In cases of chronic ileocecal valve problems, this area of the spine should be evaluated by a chiropractor.

Emotionally, ICV problems, as well as and other intestinal disorders, indicate that something inside us is causing irritation. Unexpressed emotions fester in the gut until a state of dis-ease manifests somewhere in the body, showing us that our gut feelings need to be expressed and resolved.

HEALTH TIP #10: Correction of Ileocecal Valve Problems

Ileocecal valve problems, like those of the hiatal hernia, are relatively common ailments that can be extremely troublesome, as they both elicit symptoms from a variety of body systems. Whenever the iloececal valve gets stuck, symptoms can begin almost immediately. Thankfully, the ICV correction is relatively simple and effective.

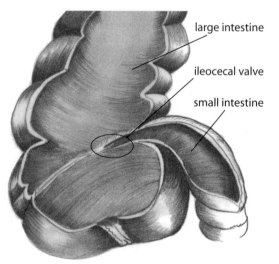

large intestine

ileocecal valve

small intestine

■ Direct Pressure on the Ileocecal Valve

1. Either sit in a relaxed position or lie down.
2. Locate your ICV, which is about 1–2 inches below and to the right of your navel (see accompanying illustration).
3. Cup your hands and place them on the skin immediately below the ICV.

Fig. 8.6: The Ileocecal Valve

4. Apply about 5–10 pounds of pressure, pushing inward toward the spine, and begin to move your hands in the direction of your left shoulder. Your fingers will barely move on the surface of the skin, but will move 3–4 inches on the ICV.
5. Pull your fingers up in the direction of the left shoulder.
6. Maintain the inward pressure as you switch directions with your fingers, pushing down now toward the right thigh.
7. Continue with the pressure until your contact is slightly past the point where you started.

Essentially you are contacting the ICV and moving it diagonally a few inches in both directions. This motion will usually free up an ICV valve that is stuck in the open or closed position. Perform the procedure three consecutive times.

Caution should be used if extremely painful areas are encountered. If this is the case, use less pressure and work more on the associated reflex points and on your diet. In cases of chronic or painful ICV, correction by a chiropractor trained in this applied kinesiology technique is highly recommended.

■ Reflex Points

Rubbing the associated ICV reflex points will assist in correction and will help to reduce associated symptoms. These reflex points may be very tender initially, but usually abate after a few days of stimulation. If severe symptoms or extreme tenderness persists, see your chiropractor or medical practitioner. To ensure beneficial results, take special care to contact your Inner Intelligence whenever performing this or any procedure outlined in *Health Is Simple*.

The accompanying ICV reflex points are of great value and are a big help in determining if an ICV problem exists. Stimulate these neurolymphatic reflex points in a clockwise direction, and use 5–10 pounds of pressure.

■ Acupuncture Tapping Points

In addition to the lymphatic points, there are two acupuncture tapping points that can be useful in correcting an ICV problem. Locate these tender points on the accompanying illustration, and tap them for about 15–30 seconds each, twice per day, until the tenderness is eliminated.

■ Diet to Correct Ileocecal Valve Functioning

A dietary solution is also necessary for the long-term correction of ICV. Even without the procedures described above, a stuck ICV can often be corrected by diet alone. For three days, avoid foods that irritate the valve. These foods include all raw fruits and vegetables, popcorn, chips, nuts, whole grains, salads, spicy foods, pepper, chili peppers and other intense spices, caffeine, alcohol, and chocolate. Fruits and vegetables can be eaten if cooked, which reduces their roughage content. Cor-

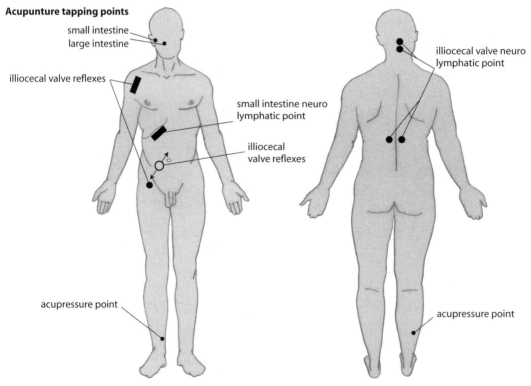

Fig. 8.7: Ileocecal Valve Reflex Point Chart

rection of a stuck ICV is also supported by taking oil-soluble chlorophyll, calcium, and magnesium supplementation (see appendix A).

The Large Intestine or Colon

To many anatomists, the internal environment of the large intestine looks as if it were designed to house bacteria. Over four hundred kinds of bacteria take up residence inside the colon, with most of them being of great benefit to the body. Disease-causing bacteria become present in the colon when the quality of the internal environment begins to degenerate. This change in the internal environment often occurs after the use of antibiotics, when incomplete digestion of protein occurs, or when abnormal levels of toxins are present in the body. These changes in the internal environment create an atmosphere in which the putrefaction of undigested matter is followed by an insurgence of bacteria associated with disease. Imbalance in the colon is often a precursor to a host of chronic disease conditions.

The colon needs as much help as we can give it, and this is especially true in an external environment riddled with toxic chemicals, pesticides, and pollutants.

How to Create a Healthy Environment in the Colon

Introduce beneficial bacterial and yeast cultures into the intestine. Sources for these cultures can be obtained from kefir, which contains both bacteria and yeast cultures, and/or nutritional supplements containing bifidus bacteria and lactic acid yeast. Sources for all supplements are listed in appendix A.

Bacteria transform dangerous toxins in the bowel into harmless carbon dioxide and water. Bacteria also reduce sensitivities to environmental toxins and help to create a beneficial environment in the colon. They contribute to our health by manufacturing at least nine essential vitamins, including B complex, thiamin, riboflavin, B12, and vitamin K, which is beneficial in the clotting of blood. It has been estimated that in the normal course of a day the average person eliminates over 100 billion bacteria from their intestines. Those bacteria need to be replaced on a daily basis. Beneficial bacteria and yeast cultures also produce lactic acid, which is essential for a healthy colon and will aid longevity. I believe we should all supplement a whole foods diet with beneficial bacteria and yeast cultures on a daily basis to support our intestinal health.

Eat a diet rich in organic whole foods, which provide an abundance of synergistic factors that aid digestion.

Reduce your consumption of red meat.

Limit your intake of refined and denatured foods and drinks.

The upper portion of the large intestine is very much like the small intestine in that it absorbs and recycles large amounts of water and electrolytes. If we don't drink enough water and become dehydrated, the large intestine still continues to recycle the much-needed water from our intestines. This is often the simple cause of constipation, which is much more common in our society today than we acknowledge.

The remainder of the colon is used for the temporary storage of fecal matter, which is moved through to the rectum by the action of peristalsis. It is estimated that the average person has well over ten pounds of excess fecal matter stored in the colon. This residue of fecal matter is one of the main causes of toxicity and disease in the body, as toxins get reabsorbed in the body with water.

The nerve system reflexes in the digestive system are designed to consistently move digested food through the system. The teeth chew our food, the stomach mixes it with acid, the liver and pancreas digest it, the small intestine digests and absorbs it, and the colon eliminates the remains. Whenever we eat food, we automatically stimulate the elimination reflexes to occur. If we repeatedly ignore the urge to eliminate, the colon distends and enlarges to accommodate the excess fecal matter, and our elimination reflexes diminish. This common condition allows for additional putrefaction and gas to occur in the intestines.

Gas is usually a sign of incomplete digestion and may signify that you need proper food combining techniques as well as digestive enzymes.

The large intestine is extremely sensitive to the variety of emotions that we often hold inside. Unexpressed emotions irritate the colon, and often lie at the core of our digestive disorders. This can lead to conditions such as irritable bowel syndrome, colitis, and a host of other intestinal diseases.

The bowels of a ship are the deepest, darkest part, lying at the very bottom of the vessel. The large intestine is the bowel of the body, where our deepest, darkest emotions lie buried until they are dredged up. Emotional stress is no friend to the large intestine, as it will let us know right away when our feelings are out of balance. Thankfully, our intestines also reveal our true feelings. Our intestines and abdomen work like a weather vane, indicating the truth in the present moment. If your belly aches during interactions with others, chances are good that something isn't quite right—on that you can depend. No matter what your thoughts say, your gut feelings usually tell you the absolute truth.

The emotional holding points presented in chapter 3, along with the emotional release points listed below, are extremely helpful in balancing your emotional health. Both are excellent tools to utilize when the emotional tide is high.

As human beings age, the effectiveness of the digestive system usually diminishes, along with the amount of digestive enzymes that we produce.

Symptoms of large intestine involvement include constipation, diarrhea, skin rashes, chronic headaches, coated tongue, excessive gas, chronic indigestion, and lower back pain.

The structural relationship for the large intestine is an important one and is centered around the transitional upper and lower lumbar spine. A subluxation or misalignment of the spine at the level of the first or fourth lumbar vertebrae is often responsible for altered colon function, and is a frequent cause of constipation.

It is always a good idea to get in the habit of cleansing your colon a few times a year. This cleansing process assists the body by removing excess fecal matter and mucus, which forms on the walls of the intestines. Colon cleansing improves digestion, the absorption of fluids, the elimination of toxic wastes, and reduces an overly acidic pH condition throughout the body. Colon therapy or colonic irrigations performed by a certified colon therapist several times a year will aid in cleansing the walls of the colon, which can be an extremely valuable health-building practice. Whenever your body manifests symptoms of toxicity, it indicates the need for cleansing.

HEALTH TIP #11: Colon Cleansing

Try over-the-counter colon cleansing products, especially those containing bentonite clay. These over-the-counter products are effective in absorbing large amounts of toxins and can be used on a semi-annual basis. Drink extra amounts of water whenever using any of these products, as dehydration can become a real problem. Colon therapy or home enemas should also be used when consuming any colon cleansing products. See your local health food store for product details.

Take probiotics to improve the nature of the flora in your intestines. Probiotics containing acidophilus bifidus bacteria can be considered an essential part of any cleansing process. Bacterial supplements can be an excellent source, too, but be aware that excessive heat renders bacterial supplements much less effective. Check for refrigerated bacterial sources, especially during shipping. Check appendix A for sources.

A kefir culture is also a great choice for improving your digestion and your elimination, and it is actually a combination of bacteria and yeast cultures. Kefir grains can often be obtained from a quality health food store and are best when grown at home.

I have used kefir for some time now, and when I began, I had trouble getting it to taste right. I learned that if I used regular milk to feed the kefir, the taste, consistency, and flavor were totally unacceptable. But when I used organic milk to feed my kefir, I noticed an amazing difference in productivity, consistency, appearance and taste, which demonstrates the vast difference between regularly produced and organically produced dairy products. A source for quality kefir grains is listed in appendix A.

Yeast cultures are also important to the colon as they produce lactic acid as a by-product. Besides kefir, I include lactic acid yeast wafers. Taken on a daily basis, they improve the quality of your internal environment. If you are plagued by candidal yeast, taking yeast cultures allows beneficial yeast to slug it out with the candida, which is usually much more productive than attacking candida yourself.

Fermented vegetables, such as organic sauerkraut from a health food store, are free of harmful chemical additives and help to culture the environment of the colon. Unfiltered apple cider vinegar is also considered fermented and can be used in small amounts to balance your internal environment. It can be used in salad dressings, or in a 5–10 percent solution (5–10 percent apple cider vinegar to 90–95 percent water) as a hot morning drink, which can be alternated with hot lemon water. In most cases, a teaspoon of unfiltered honey, used for over fifty years as a folk remedy, can be added to the apple cider vinegar, which aids in its effectiveness as a balancing agent.

HEALTH TIP #12: The Stomach Lift

The stomach lift helps to stimulate the intestines, to move its contents through your colon, and to get rid of excess weight in your belly area by strengthening the abdominal muscles. The Stomach Lift can be performed on a daily basis and is especially easy to perform in the shower.

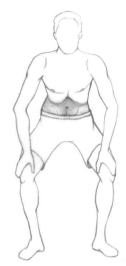

The Stomach Lift is performed while standing with your knees bent, your hands resting on your knees, and your palms against your thighs. Begin the exercise with a large inhalation, followed by a complete exhalation. Exhale all the breath out of your lungs. At this point—without breathing in—suck your stomach as far toward your spine as possible, holding your breath and your stomach for as long as you can. Release the stomach and abdomen, and breathe in a cleansing breath. The Stomach Lift can be performed 1–3 times in succession, on a daily basis, and is very helpful with digestive problems.

Fig. 8.8: Stomach Lift

HEALTH TIP #13: Abdominal Massage

Take inventory of the condition of your internal organs by massaging your abdomen at least once a week. Use the accompanying illustration as a map to determine the location of the stomach, liver, gallbladder, small intestine, large intestine, pancreas, and spleen. Massaging these organs, using about 5 pounds of pressure, will help you become aware of their location and condition, and assist you in releasing any stress or blockage that you may find. Massaging the tension from your abdominal organs will help to release congestion from your organs and improve their function. Concentrate on releasing areas of tenderness. If extremely painful areas are located, ask your health care practitioner for assistance. After your organ massage, you will be impressed at how well you sleep.

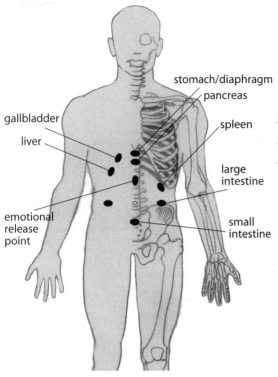

gallbladder

liver

stomach/diaphragm

pancreas

spleen

large intestine

emotional release point

small intestine

Fig. 8.9: Organ Map Chart

1. Increase digital pressure to 10–15 pounds for an Organ Release for the liver, gallbladder, and stomach. This release is similar to working the reflex points for a hiatal hernia.

2. Locate the organ on the map.

3. Find the tenderness with your fingers.

4. Slowly increase the pressure on your abdomen.

5. While maintaining constant pressure, breathe slowly throughout several controlled breaths.

6. Use the pads of your fingertips on both hands to push into your abdomen. If severe tenderness exists, decrease the amount of pressure. Slowly increase the amount of pressure in succeeding sessions until 10–15 pounds of pressure is reached. If extreme tenderness persists, see your health professional for guidance.

HEALTH TIP #14: The Emotional Release Point

The emotional release point listed on the organ map lies at the very center of your abdomen. This point has been clinically demonstrated to be a very powerful tool in releasing emotional stress in the body. This release point is especially effective when a person has not recovered from emotional trauma.

The release point is addressed in the same way as the organ release points above, using 10–15 pounds of pressure while lying on your back. You can hold the release point for 20–30 seconds, using your breath to increase effectiveness. This point is usually very tender when emotional stress is being held in the body. Pressure should be decreased if a deep pulsing is felt under the fingertips. After a few initial sessions, the procedure can be performed while lying on your stomach, with the fingers of both hands on the emotional release point to increase the effect.

HEALTH TIP #15: Castor Oil Packs

Whenever persistent abdominal pain, constipation, or digestive problems exist, make a castor oil compress. This is best done in the evening by soaking a square of flannel about the size of your abdomen (12 inches or so) in castor oil. Use only enough oil to thoroughly soak the square, as too much oil becomes messy. Place the oiled flannel directly on your abdomen, and cover it with a piece of plastic to protect your clothes and bedding. A small plastic bag usually works great. Finally, place a hot water bottle or heating pad on top of the plastic bag and wrap your abdomen with a large towel or cloth. You now have a castor oil sandwich, with you in the middle. Try to leave the compress on for at least several hours. This technique is not recommended on a daily basis, as too much heat can increase inflammation.

HEALTH TIP #16: Nutrition

Add a wide variety of beneficial bacteria and lactic acid–forming yeast, fermented foods and drinks, and whey powder, which all help to balance the internal environment of the colon and help to keep putrefying bacteria in check. A list of beneficial foods and supplements for the large intestine are listed in appendix A.

The avoidance or reduction of wheat and dairy products is an asset in restoring normal colon function.

- Kefir drink
- Fermented vegetables
- Herbs that support colon function are slippery elm, flaxseeds soaked overnight or flaxseed meal, alfalfa tablets, peppermint, and chamomile. The occasional use of buckthorn bark tea and cascara sagrada are helpful for chronic problems with constipation.

Constipation is often an indication of a poor internal intestinal environment in which healthy bacteria and yeast colonies have a difficult time thriving. Constipation is often a result of a lack of water and roughage in the diet, and the overconsumption of refined foods.

Two Digestive Systems

You may have already noticed that human beings essentially have two different digestive systems: An acid digestion that digests proteins and fats, and an alkaline digestion that primarily digests high starches and sugars, called high carbohydrates. To some degree, all food contains a combination of protein, fats, and carbohydrates, but most foods have one category that predominates, which brings us to the topic of food combining.

Our digestive system works better when the alkaline and acid systems don't have to work against each other. When fats and proteins are eaten together, our acid digestion predominates. When high starches and sugars are eaten together, our alkaline digestion becomes dominant. When a mixed meal is eaten, containing proteins, fats, and high carbohydrates, our acid digestion goes into high gear to digest the proteins and fats, followed by the alkaline digestion of starches and sugars by the pancreas and small intestine. In a mixed meal, the pancreas and small intestine have to work much harder to change a highly acidic environment into an alkaline one.

Now this may not be such a big deal when a person is in their teens or twenties, as you can do most anything during those years, but when a person has digestive-related problems, food combining can make a huge difference. I have found this to be true for myself and many of my patients over the years. Combining the right foods improves digestion and reduces many seemingly unrelated health disturbances throughout the body as well.

HEALTH TIP #17: Food Combining

Even though food combining can be made difficult and complicated, the basic principles involved are actually very simple. Here are some basic principles:

- Eat fats and high carbohydrates separately. (Example: When you are having bread or potatoes, avoid butter, cream, and protein.)

- Eat protein and sugars separately. (Example: When you eat fish, eggs, or cheese, avoid bread, potatoes, or sweets.)
- Fats and proteins can be eaten together because they support the other's digestion.
- Acidic liquids, including citrus juice, buttermilk, vinegar, and

Food Category	Description
Carbohydrates	sugars and high starches
Starches	bread, potatoes, cereals, grains, pasta, sweets & legumes
Protein	meat, fish, eggs, cheese & tofu
Fats	butter, cream, bacon, meat, etc.
Acid liquids	citrus juices, vinegar & buttermilk
High starch vegetables	lima, kidney, & navy beans, peas, corn & potatoes
High starch fruits	bananas, grapes, cherries, apples, apricots, blueberries, pears, pineapple, plums and raspberries.

Fig. 8.10: Food Category Chart

coffee, can be taken with protein and fats, but not with high carbohydrates.

Food Categories

Most vegetables are neutral and can be eaten with either a high-carbohydrate meal or with protein, fats, or acidic liquids as a protein meal. A more complete list of foods and their categories is found in appendix B.

The main principles of food combining are effective for anyone with digestive problems. Symptoms may include gas, acid indigestion, sour stomach, stomach pain (either immediately after eating, or up to three hours after eating), constipation, diarrhea, foul-smelling stools, allergies, migraine headaches, skin problems, hay fever, asthma, and general sluggishness. If digestive disturbances or any other of these symptoms are present, I recommend the food combining guidelines presented here.

For more information on classifying foods as carbohydrates/starches, proteins, or fats, utilize *Dr. Atkins' New Carbohydrate Gram Counter* or *The South Beach Diet Good Fats/Good Carbs Guide*. These books are very helpful for clarifying the categories in the food combining process. See the bibliography for more details.

Most Americans eat too many refined carbohydrates. If you are overweight or have symptoms of digestive problems, try to eat more protein combination meals than high-carbohydrate meals. When you eat a predominantly high-carbohydrate meal, follow it with one or two predominantly protein, fat, and acid liquid meals. Keep rotating back and forth to make your diet more interesting. If you suffer from digestive problems, this regime will usually help to eliminate most digestive-related symptoms.

The Other Elimination Systems

There are four eliminative organs in the body: the lungs, the large intestine, the kidneys, and the skin. Let's first take a look at the kidneys and how they function to eliminate toxic waste from the body.

The kidneys are bean-shaped organs that lie on either side of the spine at about the level of the waist. The kidneys have the big job of maintaining balance in our internal environment. Our kidneys help to balance the fluids of the body, including electrolytes, to control the acid/alkaline balance, and to reabsorb and recycle water.

The kidney has over a million little filtering units that look like miniature stills and that function together to filter out water and solids from the bloodstream. Twenty-five percent of the blood pumped by the heart passes through the kidneys each and every minute, which adds up to about 430 gallons of blood moving through the kidneys every day.

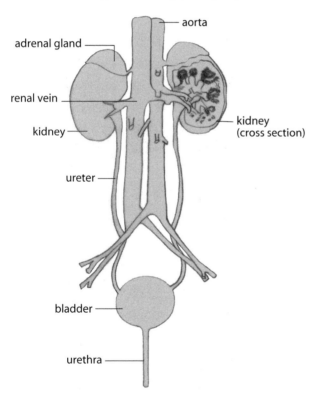

aorta

adrenal gland

renal vein

kidney

kidney (cross section)

ureter

bladder

urethra

Fig. 8.11: The Kidney, Ureter, Bladder, and Urethra

The majority of the water, electrolytes, and nutrients filtered by the kidneys returns through miles of little convoluted tubes. These tubes help the kidney reabsorb salts, sugars, amino acids, minerals, and bicarbonates into the bloodstream. The remainder of the water is used to eliminate toxic waste products through the urine. Bicarbonates are alkaline compounds that help to balance out acidity in the body.

You may remember the powerful little adrenal glands that sit perched atop each kidney. These little powerhouses help to govern the rate of kidney function. The adrenals secrete hormones that influence the amount of fluids and electrolytes reabsorbed back into the bloodstream, and how much of each substance the body wants to eliminate through the urine.

As shown in the illustration, urine passes from the kidneys through long tubes called ureters until it reaches the urinary bladder, which is composed of elastic tissue surrounded by muscle. The urinary bladder is basically a holding tank for urine. As the contents of the bladder increase, so does our urge to urinate. The urethra is the tube that runs from the bladder to the outside surface of the body.

When dehydration is present, which seems to be the norm rather than the exception, urine becomes very concentrated in the bladder. Concentrated urine is often very toxic, and can result in the irritation of the urinary track and the walls of the bladder. Concentrated urine has a deep yellow color and a strong odor, and is a great indication that we need to drink more pure water throughout the day.

The structural relationship to the kidneys centers around the eleventh thoracic vertebrae. Misalignment of this structural transition area of the spine can be responsible for causing ileocecal valve problems, small intestine and large intestine problems, and can be a major cause of interference to the function of our kidneys.

HEALTH TIP #18: Enhance the Functioning of the Kidneys

The ideal pH of urine is 6.4, but may be as high as 7, especially in vegetarians. Check the pH of your urine and saliva on a regular basis. Urine is an important component to evaluate in both health and dis-ease. As a rule, vegetarians have a more alkaline pH, due to the fact that vegetables build up your alkaline reserves, which is an excellent strategy for health. Those of us who eat meat and refined carbohydrates will usually have a lower, more acidic pH.

If our urine becomes too acidic, or too alkaline, as is the case with bladder infections, colds and flu, these problems can be alleviated by utilizing the acid/alkaline food list to balance our pH. For kidney and bladder infections, use natural cranberry juice or tablets, without sugar, to help change your pH. Cranberry juice helps to support the bladder and kidneys and also contains specific tannins that help fight bacteria. Detrimental bacteria in the kidney don't like lemon or cranberry juice, as these juices when taken on a regular basis help to keep bacteria in the kidney and bladder in check.

Alcohol, cigarettes, and caffeine stress the kidneys and the adrenal glands. The kidneys love parsley tea, celery juice, cornsilk tea, and the herb uvaursi.

Kidney function is also enhanced by lecithin, kelp, the mineral magnesium, and the natural, whole food vitamins A, B complex, C, and E. Regular exercise aids the body to move fluids easily through the kidney.

Stimulate the neurolymphatic reflex points for the kidney and bladder, which are located on the Neurolymphatic Chart in chapter 5.

Use the vascular holding points for kidney and bladder, which are located on the Vascular Holding Point Chart in chapter 6.

The Skin

The skin is the largest organ in the body, covering over 3,000 square inches of surface area and weighing about six pounds, which is more than the liver and the brain combined. The skin receives about 1/3 of the body's blood supply, and is a great regulator of body temperature, as it releases sweat when we get overheated and creates goose bumps and shivers when we get cold. The skin is a waterproof envelope that allows the body to interface with the external environment, yet it protects us from harmful physical and chemical agents. The seven layers of the skin keep our body contained. The skin is tough yet soft, it expands and contracts to accommodate the shape of the body, and it regenerates and repairs itself when cut or injured. The skin is the perfect container for the body.

The skin also functions like a third kidney, as the body will eliminate waste products through the skin when the kidneys are overloaded with toxins. Skin problems and eruptions are usually an indication that our normal elimination channels have become overburdened, and the body is now using the skin as a backup route for eliminating toxic wastes. Improve your digestion and elimination, and the body will usually stop using the skin as a toxic escape route. This idea puts dermatology in an entirely new light.

The skin is also our means for sensing the outside world. The skin has billions of sensory organs for touch and pressure that are direct extensions of our nerve system. Our brain depends on information collected by the skin to let our Inner Intelligence know when we are cold, hot, in danger, or in pain. Our skin is directly wired to our brains, and even responds to conditions of mental or emotional stress, at which point we can break out in a cold sweat.

The outer layer of the skin is called the epidermis, which is composed of five thin layers. The epidermis acts as a barrier to light waves, heat waves, microorganisms, and many harmful chemicals. Our skin absorbs water, and when it does, it absorbs the toxic chemicals that we typically add to it. For instance, most of the chlorine that is absorbed in the body is absorbed through the skin when we bathe or shower. The epidermis is the thickest over the palms of our hands and the soles of our feet.

Melanin is the pigment that colors our skin and is responsible for skin differences among races. The more the skin is stimulated by the sun, the heavier the pigment appears in the skin. The heavier the skin pigment, the darker the skin and the more protection it offers from the elements.

What is the best protection from the sun? It's not sunblock, but rather sufficient amounts of essential fatty acids in your diet. It's true: the best protection from the powerful rays of the sun is internal protection through building up the level of EFAs in your body. Taking omega-3 supplements, in addition to omega-6 fatty acids contained in extra virgin olive oil, will help protect you from the sun.

Using EFAs allows melanin to effectively darken your skin, which provides the best protection from the sun's rays. Sunscreens, on the other hand, actually keep melanin from being formed in the epidermis.

Contrary to most popular beliefs, the sun's rays are beneficial to the human body, and like all good things, they need to be experienced in moderation. After all, the sun is our major source of vitamin D. Most sunscreens contain several harmful chemicals that may be the cause of our increased rate of skin cancer. These chemicals have been found to stimulate tumor growth

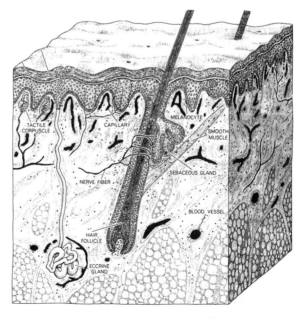

Fig. 8.12: The Skin

in mice. Let EFAs be your natural sunscreen, and expose yourself to the sun in moderation. This process will slowly let your skin get dark enough to protect you from harmful rays. A few good sources of natural sunscreen are included in appendix A.

As illustrated, the dermis is a much thicker layer of skin that consists of semi-elastic connective tissue, blood vessels, lymph vessels, nerves, hair follicles, sweat glands, sebaceous glands, and even tiny little muscles that make our hair stand on end. The sweat glands are found almost everywhere in the skin, and are most prolific in the soles of the feet and the palms of the hands. It is estimated that there are over 3,000 sweat glands per inch in the palms of our hands alone. These sweat glands let us know when we are getting into a potentially stressful situation.

Sweat comes from below the level of the skin and has the same basic composition as all other body fluids. Basic sweat also contains urea, uric acid, amino acids, lactic acid, ascorbic acid, and sugar. The smell associated with sweat is produced by the action of bacteria. The more toxic the body, the smellier the sweat. If your sweat really smells, it signifies that it is high time for the benefits of a cleansing diet. Sweating is also the body's primary means of lowering our body temperature.

Sebaceous glands are associated with the hair follicles, and produce an oily substance that lubricates the surface of our skin. The oil, called sebum, has antibacterial and antifungal properties, and helps to maintain the soft, pliable texture of the skin. Sebaceous glands are under the direction of endocrine hormones, and begin to secrete oil at puberty and recede with advancing age.

Oil is always associated with essential fatty acids in the body. Those of us that have healthy, well-lubricated skin with great texture will usually have an abundance of beneficial EFAs in our diets. If we eat a lot of denatured fats and hydrogenated oils, which are present in most refined carbohydrates and snack foods, we usually will have more dry, lifeless skin. Denatured fats and oils eventually end up on our faces, where we least want them to show up.

The acid mantle of the skin is a characteristic that protects our skin from bacteria and chemical irritants. This acid mantle often begins to break down with the continued use of soap and other harsh skin-cleansing products. In many cases of chronic skin problems, I have found it necessary to help people restore the acid mantle of their skin (see health tip #19 below).

HEALTH TIP #19: The Skin

Reestablish the balance of essential fatty acids in your diet, and add the oil-soluble vitamins, A, D, E, and K, which are present in oil-soluble chlorophyll.

Restore the acid mantle by completely eliminating the use of soap and using a 5–10 percent dilution of apple cider vinegar applied directly to the skin (5–10 percent apple cider vinegar to 90–95 percent water). In a few short weeks, the protection provided by the acid mantle is usually restored.

Use a natural skin cleanser in place of soap, and add antioxidants such as picnoginol, CoQ10, or alpha-lipoic acid to your supplement regime. These will usually succeed at improving the anti-aging abilities of your skin.

Therapeutic baths, steam baths (without fluoride and chlorine), dry saunas, infrared saunas, and the detoxifying foot bath can assist the removal of waste products through your skin.

In addition to the nutritional support listed above, try dry skin brushing. It is the best care possible for the skin. The skin builds new cells from the inside, which requires that the old layers of skin peel off before healthy new skin appears. Dry skin brushing helps move out your old skin, release toxins, and stimulates the creation of new skin cells.

Skin Brushing Technique

Skin brushing is usually performed when the skin is dry. Stand on a towel to catch the sloughing skin, and begin brushing from head to toe with a semi-stiff dry skin brush. Brush both sides of your neck, arms, chest, legs, and back. Skin brushing should certainly make your skin feel stimulated, but in no way should it feel irritated. Skin brushing assists the elimination system by removing dead skin cells from the skin and stimulating the growth of healthy new skin cells. Skin brushing several times per week is beneficial.

Hair and Nails

Hair is an integral part of the skin. Most of our body is covered with it. Hair is similar to the skin in both its growth patterns and its nutritional needs, with essential fatty acids and oil-soluble vitamins at the top of the list. Hair is especially dull without sufficient amounts of vitamin A complex.

Hair problems can also point to problems with digestion or with the thyroid gland, as the thyroid is needed for the conversion of vitamin A from beta-carotene. Without good digestion, hair will not receive these important vitamins and nutrients and will show the deficiency. Surprisingly, digestive enzymes, especially those associated with fats, will often improve the health of your hair.

Healthy hair is also dependent on the action of B complex vitamins, preferably from whole food sources, a deficiency of which is the suspected cause of prematurely graying hair. Adequate protein, in the form of amino acids, is also necessary for normal hair growth, as the hair follicle is primarily composed of protein. Thinning hair may be an indication of poor protein utilization or a lack of protein in the diet.

Because the hair follicle is alive, it reflects the mineral content in the entire body, which is why hair analysis is used to detect mineral deficiencies in the body, mineral excesses, and the presence of heavy or toxic minerals that can cause serious health problems in the body. It's also why adequate minerals are so important for healthy hair.

The last component of the skin is the nails. The condition of the nails is a true reflection of the state of health that exists in the body. For example, the pink color in the nail beds indicates a healthy circulatory system, while a bluish tint indicates poor circulation. The condition of the half moons that normally reside on the finger side of the nails indicate the depth of your constitution, which is your ability to create health in the body. Large half moons are a sign of good energy reserves and a good constitution, while small or absent moons indicate a lack of reserve power in the body.

Ridges or rough spots on the nails usually indicate an EFA deficiency, while spoon-shaped nails often indicate an iron deficiency and an overworked circulatory system. White spots on the nails indicate mineral deficiencies, especially zinc, while brittle or peeling nails indicate a need for whole food nutrition. Overall, the health requirements for our nails are very similar to the requirements for healthy hair. Adequate nutrition, which includes a whole foods multivitamin and multi-mineral supplement, and the addition of extra calcium, magnesium, and silica usually make for strong, healthy nails and skin.

HEALTH TIP #20: For Nails

To restore strength and durability to your nails, take a natural whole food multiple vitamin and mineral supplement; add brewer's yeast or rice bran syrup as a whole food source of the B-complex vitamins; include a healthy source of bonemeal; and use horsetail and oat straw teas to improve your silica content. Avoid sugar, refined carbohydrates, and caffeinated beverages.

If dull hair and weak nails are part of your health picture, make sure to include a full-spectrum digestive enzyme in your diet, because a poor digestive system can keep you from absorbing the nutrients you do eat. It is also important to realize that nails grow slowly, only about two inches a year, so give yourself enough time for the results of your good nutrition to show up.

Conclusion

The digestive system lies at the core of the body and is the system that allows us to break down and assimilate the nutrients of life. It acts as the hub of a wheel, and has the ability to bring either health or disease to the systems of the body. If we take care of it, our digestive system will function effectively for a lifetime. If we abuse it, it will likely be the cause of our demise.

In natural health circles, it is often said that degenerative disease begins in the colon. If you keep your digestive and elimination systems functioning at optimal levels, your chances of experiencing increased longevity and freedom from chronic disease become vastly improved.

This is most easily accomplished by improving the health of these vital systems before problems arise, and by taking the initiative to learn how these vital systems work. In this way, you can decipher what your Inner Intelligence is trying to tell you through your signs and symptoms. This understanding will help you determine how you can help right now, which means avoiding the things that compromise your digestion and elimination, and incorporating new habits that will improve it. Use the functioning of these two systems as a barometer for change.

Chapter 9

The Immune System

THE IMMUNE SYSTEM has to be one of the great miracles of the human body. It is the most sensitive and extensive surveillance system ever contrived. In fact, it is so sensitive that it can hear a biochemical pin drop. In relationship to our immunity, this awareness is ultimately translated into a recognition of what is self and what is not self. Our Internal Intelligence has the ability to observe and analyze myriad events that occur simultaneously throughout the body, and to take immediate action when a problem is perceived.

Our Internal Intelligence also has the ability to assess, analyze, evaluate, and perceive the current condition of every cell, tissue, organ, and system throughout the body, and then make any necessary changes to maintain the balance of our internal environment. Even the feeling tone that we express has a positive or negative effect on the way our immune system functions.

To mobilize its defense system effectively, the Intelligence of the body requires feedback from the integrated array of healthy functioning systems, especially the neuroendocrine system, which acts as systems control in the body.

From my perspective, immunity contains both an offensive and a defensive strategy. The offense represents the ability of the body to monitor an incredible amount of information with state-of-the-art surveillance technology. Problems arise in the body when this surveillance system either becomes ineffective in certain areas or simply breaks down.

Because our health exists multidimensionally, an increase in stress on one or more levels of our experience significantly reduces the ability of our immune system to resist dis-ease. Mental or emotional stress, for example, prompts the adrenal glands to secrete cortisol, which inhibits immune system function and begins to shut down our surveillance system. If, for example, the fight-or-flight mechanism is triggered in the body, the immune system is temporarily shut down in order to save our life, as all of our energy is channeled into our muscular system in order to make a quick exit. In the past, this fight-or-flight mechanism was rarely used. Unfortunately, high levels of stress exist on all levels of experience now. For many, this fight-or-flight mechanism becomes triggered on a daily basis, and for some it remains activated for most of the day. This simple fact translates to an overall decline in our immunity, and is one of the major reasons why chronic disease is so rampant in our society.

When high levels of stress exist in the body, our immune system loses some of its ability to assess the condition of certain areas of the body. These stress levels can also interfere with the ability of your body to create an effective strategy against foreign invaders.

Most of us buy the popular belief that health is regained by fighting bacteria, viruses, and disease, as if they were the enemy. But they are not the enemy. There are times when the body needs our assistance in this regard, but for the most part, we need to learn how to support our body to regain the health it has lost. Creating a healthy immune system lies not in warding off foreign invaders, such as bacteria and virus, but in learning how to enhance the body's ability to resist them. An immune system that is compromised provides an open door to myriad agents of disease. A completely healthy immune system will not give foreign invaders access to the body in the first place.

Our Amazing Defense System

When a healthy immune system senses the presence of foreign invaders, it rapidly springs into action with all the power and might of nature. When provoked, the immune system is ruthless, employing an array of weapons designed to render any enemy helpless. Our amazing system acts quickly and furiously to overcome an endless array of invading organisms, which, if left unattended, would overrun the body.

We know the thymus gland is the director of our immune system. When foreign invaders are detected, the thymus stimulates the lymphatic organs throughout the body to develop specific antibodies in response to specific foreign invaders. These lymphatic organs include the thymus, spleen, tonsils, adenoids, appendix, small intestine, lymph nodes, the skin, and the inner marrow of our long bones.

The thymus is an integral part of a one-two punch provided by the immune system, with the second punch coming from the marrow of our long bones. Let's take a look at how these two facets of our immune system are designed to work together in perfect harmony.

The thymus creates, nurtures, and develops T cells. The "T" stands for thymus. The bone marrow develops B cells ("B" for bone marrow). See how easy this is? When foreign invaders are detected by our surveillance system, they are first detected by ground troops called monocytes.

Monocytes, as the name suggests, are single cells that originate from bone marrow and circulate throughout our bloodstream. When they are fully developed, monocytes migrate into the tissues of the body and become macrophages. Now, macrophages are cool. They are huge Pac-Man–like cells that gobble up foreign invaders and use powerful enzymes to digest the enemy.

After a macrophage eats an invader, it has the ability to determine exactly what type of invader it just ate, and quickly pass that detailed information on to the thymus gland. The thymus gland in turn seeds the entire lymphatic system with the exact formula needed to create antibodies for that specific invader.

It is the macrophage that starts the immune system response, by transferring information to the thymus, which in turn downloads that same information to the entire lymphatic system.

Macrophages are like advance scouts that alert headquarters about the type of enemy they encounter, and where that enemy is located. Macrophages are capable of detecting a wide range of foreign invaders that roam aimlessly in our tissues, including a host of microorganisms, pollen, and even cancer cells. Macrophages are also important players in the inflammatory process, as they secrete a variety of enzymes and other substances that promote growth and healing. The healthier our immune system, the more macrophages we have in our tissues; the weaker our immune system, the more scarce is the macrophage.

Other types of monocytes are an integral part of our army of defense, many of which you may be familiar with from routine blood tests. These include neutrophils, basophils, eosinophils, and leukocytes, which comprise our white blood cells (WBCs). If our white blood cell count is elevated, it indicates that an infection is present somewhere in the body. An elevated white blood count indicates that a battle is currently taking place between foreign invaders and the ground troops of the immune system, the WBCs.

Other cells that are players in the immune system include mast cells, which are associated with the production of immunoglobulin, an immune system enhancer; platelets, which attract WBCs to the battleground or injury site; natural killer cells, that are specifically designed to neutralize cancer cells and viruses; and the ever popular stem cell, which are blank cells that can be used for whatever function the body deems to be most pertinent. Stem cells can be used as lymphocytes that carry specific antibodies exactly where they are needed, as white blood cells that are utilized at the point of attack or injury, or they can be made into red blood cells that carry oxygen in the body.

All the cells of our immune system have separate functions that allow them to fit perfectly into the needs of our immune system. Some cells are designed simply for communication, while others secrete substances that halt the enemy in its tracks. Some cells act as trained killers, while others dispose of the dead bodies. Some cells are designed simply to speed up or slow down the action, while others are designed to remember the confrontation for years to come. Some immune system cells initiate the battle, while still others signal that the war is over. Our amazing immune system is perfectly designed offensively to maintain our health, and defensively to keep foreign invaders at bay.

Initially, you may not recognize the signs and responses of a normally functioning immune system. For instance, whenever our WBCs are at war, the battle is usually accompanied by a fever. This fever is purposefully created by the body to assist in the global healing process. Our Inner Intelligence knows that an elevated temperature doesn't hurt the body; rather, it has a devastating effect on foreign invaders such as bacteria and virus.

Although a temperature of 98.6 is considered normal, the range of normal temperatures can include lower temperatures in the 97 range, and higher ones in the range of 101 degrees. Just for fun, take your temperature throughout the course of a day, especially when you are feeling great. You may be surprised at the variation. In a static world, our temperature will always be 98.6; in the dynamic world we actually live in, nothing is ever stagnant. In times of biochemical warfare, our normal temperature can range from 98.6 degrees up to 103 or 104.

In times of an all-out invasion, our body temperature may even increase to 105 degrees or higher. These higher temperatures may only happen once or twice during one's lifetime, and they indicate extreme conditions. They are an indication that the immune system is in trouble and desperate measures are underway. If you experience temperatures as high as these, you need the services of a physician who understands the natural workings of the body. For the record, brain damage doesn't occur until fevers reach 110 degrees.

The higher the temperature the body creates, the more desperate the immune system has become. The bigger the battle, the larger the biochemical imbalance. If our immune system is frequently under attack, it is an indication that it is significantly compromised and is in desperate need of our support.

Does Chicken Soup Really Work?

In increasing numbers of cases, the body loses its ability to distinguish between what is us and what is a foreign invader, and begins to attack its own tissues. We literally become allergic to ourselves. This indicates that the immune system has become so hypersensitive that it is triggered at the drop of a hat. This is called autoimmune disease.

This hypersensitive condition indicates that the immune system has been overworked, undernourished, and is in desperate need of repair and rejuvenation. The surveillance portion of our immune system has become so excessively vigilant that our neuroendocrine system stays stuck on constant alert, and our poor adrenal glands are in a perpetual state of emergency.

This situation does not develop overnight, but usually builds up over a period of time. During the years preceding the onset of autoimmune disease, the body simply begins to wear itself out. This usually occurs because we demand too much from our body, have an enormous amount of multidimensional stress in our lives, live in a biochemically hostile and toxic environment, or, most likely, a combination of all three. We tend to push ourselves to the limit and don't replace the resources that we use up. When our immunity degenerates to this point, most of our internal organs become too weak to do anything about it. The solution is now difficult, but not impossible.

It helps to understand why the body is attacking itself. This mystery was actually solved in the 1930s by a nutritionist named Dr. Royal Lee. Dr. Lee, who founded Standard Process Laboratories, discovered that weakened organs leave behind a trail of cellular debris when they break down. Initially, it is this trail of cellular debris that the immune system traces back to its origin. The immune system correctly determines that it is one of our organs that is causing the cellular debris. At this point, our immune system tries to resolve the problem by attacking the cause—in this case, its own organ.

This weakened organ continues to break down, creating even more cellular debris, while the immune system continues to attack the source of the problem. It is like a catch-22 in the body for which there is no real solution.

Believe it or not, this is where chicken soup comes in. Chicken soup creates additional cellular debris from the tissues and bones of the chicken, and our immune system leaves the weakened organ alone, focusing instead on the debris created by the chicken soup, which is much greater in degree than the weakened organ in question.

We can take advantage of this internal mechanism by using what is called a protomorphogen. Like the chicken soup, a protomorphogen acts as a decoy, so that the immune system attacks it and leaves our weakened organ alone. Meanwhile, we use the time we gain from this distraction to rebuild the weakened organ. In the short span of a month or two, the organ regains its strength and ceases leaving a trail of chemical debris, and our immune system stops its attack.

Your grandmother was right: Chicken soup does have magical powers!

A list of protomorphogens for a variety of organs is included in appendix A, and can be used to help our depleted organs without any side effects. It is interesting to note that the most common organs involved in this scenario are the organs of the endocrine system, especially the adrenal glands and the thyroid.

If you take a protomorphogen for a weakened organ, it is also important that you take specific nutritional support to rebuild that organ at the same time. The combination of protomorphogen and nutritional support can usually get the job done in a few month's time.

The Lymphatic System

Another system integrally linked to immune function is the lymphatic system. It also has a number of its own functions. The lymphatic system is an extensive system that infiltrates all the tissues of the body and has been described as the body's sanitation system. Lymph fluid travels through this extensive system carrying the remains of bacteria, virus, microbial parasites, and toxic wastes. The lymph tissue, especially the lymph nodes, filters out these waste products in order to keep them out of your blood.

As the accompanying illustration indicates, the lymph system and blood system are intimately connected, and have many similarities in function. In reality, these two systems function together as parts of a grand circulatory system.

The lymph system cleanses, and the blood system nourishes. The circulatory system has a pump—the heart—while the lymph fluid is squeezed out by the contraction of our muscles as we move. The lymph system uses the spleen to create cells for the immune system, and the circulatory system uses the spleen to rejuvenate and store the red blood cells that carry vital oxygen to all our tissues and cells. The basis of lymphatic fluid and blood plasma are essentially the same, and ultimately, lymphatic fluid is dumped into our bloodstream.

Lymphatic fluid travels through a series of one-way valves that purify the lymph so that it can eventually become the basis for our blood. However, if our lymph fluid gets too thick, our blood will too. If our body becomes too toxic, lymph fluid becomes sluggishly thick and doesn't flow through

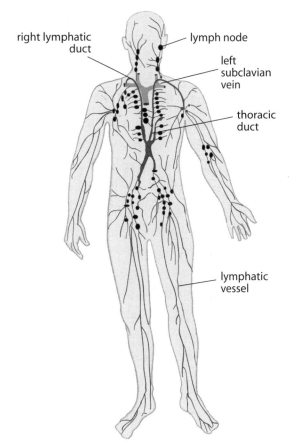

Fig. 9.1: The Lymphatic System

our tissues as easily. This can cause a number of problems in the lymph system, as some of the debris in the lymph nodes begins to fester and breeds harmful strains of bacteria and virus, which can weaken our immune system even more.

When we don't exercise enough or drink enough pure water, and overconsume refined carbohydrates, dairy products, and other foods with a high gluten content, our lymph fluids become thick, slow moving, and excessively toxic, which has a direct influence on how well the tissues of the body drain themselves of the toxic wastes created by normal cellular activities. When this scenario is in place, the toxic levels of the tissues gradually increase, our pH becomes too acidic, muscular activity becomes sluggish, our blood begins to carry too many toxins, and our immune system becomes significantly compromised.

Unfortunately, these conditions are all too commonplace in our society, which is why our lymph system needs to become a focus for cleansing, exercise, and repair.

HEALTH TIP #1: Lymphatic Drainage Technique

The lymphatic system, which can be described in part as our sanitation system, occasionally backs up due to dietary indiscretions, a lack of water intake, and a general lack of exercise. Its drainage can be aided by a gentle self-massage using three or four fingers. This massage is directed in a circular motion along the lymphatic channels, in the direction of lymph flow, as outlined in figure 9.1 on page 269. Evaluate the areas in which lymph nodes or lymphatic filters are concentrated by checking them for tenderness and/or swelling. A lymphatic massage can also be performed by a massage therapist trained to assist the function of the lymphatic system. See your local listings for details. The areas of lymphatic concentration are located in the following areas: along both sides of the neck, along the base of the skull at the top of the neck, under and around both armpits, the muscles across both sides of the chest, and in the inguinal or groin region on both sides of the body.

Immunity and Emotions

The thymus is the heart of our immunity, and it lies at the heart of the endocrine system. There are three endocrine organs above thymus: the pineal, pituitary, and thyroid. And there are three endocrine organs below the thymus: the pancreas, adrenals, and gonads. The thymus not only centers the immune system in the body, but it is the endocrine organ that centers the respiratory function of our lungs and the circulatory function of our physical heart.

Emotionally, the thymus is connected to our heart center. The thymus is so sensitive to emotions and feelings that it shrivels up in the presence of caustic emotions. When we embrace feelings of love and joy, the thymus boosts the function of its related organs and systems. When we are in the throes of negative emotions like anger, rage, or fear, these same systems begin to shut down. Because the thymus is at the heart of our endocrine orchestra, any compromise to it tends to sour its otherwise sweet music. Have you ever noticed that when you are angry, you don't breathe? Or that when you give over to rage, your face gets red? When we are enraged, our circulatory system becomes so amped up that our eyes pop out of our heads. Whenever we allow negative emotions to take control of our bodies, they wreak total havoc. Fortunately, the opposite is also true.

The resonant frequency of love is so contagious that it spreads throughout the bodies of both the giver and the receiver. Love is the most powerful cure available to us in any moment of our lives. Want to enhance the function of your immune system? Share some love.

How to Create a Healthy Immune System

To successfully build an effective immune system, we must consider both its offensive and defensive sides. The offensive component consists of supporting an immune system that is already working effectively by rejuvenating its organs and related systems, reducing our multidimensional stress levels wherever possible, eating an optimal diet, drinking sufficient amounts of pure water, and cleansing the tissues of the body on a seasonal basis.

The defensive component consists of rebuilding weakened organs, reducing stress, building up the level of antioxidants in our tissues, avoiding food and water with chemicals and pesticides, and helping our bodies fight the agents of dis-ease.

Immune System Relationships

HEALTH TIP #2: Build the Health of Your Immune System

Support your adrenal glands. Follow the guidelines for healthy adrenal glands as outlined in chapter 6.

Overdoing it seems to be the downfall of the adrenal glands. Evaluate your multidimensional stress levels and your lifestyle to determine whether or not all the things you currently do are absolutely necessary. If the fight-or-flight mechanism is a regular visitor in your home, you may want to create a healthier lifestyle for yourself, your family, and your adrenals. If your immune system is always on the defensive, it is important not to overstimulate your adrenals. Initially, this can be accomplished by drinking licorice root tea (unless you have high blood pressure), and avoiding the things that overstimulate the adrenals, such as caffeine and sugar.

Support and cleanse your lymphatic system using the Lymphatic Formula in appendix A, as well as implementing nutritional support for the thymus and spleen. These remedies can be self-tested, or tested by a chiropractor trained in the art of muscle testing.

Techniques for lymphatic massage and skin brushing are outlined in chapter 8. To improve immune system function, rub the neurolymphatic reflexes for the thymus, spleen, and adrenal glands, located in the accompanying illustration.

Avoid the following substances, which drag down immune function: alcohol, stimulants of all kind, caffeine, the chemicals and additives in foods and drinks, carbonated soft drinks, refined carbohydrates, dairy products, and the overconsumption of wheat, trans fatty acids, hydrogenated fats, vegetable oils, over-the-counter and recreational drugs.

For diet and cleansing, consume six vegetables, two fruits, one starch, and one protein on a daily basis to provide the body with all the necessary buildings blocks for health. The natural

Immune System Relationships	
Organs related to the Immune System	thymus, spleen, heart, lungs, adrenal glands, adenoids, appendix, small intestine and numerous structures within the lymphatic system.
Signs & symptoms of Immune System dysfunction	frequent colds & flu, allergies, continual fatigue, painful muscles & joints, psoriasis or excema, inflammatory disorders & frequent cold sores.

Fig. 9.2: Organs related to the Immune System/Signs and Symptoms of Immune System Dysfunction

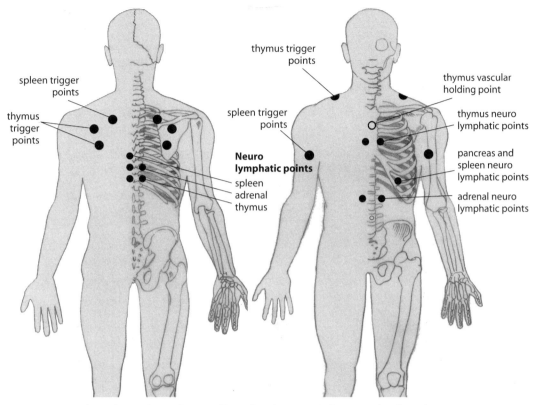

Fig. 9.3: Neurolymphatic Stimulation Chart for Thymus, Spleen, and Adrenals

antioxidants contained in whole foods such as broccoli, cauliflower, Swiss chard, and kale reduce the effects of free radical oxygenation in the immune system and throughout the body. Super foods, including spirulina, blue-green algae, green drinks, and certain mushroom formulas, greatly improve immune system function as well.

Beneficial plant fats contained in organic fruits and vegetables provide the immune system with the basic building blocks it needs for normal hormone production. Sources for these beneficial fats include flaxseed oil and meal, raw sesame seeds, sunflower seeds, almonds, and almond butter.

Fruit sources of EFAs include figs, oranges, apricots, apples; vegetable sources include peas, squash, olives, potatoes, and unadulterated soybeans (not genetically modified). Other food sources include rice bran syrup, buckwheat, wheat germ oil, and wheat germ.

Animal sources of essential fatty acids are found in fish, seafood, scallops, oysters, crab, shrimp, and lobster. It is important to note that fish sources may contain mercury and other toxic elements that have been dumped into our oceans.

Try also the cleansing guidelines provided in chapter 7. If your immune system is severely compromised, only mild cleansing is recommended.

Immune system supplementation includes a whole food multiple vitamin and mineral supplement, sufficient amounts of real vitamin-C complex, vitamins A, D, E, and K (contained in oil-soluble chlorophyll complex), low potency and full spectrum vitamin B complex, thymus extracts, echinacea to enhance spleen function, mercury-free fish oils, and essential fatty acid supplementation in the form of flaxseed oil.

Drink sufficient amounts of pure water (half your body weight in ounces every day). If digestive problems exist, take a full-spectrum digestive enzyme. Sources and guidelines for all whole food nutritional supplements are listed in appendix A.

Moderate amounts of exercise facilitate increased flow of lymph fluid throughout the body. Exercise options include yoga asanas, or poses, the Slant Board Exercise, the mini trampoline, Yoga Swing Exercises in appendix B, and the breathing techniques presented in chapter 10.

Practice techniques for stress reduction, including meditation (see chapter 11).

Use techniques for emotional clearing (see chapter 12).

The Agents of Dis-ease

As we look at the external factors that drag down the function of our immunity, it is important to understand that disease cannot exist in a healthy body and can only exist in one that has broken down first. Maintaining this elevated perspective is essential, as the tendency exists to look outside of ourselves for the cause of our problems. This tendency has led human beings to look in all the wrong places for the causes of disease.

Both health and dis-ease come from within. Only after our body starts to break down do the external agents of dis-ease—bacteria, viruses, yeast, parasites, toxic chemicals and metals—become a factor.

In the remaining portion of this chapter I wish to discuss these agents of disease, how they effect our health, and what we can do to minimize their presence. Along with improving the ability of our body to resist disease, addressing the agents of disease can also be a successful part of enhancing our immune system function.

Bacterial Infections

Bacteria are an essential part of the continuum of the natural world. They fill a niche in the external environment and assist nature in the essential recycling process of decay and degeneration. In the human body, there are over four hundred different kinds of bacteria that contribute to our health. Bacteria are significant players in the renewal process of nature. It is important to note that less then 10 percent of all bacteria contribute to the disease processes, while over 90 percent are here to help us. As a matter of fact, without their help, we would not be able to live successfully on planet Earth.

Bacteria have the ability to transform and mutate quickly, constantly adapting to the changing internal environment in the body. If the defenses of our body weaken or begin to degenerate, detrimental bacteria gain an opportunity to overcome our immune system, which leads us further into a state of dis-ease.

In the medical war on bacteria, the overuse of antibiotics has created resistant strains in virtually every class of bacteria, which pushes our body's defense system to the limit. Essentially, we have forced bacteria to mutate into rebel strains in order to survive. These strains now have the ability terrorize any immune system that operates at less then 100 percent. This is why it is so important to have an immune system that works at peak performance levels.

HEALTH TIP #3: Bacterial Infections

In observing patterns of health and dis-ease in my patients over the years, I have observed three necessary steps for ridding the body of harmful bacteria.

Locate and correct weakness present in the immune system. You can begin this process by using the self-test procedures presented later in this chapter, and follow up with an evaluation by a chiropractor or other natural health care practitioner. This important step enhances and empowers the immune system to take better care of bacteria by itself. When we remove the interference that exists on the structural, biochemical, mental, emotional, or spiritual levels, the body is more capable of intensifying its own defenses.

Introduce a natural antibacterial substance (listed in appendix A) that does not adversely effect the body. This will render the internal environment unsuitable for bacteria, as they only flourish within a certain temperature range and within a specific range of pH. Antibiotics are commonly used for the purpose of reducing the effect of detrimental bacteria in the body, but they do so at the body's expense. If you want to eliminate a fly that is on your piano, you can either use a flyswatter or a hammer. Both of these techniques will kill the fly, but using a hammer also damages the piano. When they are necessary, antibiotics save lives, and they should be reserved for life-threatening situations only. Less invasive solutions should be tried first, drugs second, and surgery absolutely last.

Introduce beneficial bacteria into the body for hand-to-hand combat. Introducing billions of beneficial bacteria into the digestive tract will reduce the number and the virulence of disease-related bacteria in the body. The sheer number of these beneficial little critters helps to overrun the competition. When dealing with microorganisms inside the body, it is always preferable to let beneficial bacteria do as much of the dirty work as possible.

If disease-producing bacteria have taken up residence in your body, you will experience recurring bacterial infections. Following these three simple steps will reduce chronic infections, improve overall immune system function, and provide increased energy levels because the immune system isn't busy fighting bacteria anymore.

HEALTH TIP #4: Self-Testing to Detect Disease-Causing Bacteria

Locate a natural health care practitioner near you who can evaluate the presence of bacteria either through muscle testing or stool samples. See the resources listed in appendix A.

You can also test yourself to evaluate the conditions in your body. Muscle self-testing is used for testing nutritional remedies, but it can also be used to evaluate any situation in your body. Muscle self-testing uses yes-or-no questions to help you determine which remedies are right for any system in the body. This process can be used to determine your dietary needs, cleansing options, food choices, organ vitality, structural areas of need, color and lighting preferences, and answers about beliefs and feelings, etc. Although there are several options, I employ the following finger muscle-testing procedure.

Test your index finger by using the strength of your middle finger as illustrated.

1. Actively point your index finger.
2. Place the pad of your middle finger on top of the nail of your index finger.
3. Keeping your index finger active and straight, push down with your middle finger to meet the resistance of your index finger.
4. A positive response (a "yes" answer) is indicated when your index finger remains strong in the extended testing position.
5. A negative response (a "no" answer) is indicated when the resistance provided by your index finger is eliminated. The straightened index finger will flex downward, toward your palm, as if the muscles have been switched off.
6. Practice testing for positive and negative responses for several days before asking specific questions or testing any remedies. Relax, and let your Inner Intelligence show you how it is done. After all, a muscle test is a way to communicate with the wisdom of your Inner Intelligence.

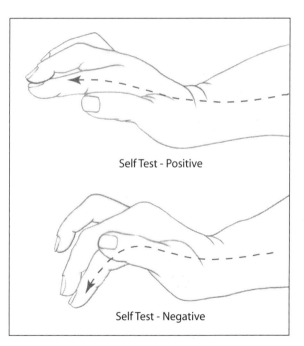

Self Test - Positive

Self Test - Negative

Keep in mind that any muscle test is specific to the present moment, and it can be influenced by your mind. To be successful in using this valuable tool, it is essential that you find a way to shut off your questioning mind.

Fig. 9.4: Muscle Self-Testing

HEALTH TIP #5: Antibacterial Remedies

There are many natural antibacterial remedies. Herbal preparations include a combination of echinacea and goldenseal, garlic, olive leaf extract, lomatium, oil of oregano, propolis, and gentian violet. The tincture form of herbs is usually the most effective. Cranberry juice can be used to acidify the pH of the urinary tract and is the first course of action for urinary tract infections. Concentrated cranberry tablets are also available at your local health food store.

For antibacterial vitamin preparations, see appendix A.

For whole foods remedies, including Morinda Supreme, see product in appendix A.

Many sources of beneficial bacteria especially those that are not refrigerated, don't survive the manufacturing or shipping process. Be careful to buy from the most reputable sources.

Important strains of beneficial bacteria to include in a probiotic are acidophilus bacillus, bifidus, lactobacillus sporogenes, lactobacillus infantis for children, and soil-based organisms (SBOs), which can be difficult to find.

Soil-based organisms are beneficial bacteria that normally live in healthy soil, and ultimately find their way into our digestive systems. SBOs rarely exist in today's depleted soil, but nutritional products do exist and are of particular benefit to the small and large intestines. Suppliers for these vital products are included in appendix A.

Utilize a kefir culture on a daily basis to combat the effects of bacterial imbalances as described in chapter 8.

Viral Infections

Viral problems fall into the same category as bacteria, but viruses have a slightly different role in the overall scheme of the natural world. Although much of the role of the virus still remains unknown, it appears that one important function is to communicate to bacteria any important changes that occur in their immediate environment. A virus actually transfers information on contact to bacteria, informing them of the latest changes in the internal and external environment, which enables bacteria to mutate quickly.

Utilizing drug therapy to fight viral infections, especially antibiotics, is not a health-producing strategy, as antibiotics are useless against viral infections. Using the gift of natural herbs and natural remedies actually supports the body to stay in control of the battle against the virus. This shows us the difference in strategies.

Following the same three steps that are outlined for the treatment of bacteria will usually ensure success in the treatment of viral problems as well. Keep in mind that the purpose of any treatment program is to rebuild the effectiveness of the immune system so that it can be more effective in fighting viral invaders. A healthy body is always more effective than any drug in fighting bacteria and virus, and it does so without creating a chronic immune system weakness. Make no mistake about it: In the medical model, the war on microbes will eventually be won by the microbe.

HEALTH TIP #6: Antiviral Remedies

There are many similarities between viruses and bacteria, and many similarities in their remedies.

Herbal remedies include oregano oil, olive leaf extract, a tincture of echinacea and goldenseal, lomatium, and garlic, which has the effect of a broad-spectrum antibiotic without any of the side effects.

For antiviral vitamin preparations and their suppliers, see appendix A.

For whole foods remedies, including Morinda Supreme, see sources located in appendix A.

Beneficial bacteria or probiotics are also an important factor in all conditions involving viruses. The important strains include acidophilus bacillus, bifidus, lactobacillus sporogenes, acidophilus infantis for infants, and soil-based organisms that help to change the inner terrain of the intestines.

Yeast Intolerance

Yeast and fungal infections are commonplace in the body and can be extremely difficult to eliminate. These infections, which are not only confined to women, often involve several strains of yeast and fungus, the most famous of which is *Candida albicans*.

Candida is a systemic yeast infection that can cause myriad symptoms and health problems. Some of the signs and symptoms of candida include digestive system problems, diarrhea, constipation, fatigue, allergies, acne, migraine headaches, PMS, menstrual disorders, endocrine system imbalances, respiratory problems, joint pains, insomnia, chemical sensitivities, memory loss, mood swings, and depression. I have seen severe cases of depression completely eliminated when the cause of candida had been resolved.

There are several causes for a candida or yeast overgrowth in the body, and the primary one involves the use of antibiotics. Antibiotics usually kill all bacteria in the intestines, both good and bad, but have no effect on yeast or fungal organisms. When bacteria are eliminated in the intestines, a rapidly escalating yeast population simply takes over their place.

Nutritionist Roger Williams explains how fast yeast can multiply in the intestines when given an unlimited growth environment: "If a single yeast cell were given the perfect environment for growth, within 24 hours it could produce a colony of over 100 cells. At this rate of reproduction, within a week, it would continue to produce a yeast colony weighing one billion tons." Of course, this can't happen inside a human being, but it gives a good indication of the hardy growth rate of yeast cultures.

Perhaps you think you hardly ever use antibiotics. Unfortunately, that is not true for most of us. If we don't take them to support our immune system, we are consuming them in our foods. Antibiotics are routinely injected into the animals we eat, are present in their feed and water, and are legally allowed in our milk and dairy products.

Although we receive these antibiotics secondhand, they slowly wipe out the strains of beneficial bacteria in our intestines. As the number of bacteria is reduced, ambitious yeasts, such as candida, quickly inherit their territory.

Other causes of candidiasis, as it is also called, include the contraceptive pill, which negatively effects over 25 percent of its users; the use of steroid hormones; pollution, which raises the amount of free radicals in the body; inadequate nutrition; stress; and inherited genetic weakness.

As the immune system gets weaker, it begins to tolerate yeast and fungus, and no longer tries to eliminate them. The body begins to perceive yeast and fungus as a normal part of self.

Most yeasts are dimorphic. They have two different forms, a yeast form and a fungal form. The yeast form described above is more easily treated, while the fungal form is more difficult. The fungal form is root-like in nature, and grows on a stalk that is rooted directly into our intestines. Fungal infections are usually long-standing and include problems like athlete's foot, jock itch, chronic rashes, and toenail fungus. Unless aggressive treatment and lifestyle changes ensue, these fungal infections often stick around for life.

By-products of Yeast and Fungus

The good news is that beneficial organisms secrete or manufacture substances that support a huge list of functions in the body. Bacteria, for example, manufacture a host of vitamins and enzymes that assist the body to break down toxic waste products in the intestines. Beneficial bacteria love to eat acid wastes; after all, acidophilus means "acid-loving."

However, yeast and fungus manufacture toxic waste products. These waste products pollute the intestines and create an alkaline pH in the intestines. These changes in the intestinal environment create a host of problems throughout our digestive and elimination systems.

There are over a hundred different forms of yeasts and fungi that create forms of alcohol and aldehydes as their waste products.

Formaldehyde, for instance, is used to preserve organ parts by the undertaker to preserve corpses. Aldehydes created by yeast and fungal infections start to preserve our own bodies while we are still living in them. Aldehydes are extremely toxic to the body and are usually an important component of environmental illness.

The most common aldehyde produced by *Candida albicans* is acetaldehyde. A toxic irritant to the body, acetaldehyde also inhibits the growth of beneficial bacteria, making even more room for aggressive yeasts and fungus. You can smell aldehydes in a new car or carpet, in perfumes and cigarette smoke. If you are particularly bothered by these smells, you should suspect a candida overgrowth.

The most common form of alcohol produced by yeast and fungus is ethanol. Ethanol may be fine for powering your car, but it wreaks havoc when introduced into your body. Aldehydes and alcohol weaken the immune system, create allergic reactions, are extremely toxic, and produce degeneration and disease in the body.

How Yeast and Fungus Multiply

Yeast and fungus usually reproduce by forming spores in the body. These spores are difficult for the immune system to neutralize. If the digestive system is not producing enough stomach acid, for instance, yeast and fungal spores make it through the digestive process and attach themselves to the walls of the intestines.

As is the case with all organisms, yeasts and fungi need to eat food in order to survive. Yeast and fungus love to eat sugar and sweets of all kinds, including fruits and their juices. If you suspect a candida overgrowth in your body, observe how your body reacts to any of the foods listed below. If your symptoms get worse after eating these foods, candida overgrowth is the main suspect. To make sure, take the candida assessment in appendix B.

Foods that feed yeasts and fungus include fruits, dried fruits and their juices; all types of sweeteners, including honey, maple syrup, refined sugar, and corn syrup; cheese; and any foods containing yeast, alcohol, or vinegar (except apple cider vinegar).

For achieving the best results in decreasing candida overgrowth, avoid these foods for a period of at least three weeks, and up to six weeks for severe cases. During this time, use the appropriate antifungals and supplements to restore the digestive track.

Candida poses a serious health threat to millions of people throughout the world. It is estimated that over thirty million women suffer from problems related to *Candida albicans.*

Treatment alternatives include the use of cellulose enzymes that digest the cell wall of the candida organism, and an antifungal regime that directly attacks yeasts and fungi. I recommend the cellulose treatment initially, which can quickly resolve a majority of candida problems. If symptoms of candida persist, start an antifungal regime. In severe cases of candida, it may be necessary to treat the yeast in your sexual partner as well.

HEALTH TIP #7: Treatment for Yeast and Fungus

Cellulose treatment for candida is a relatively simple solution to a difficult problem. Several products listed in appendix A contain beneficial bacteria and cellulose enzymes that destroy the cell walls of yeast and fungus. Treatment in many cases lasts for only two to three weeks.

Herbal remedies include antifungal herbs for yeast and fungus, including Pau d'Arco, garlic, quaw bark, spilanthes, and black walnut hulls.

Antifungal vitamin preparations include specially prepared yeast and fungi formulas including those listed in appendix A.

Whole food remedies include Morinda Supreme. Resources for all antifungal preparations are listed in appendix A.

Foods to avoid during treatment include all sugars and sweeteners, fruit juice, dried fruit, vinegar, cheese, yeast, alcohol, soy sauce, all fermented products, and refined carbohydrates. These foods should be avoided for at least three weeks in order to strengthen the immune system and starve out yeast and fungus.

After three weeks, slowly return to a diet that includes significantly fewer sweeteners, fruits, and refined carbohydrates, and substantially more whole foods and raw vegetables. Use your symptoms as feedback to indicate the need for dietary changes or the continued use of antifungal agents. You can use the self-test to determine which foods should still be avoided and which can be reintroduced into your diet (see page 277).

General nutritional support includes a whole food multiple vitamin and mineral supplement, essential fatty acids (omega-3 and omega-6), and low-potency, whole food source vitamin B and C complexes. You can use the self-test to evaluate the necessity of taking any of these supplements.

Beneficial cultures of bacteria and yeast in the form of probiotics are also extremely important to include in the treatment of yeast problems, especially the bifidus strain, which is particularly evident in conditions of candida overgrowth.

The ingestion of beneficial yeast cultures will support the formation of beneficial yeast colonies in the intestines, which will help combat *Candida albicans*. This is facilitated by several beneficial yeast supplements, live kefir culture, and fermented food sources, such as healthy sauerkraut. Sources for these foods and beneficial yeast supplements are listed in appendix A.

Self-test to evaluate the need for cellulose treatment, herbal remedies, and antifungal preparations. Practice the self-test on a regular basis.

Parasites

We think of parasites as a Third World problem, but they exist right here in the U.S., causing significant health problems throughout our population. Many experts in the field estimate that 70 percent of the population has some form of intestinal parasite, while other experts insist that the number is closer to 100 percent. In any case, the possibility of having parasites is significant; if you have a pet around the house, the odds are definitely not in your favor. Children are very likely to have parasites because they tend to put everything in their mouths. Raw fish is also very likely to contain some form of parasite.

I find that the presence of parasites in the intestines is a real threat to our general health and significantly reduces the effectiveness of our immune system. Parasites reside in the intestines, along with detrimental bacteria and yeasts, and further disrupt the internal ecology of your intestines. Parasites can create serious health problems by stealing your nutrients, creating vitamin deficiencies, and damaging the walls of your intestines. Parasites come in a wide variety, ranging from simple pin worms to serious forms of amoebas, which can be life-threatening.

Parasite Testing

Most labs test for parasites. Unfortunately, most of them don't usually find much, as it is not their primary area of interest. Natural health providers that are effective in testing for parasites are listed in appendix A. A good lab can determine which parasites are present and can even recommend an effective natural remedy. Whenever chronic health problems persist, a stool analysis is a highly recommended course of action. The downside of these tests is that they are fairly expensive.

If you have traveled to a developing country and are experiencing chronic health problems, you may want to test for amoebas in a reportable laboratory. If amoebas are present, you will need to take stronger pharmaceutical measures to get rid of them, and deal with the side effects later. See your medical doctor, as amoebas can be deadly.

Some signs and symptoms of parasites taking up shop in your intestines are diarrhea, constipation, abdominal pain, intestinal gas, intestinal cramps, foul-smelling stools, blood or mucus in stools, weight loss, excessive appetite, fatigue, recurring fevers, allergies, chronic hair loss, and chronic itching in the nose or anus.

Bacterial parasites can also be contracted by drinking unsafe water in mountain streams, spoiled wells, or drinking water that has come in contact with sewage.

Parasitic problems can be difficult to treat, because every few weeks parasites produce offspring (eggs), which also need to be treated. Treatment requires a persistent effort and one that matches the right remedy to the right person. This can be successfully determined through the use of the self-test. A chiropractor or natural health practitioner trained in the art of muscle testing can also determine the correct remedy and the right course of treatment.

As is the case in the treatment of yeast and fungus, parasites feed themselves on sugar and refined carbohydrates. Avoiding these substances during treatment and reducing their intake thereafter will produce much better results. Parasites can be contracted when one is in close contact with other people or pets infested with parasites. All people and involved pets should be treated on an annual or biannual basis.

Traditional medical treatment for parasites is highly toxic to the body as well as to the parasites, and should only be used for amoebas or other life-threatening parasites. Although these treatments may be necessary, it can take many months for your body to recover from the effects, which can be supported by natural remedies.

HEALTH TIP #8: Natural Methods of Treatment for Parasites

This safe and effective treatment consists of four to six weeks of using an antiparasite remedy, followed by a two week break, followed by two more weeks of treatment. Natural antiparasite remedies include the following:

- Herbal remedies include raw garlic for the brave of heart, tinctures of black walnut hulls, wormwood, artemisia, quassia bark, or cloves.
- Vitamin preparations include several combination remedies are listed in appendix A, along with a detailed protocol.
- Whole foods remedies include Morinda supreme.
- General nutritional support during treatment includes beneficial bacteria; aloe vera gel, which helps to heal the walls of intestines; and vitamins A and C, for healing and nutritional preparations to balance the intestinal environment. See appendix A for more product details.

Toxic Chemicals

Make no mistake about it: we are all immersed in an sea of toxic chemicals. These toxic chemicals are placed in our soil, our water, our beverages, the processed foods we eat, and are expelled into the polluted air that we breathe. Toxic chemicals come in the form of pesticides, herbicides, toxic cleaning agents, solvents of all kinds, additives in foods and drinks, and a host of environmental poisons too numerous to mention.

Toxic chemicals present a real problem to the body, and one that is not easily remedied. We can learn to avoid some of these chemicals, but others are so deeply embedded in our environment that it is nearly impossible to avoid them. We must change the things that we can change, and try to neutralize the things we cannot.

Toxic chemicals in our food and water are perhaps the most significant problems, and may be the ones most easily rectified. Most of the water we drink and use contains two very toxic chemical waste products, chlorine and fluoride. We are told that these chemicals are fit for human consumption and do not cause any health problems, but this is far from the truth. In my experience and the experience of countless other health professionals, eliminating these two toxic chemicals from your water should be your top priority. If you are currently utilizing a city water supply in either your home or workplace that contains these very toxic chemicals, it is time for a change. These harmful chemicals can easily be filtered out of your drinking water, shower, and bath water. See appendix A for a list of suitable water-filtering products.

Purchase spring water to drink if filtering is not possible, or drink water treated by reverse osmosis. Reverse osmosis water is chemically dead, so mineral supplements must be added. Because we absorb most of our chlorine in our shower or bath, it is important to use a shower or bath filter as well. Chlorine is easily absorbed by the body when showering, bathing, and wearing clothes washed in chlorinated water. I see many patients with allergic reactions, skin irritations, and general toxicity problems that are completely resolved by removing these toxic chemicals from their water supply.

Processed food also contains a significant amount of toxic chemicals. Processing our food involves fragmenting a whole food, preserving it with chemicals so that it lasts longer on the shelf, and coloring it with toxic additives to make it more appealing. Real food doesn't last for six months on a shelf without spoiling. If a food item does last that long, either something very vital is missing, or something very toxic has been added. With processed foods, it is usually a significant amount of both.

Unfortunately, as far as our supermarket food is concerned, chemical additives are commonplace. Switch to whole foods or organically produced foods and beverages whenever possible.

Dairy Products

Whole milk straight from a cow, like our parents and grandparents used to drink, is actually a wonderful food. Today, that kind of milk is actually illegal. The milk that you see most often in grocery store has been drastically altered. It has been homogenized, pasteurized, and pumped full of artificial vitamins and minerals in a feeble attempt to replace the natural ones that have been destroyed. Toxic chemicals are added so that it lasts far longer on the shelves than it should. As a matter of fact, we have altered milk so much that it doesn't really spoil anymore; it rots. Cows are given toxic chemicals in the form of antibiotics, pesticides, hormones, and other drugs, which are passed on to us through their milk.

One of the magical things about whole foods is that they normally contain all the essential enzymes and hidden elements that assist the body to digest and utilize them. Real whole milk—the illegal kind—contains a wide variety of enzymes, valuable fat-soluble vitamins, essential minerals, and beneficial bacteria that are, for the most part, destroyed in the superheated pasteurizing process. Pasteurization also creates a breeding ground for the wrong kind of bacteria. Many of the allergy patients that I see in my practice have reactions to the type of milk widely available today. Many of us are allergic not only to milk but to dairy products in general, including pasteurized cheese, yogurt, cream, and half-and-half. Most of us would do well to stay away from dairy products altogether. If fresh goat's milk is available in your area, by all means feel free to use it. Goats are nearer our size than a two-thousand-pound cow, so the nutrients in their milk are much better for us. Besides, the milk is homogenized by nature.

Air Pollution

Another source of toxic chemicals is air pollution. If you live and breathe in a particularly toxic place, air pollution can be a huge factor in weakening your lungs and your immune system. If you live in a big city with big air pollution, you won't be able to influence much except in your own home. The air inside your home doesn't have to be polluted. Air filters, ozonators, and ionizers are readily available to make the air you breathe at home more conducive to health. Sources for several air filtration products are listed in appendix A. If the quality of the air you breathe is poor, filter it in your home and, if possible, in your workplace.

Toxic chemicals in the workplace are a real hazard. These toxic chemicals and hydrocarbons can take a significant toll on your body. When necessary, use a filtration mask whenever possible. The body will put up with working in a toxic environment for only so long, and eventually reaches a point of saturation when it will be unable to process any more toxic chemicals without significant side effects. At that point, the body will begin to develop some kind of chronic disease process. If you have to work around these toxic chemicals, check to see that your workplace is properly ventilated. Stay ahead of the game and try to work your way into a less toxic job if possible.

Drugs

Another source of chemical toxicity is drugs. Whether recreational, over the counter, or prescribed, drugs are toxic chemicals. Drugs may contribute a beneficial action somewhere in the body, but they always contain toxic elements that negatively effect the body somewhere else. In the body, drugs always have side effects. According to the *Journal of the American Medical Association,* hardly a radical rag, every year there are over two million drug reactions that cause approximately 100,000 deaths. This makes deaths from prescription drugs the fourth leading cause of death in the United States.

If you need to use drugs, ask your doctor to prescribe as low a dose as possible, and make sure your physician knows all of the other medications you are taking. When a person has more than one doctor and is taking several prescribed medications, no one physician is really monitoring all the prescriptions. Some patients in my practice are taking a half dozen or more medications. In my experience, taking this many toxic chemicals on a long-term basis is a recipe for disaster.

If you are consistently exposed to toxic chemicals, don't wait until it is too late to do anything about it. Be proactive now.

Eating and drinking organic whole foods will provide your body with antioxidants and other healthful substances, which in turn will help protect your body from the effects of a toxic chemical environment. Having pure water to drink and bathe in, and clean air to breathe, will give your body the best possible chance of processing these chemicals.

Environmental toxins are part of a large global problem with immense ramifications. All we can do about it as individuals (besides political action) is to control the environment of your own home. This includes monitoring the kind of products that you purchase, including paints, carpet, furniture, wood products, and cleaning products. Any and all of these chemical toxins disrupt the biochemical balance and function of your body, especially in your immune system. The subject of environmental toxins is vast and requires some sleuthing on your own. There are many books on the subject, a few of which are included in the bibliography. I know this all sounds daunting, and I encourage you to be creative in protecting yourself and your family from the side effects of toxic chemicals, and in creating a healthy environment both at home and at work.

Environmental Toxins

Environmental toxins create free radicals that cause tissue damage and aging. This damage results from burning up oxygen in the body in a process called oxidation. Antioxidants are substances that combat the ill effects of oxidation and reduce the amount of free radical damage to your cells.

Free radical damage can be offset by a variety of nutritional substances, the best of which are phytonutrients found in whole fruits and vegetables. For most of us, a whole foods diet containing six vegetables, two fruits, one starch, and one protein each day will provide a sufficient amount of antioxidants. For those with extra stress, whether mental, emotional, structural, or chemical, antioxidant supplementation is highly recommended.

HEALTH TIP #9: Antioxidants and Phytonutrients That Help Balance Toxic Chemicals

- Whole foods like broccoli and kale contain the largest amount of natural phytonutrients and are effective antioxidants. Whole food phytonutrient products are also available from several sources listed in appendix A.
- Herbal antioxidants include green tea, turmeric, ginkgo, licorice root, ginseng, ginger, rosemary, thyme, milk thistle, pycnogenol, grape seed extract, and spirulina.
- Other antioxidants include vitamins E and C, essential fatty acids, L-carnitine, glutathione, CoQ10 , beta-carotene, alpha-lipoic acid, selenium, copper, manganese, and zinc. Sources for all antioxidants are discussed in appendix A.
- Eating a whole foods diet low in refined carbohydrates and high in essential oils, raw fruits and vegetables provides an abundance of antioxidant protection against a variety of environmental toxins.
- Exercise is also an essential component in combating free radical damage and reducing chemical stress in the body. Exercise increases the efficiency of the body's metabolism and allows our eliminative processes to work more efficiently.
- Dry skin brushing, dry and infrared saunas, and steam showers (with nonchlorinated water) are all excellent ways to reduce and eliminate toxic chemicals from the body. The cleansing diets in chapter 7 are also a big help.

Toxic Metals

Toxic metals poisoning is also becoming a serious health threat and can be the underlying cause of a multitude of metabolic disorders. Toxic metals also seem to be a major contributor to the current surge of autoimmune diseases.

Whether we know it or not, toxic or heavy metals are commonplace in our lives. They are in our environment, in our foods and drinks, in our homes, in our air and water, in our workplaces, even in our mouths. Although some of these metals are important to the function of the body, most of them cause serious health problems.

Iron, for example, is an essential component of our blood, and it is a mineral we need to consume on a regular basis. Problems arise when we consume large amounts of inorganic iron.

Nails, for instance, are made of iron, and are great for building a house, but that type of inorganic iron doesn't go far in building a healthy body. As a matter of fact, one of the major causes of iron poisoning these days is inorganic iron nutritional supplements. The iron that is added to synthetic vitamins, and so-called fortified cereals and foods, is for the most part inabsorbable.

According to the National Center for Disease Control and Prevention, no amount of lead ingestion is safe for the body, as lead has an affinity for the gray matter and goes straight to the brain. Lead poisoning effects some three million children and is still considered the number one threat to children's health. Many children's toys still contain lead; it seems that we will sell anything if we can get away with it. The symptoms of lead poisoning include a host of brain and nerve system diseases, a reduction in intelligence, memory loss, and deteriorated thinking that ultimately leads to dementia.

At the turn of the nineteenth century, British workers in the hat industry used quicksilver (mercury) in the process of making hats. After years of direct contact with this extremely toxic heavy metal, the entire industry experienced symptoms of mental deterioration. The expression "mad as a hatter" comes from the fact that direct exposure to toxic levels of mercury causes mental illness. This madness was also true for mirror makers and goldsmiths who were exposed to mercury on a regular basis.

Dentists and their assistants also handle mercury, which may account for the fact that dentists have the highest suicide and divorce rate of any profession. Even though the American Dental Association refuses to acknowledge or talk about it, toxic metal poisoning caused by amalgam tooth fillings containing mercury continues to be a very real threat to a healthy immune system.

Dental Fillings

In my clinical experience, I have found that dental amalgam fillings, and immunizations, which both contain mercury, are serious threats to our physical and mental well-being. These two common health procedures may also be part of the cause of the vastly increased levels of autoimmune disease and learning disabilities in our children today.

This is an area that is still very controversial, and many dentists and health care providers are still skeptics. Check out the research books in the bibliography, or look for yourself on the Internet. After you have done some reading on your own, tell your dentist what you want. If you run into a wall or your dentist tells you there is no real research that proves this to be true, seek out a holistic dentist for another opinion. Holistic dentists are very much aware of toxic metal problems and their solutions.

I usually recommend plastic composite dental fillings, lava, or Bell glass for my patients, all of which are much less toxic to the body. Many dentists use gold fillings, but gold can also have a toxic effect on the body.

You'll have to educate yourself. Many toxic metals in dentistry are hidden behind familiar and unfamiliar names. Porcelain, for example, is over 50 percent aluminum. Other toxic metals used in dentistry include mercury, silver, titanium, gold, copper, chromium, barium, and disguised aluminum.

A good holistic dentist will be able to advise you properly. Chiropractors who utilize the art of applied kinesiology can also evaluate and identify the problem.

A few words of caution: Removing mercury amalgam fillings is not without its own repercussions. Many autoimmune diseases begin or are greatly accelerated by removing amalgam fillings incorrectly. Before attempting to remove the mercury in your mouth, be sure your dentist uses a dam and is trained in healthy amalgam removal procedures. Allow several months, or even a year, to complete the process, as the body needs time to recuperate. Take your time, read the books, check the research, and find a health care practitioner who can evaluate if mercury is a real problem for you, and if so, which teeth are priorities.

Aluminum

There are many toxic metals, but aluminum is the metal of greatest concern.

Scientific research demonstrates that the more aluminum we ingest, the greater the cell damage in the brain. Diseases such as Alzheimer's, dementia, ALS or Lou Gehrig's disease, Down's Syndrome, and other brain and central nerve system–related diseases seem to be significantly connected to aluminum toxicity. Research in the United Kingdom indicates a correlation between Alzheimer's disease and aluminum in drinking water. The Brits found a 50 percent increase in Alzheimer's in areas where aluminum concentrations in drinking water were high, and the evidence continues to mount between the connection of toxic aluminum and dementia.

Recent research has also shown that using aluminum cookware with the toxic chemical fluoride, the toxic metal regularly added to our drinking water, increases the amount of aluminum that leaches out of our cookware and into our food.

Cow's milk also contains high levels of aluminum. This seems to be especially true of milk formulas for infants, those derived from both cow milk and soy milk. Goat's milk, on the other hand, does not contain aluminum. You will find a goat's milk formula for infants in chapter 9, appendix B. I have used this formula in my practice (and with my own children) for over twenty-five years. It is simple, safe, and extremely effective.

Cadmium toxicity is also significant in our environment. It has no known nutritional value, accumulates in the kidneys, and contributes to high blood pressure, heart problems, liver damage, kidney disease, anemia, brain and bone disorders, and chronic fatigue. Eating refined foods such as white flour, white rice, and white sugar also increases the risk of cadmium toxicity, as the mineral zinc, which helps to balance cadmium intake in the body, is absent in refined foods.

The hazards of toxic heavy metal poisoning are very real in our society today. Heavy metals have worked their way into our kitchens and our homes. For anyone interested in maintaining their health, ignoring toxic metal poisoning is no longer an option.

Find out which toxic metals you and your family are living with on a daily basis, and discover a healthy way to eliminate them.

Sources of Toxic Metal Poisoning

Aluminum: Cookware, antacids, antiperspirants, tea, aluminum cans, aluminum foil, milk, drinking water, kitchen utensils, paints, and dental composites.

Arsenic: Poisons, pigments, dyes, wood preservatives, insecticides, wine, well water, burning coal, seafood (shellfish), and treated lumber.

Barium: Explosives, filler in paper, paints and plastics, radiology (contrast studies), and dental composites.

Cadmium: Water from galvanized pipes, softened water, coffee, evaporated milk, shellfish, cigarette smoke, sewage sludge, paint, black rubber pigments, and air pollution.

Chromium: Dyes, pigments, air pollution, and dental crowns.

Copper: Copper plumbing, sewage sludge, beer, swimming pools, copper cookware, inorganic mineral supplements, and dental crowns.

Gold: Dental fillings, jewelry, and injections for arthritis.

Iron: Dyes, inks, paints, pigments, well water, and poor inorganic mineral supplements added to our foods.

Lead: Car exhaust, paint, plumbing, canned food, hair dyes, newsprint, and tap water.

Manganese: Ceramics, antiseptics, dyes, medicines, steel products, air pollution, and water supply.

Mercury: Dental fillings, immunizations, mercury vapor lamps, seafood, polluted water, skin-lightening creams, and sewage sludge.

Nickel: Cigarettes and dental crowns.

Silver: Dental fillings and jewelry.

Tin: Canned foods.

Titanium: Pigments in paints, preservatives in medications, tap and well water, dental crowns and implants.

Zinc: Poor, inorganic supplements in foods.

HEALTH TIP #10: Eliminate Toxic Metals

General nutritional support for the elimination of toxic metals: Spirulina, cilantro, Brussels sprouts, cabbage, kale, filtered water, and sunshine. Ascorbic acid and organic trace minerals are also helpful. Sources for toxic metal-related nutrients are found in appendix A.

Heavy metal detoxifiers: Detoxifiers for specific heavy metals can be tested by a chiropractor trained in applied kinesiology, a holistic laboratory such as Genova Diagnostics (formally Great Smokies Lab), and through hair-analysis testing, which also indicates your levels of toxic metal poisoning. Care must be taken with heavy metal removal, and it is best that these procedures be done under the guidance and direction of a qualified chiropractor, naturopath, or other health care practitioner.

Allergies

Even though allergies are not a specific agent of disease, allergic reactions often occur in response to them and effect some fifty million Americans as a result. It is interesting to note that a weakened immune system, which is the underlying cause of allergies, is further weakened by allergic reactions.

In any allergic reaction, the level of physical, mental, emotional, and thermal stress experienced by the allergy sufferer is an important part of the problem, as stress brings out whatever weaknesses are already present in the body. It is important to recognize and strengthen these underlying weaknesses before they lead to major problems.

As with any health problem, to be successful in treating allergies one must correct the underlying cause. Maintaining this perspective can be difficult, as getting instant relief is so satisfying.

Treating allergy symptoms with medication gives temporary relief at best, and in most cases contributes to a further weakening of the involved tissues, setting you up for even more severe allergic reactions and long-term immune system decline.

For example, nasal sprays may give temporary relief to stuffy nose and congestion, but they often irritate and weaken the mucous membranes of the nasal pharynx, creating a more serious problem for the body to handle.

Steroids also give temporary relief to allergy sufferers but create additional weakness in the endocrine system, especially for the already exhausted adrenal glands. There are several different types of allergies, all of which point to a weakened immune system as their cause. Allergic reactions can be caused by toxic chemicals, toxic metals, airborne and environmental substances that we breathe, drugs (which comprise 20 percent of all allergic reactions), and foods.

While the focus of this section has been on toxic metals, it is just as important to understand the underlying weakness causing any of these other types of allergies as well. When the underlying cause is corrected, the Intelligence of our body will, as a rule, correct the symptoms at the same time.

Food Allergies

Food sensitivities or allergies are usually caused by repeatedly eating the same foods or types of foods for long periods of time. If you suspect that you suffer from a food allergy (if you experience a lot of gastrointestinal distress or skin conditions), try to find a chiropractor or applied kinesiologist who can help you determine the possible trigger foods. This can be done through muscle or blood tests, or through the pulse test.

The following foods are worth testing: bread (wheat), milk, cheese, orange juice, two tablespoons of sugar in water, eggs, potatoes, corn, black coffee, raw vegetables and fruits, chocolate, dried fruits, and soy milk. You may even want to evaluate your toothpaste. Pay particular attention to testing the foods that you crave or eat often.

As a culture, we especially eat too many wheat and dairy products, which are usually at the top of the problematic foods list. If you begin to rotate other grains in your diet, wheat usually becomes less of a problem. Try substituting rye, oats, buckwheat, barley, millet, quinoa, and spelt. Dairy products, on the other hand, are a more serious problem for many individuals, and for several good reasons. The way that cows are raised, injected, and fed—and the way that milk is processed—make dairy products difficult for the body to handle. If you absolutely need to have dairy, limited amounts of organic raw milk and their products, as well as fresh goat's milk, may not cause a reaction.

Other foods that are likely to trigger allergic reactions include coffee, alcohol, soft drinks, chocolate, any type of sugar, tobacco, grains, spices, lunch meats, corn, and plants in the nightshade family such as eggplants, tomatoes, green peppers, and spinach.

If you suspect certain trigger substances, try avoiding them for a three-week period while you build your immune system. You can build immune system strength by supplementing with any of the immune system builders listed in appendix A. Whenever possible use the self-test to determine the most beneficial nutritional supplements.

When the cause is located and corrected, you can slowly reintroduce any suspected trigger foods one at a time, carefully observing the feedback that your body is giving you. Avoiding these foods give your immune system a break from the constant allergic reactions. This alone will allow the immune system to strengthen.

If further reactions or any other symptoms do occur immediately after eating, such as a stuffy or runny nose, congestion, coughing, gas, signs of digestive discomfort, or fogginess, discontinue the food for a longer period of time.

After a three-week period of avoidance, a trigger food can usually be eaten on a rotational basis. This involves eating small amounts of the suspected food every four or five days. If on the fifth day that food still triggers a reaction, eliminate it from your diet.

HEALTH TIP #11: The Pulse Test

A good method for determining reactions to the foods we eat and drink is the Coca pulse test. As its name suggests, the pulse test uses your pulse rate as a barometer. This is yet another way of becoming aware of what the Intelligence of your body is trying to tell you.

The pulse test looks at your pulse rate before and after meals as an indicator of problem foods. You are looking to identify foods that elevate or diminish your pulse rates. It is important to refrain from smoking during this time, as smoking cigarettes interferes with the results.

1. Count your pulse for one full minute first thing in the morning before getting out of bed. Write down your result. This provides a baseline for your normal pulse rate.

2. Count your pulse rate for one minute just before you eat. Record your result.

3. Record everything you eat at that meal.

4. Check your pulse again three times after each meal at half-hour intervals, and then once at bedtime. Always record your results.

5. Notice whether your pulse rate changes significantly from normal, think about what you ate, and see if you can identify the trigger food.

The next step is to perform single food testing.

1. For two days, consume small amounts of different (single) foods every hour. Check your pulses before and after the meal.

2. Notice any change in your pulse rate, or if patterns are emerging with certain food groups, such as grains, dairy, nightshades (eggplant, tomatoes, green peppers, potatoes), sugar, alcohol, or refined carbohydrates. Any foods that elevate or diminish your pulse should be avoided.

You can use the pulse test to determine if the reactive foods can be eaten on a rotational basis (every five days). If not, eliminate the food from your diet. Retest the food in a few months. Keep tabs on any questionable foods by evaluating that food whenever it is eaten.

Other substances that can cause allergic reactions and can be tested by checking your pulse include dust from your bed, perfume, cleaning agents, or even newspaper print. Perform a sniff test to evaluate these substances. Take your pulse before and after exposure. If dust from your bed is the problem, your pulse will be elevated in the morning but most likely not before bed. Dust mites can also be a real problem. See appendix A for more information.

Health Problems Caused by the Agents of Disease

- Dysbiosis is an abnormal intestinal environment that breeds disease-causing bacteria.
- Leaky gut syndrome occurs when substances such as yeasts, bacteria, toxins, and proteins, which are normally contained by the membranes of the intestines, are allowed to pass through the intestinal barrier, past the body's defenses, and deeper into the circulation.

- Irritable bowel syndrome occurs when the intestines are so inflamed that elimination and absorption are adversely effected.

- Autoimmune diseases are a relatively new category of illness in which the immune system begins to attack the body.

- Chronic fatigue syndrome, irritable bowel syndrome, malabsorption syndrome, arthritis, asthma, eczema, psoriasis, and colitis are some pertinent disease conditions that are the result of biochemical imbalances caused by a weakened immune system, aggravated by multidimensional stress, and initiated by the agents of disease. All of these relatively new disease conditions have a strong emotional component.

HEALTH TIP #12: For Allergies
General Nutritional Support

Natural antioxidants and phytonutrients help the body to process free radical activity that destroys the body's cells and tissues. Antioxidants and phytonutrients are also major factors for anti-aging.

A natural antihistamine, Antronex, provides symptomatic relief while you are getting to the cause of your problem.

A natural whole food multiple vitamin and mineral supplement is also of value in supporting overall nutritional needs. Use low-potency, whole food sources of B-complex vitamins, especially pantothenic acid; vitamin complexes A, C, and F, which are extremely supportive to the immune system; antioxidants, such as vitamin E and C; ascorbic acid; EFAs; L-carnitine, glutathione, and CoQ10; beta-carotene; alpha-lipoic acid; and whole food source minerals selenium, copper, manganese, and zinc.

Synthetic supplements do not begin to support the body as well as natural ones. See appendix A for sources of natural whole food supplements.

Herbal antioxidants include green or white tea, milk thistle, pycnogenol, and spirulina. Herbal allergy remedies also provide general support for the immune system. These include echinacea, burdock, astragalus, aloe vera, mushroom formulas, and goldenseal. Pay particular attention that you are not just treating symptoms with herbs or nutritional products, but are getting to the underlying cause of your problem. You'll want to locate the source of toxicity to your body, strengthen your immune system, and cleanse your digestive system (see chapter 7 for cleansing guidelines).

Digestive enzymes including HCl (hydrochloric acid) should be used if digestive or elimination problems persist. Achlorhydria is a common condition caused by a lack of hydrochloric acid and lies at the root of many digestive problems. This is especially true as we age and for conditions related to hiatal hernia and reflux disease.

If constipation persists, additional amounts of pure water and fiber may be beneficial. The addition of eliminative herbs such as cascara sagrada, buckthorn bark tea, or psyllium is recommended. Senna tea is not recommended.

Eating a whole foods diet that is low in refined carbohydrates and high in essential oils, fruits, and vegetables is always a great way to improve the efficiency of your body. Green leafy vegetables, apples, celery, garlic, and onions help to purify the blood and detoxify the body.

The beneficial bacteria discussed earlier in this chapter are also important.

Essential fats and oils (EFAs) should be an integral part of everyone's fundamental nutrition. Using unheated extra virgin olive oil or flaxseed oil daily on salad or steamed vegetables, and a few capsules of fish oil each day, is an excellent way to assure the proper balance of essential fatty acids in the diet.

Generous amounts of pure spring, filtered, or purified water is also an essential nutrient, and perhaps one of the most important factors in improving both the elimination of toxins and reducing the effect of allergic reactions.

Exercise is another essential component in combating allergic reactions and free radical damage in the body. Exercise helps in reducing physical, mental, and emotional stress in the body, and increases the efficiency of the body's metabolism. See chapters 3 and 4 for recommended exercises.

Dry skin brushing, dry and infrared saunas, and steam showers are excellent ways to reduce allergic responses in the body and to improve elimination routes.

Conclusion

Our immune system is sensitive to foreign invaders of all kinds, and it works relentlessly to keep us healthy, even in our toxic world. As researchers have been discovering for the best part of a decade, our immune systems are especially sensitive to emotions and feelings, and are responsive to the tonal frequencies that we express in our daily lives.

Simply stated, when we express positive thoughts and feelings, our immunity becomes stronger. When we embrace and express negative thoughts and emotions, our immunity becomes depressed. Expressing negative thoughts and emotions specifically shows up in the immune system as a decrease in the overall number of white blood cells, especially phagocytes such as the macrophage. When our immune system becomes depleted, our ability to resist disease also becomes diminished, and virtually any agent of disease can penetrate our weakened defense system.

On the other hand, expressing positive thoughts and feelings directly increases our army of white blood cells.

We have been taught that germs cause disease in the form of bacteria and virus, but nothing could be further from the truth. If we catch the flu, for example, it is not because the current version of the flu bug broke down the door to our immune system. Rather, it is because our weakened immune system left the door open to the flu bug. Build the health of your immune system, and the flu bug doesn't stand a chance of getting through your defenses. Wear down your immune system by stressing yourself physically, mentally, or emotionally, and there will be a waiting line of foreign invaders at the door.

Our current medical practices have challenged bacteria and virus to mutate into stronger and more virulent forms. In response, we need to use all the resources at our fingertips to actively build super immunity. Building immunity in our toxic world requires maintaining structural alignment, nutritional and biochemical balance, a positive mental attitude, an open heart, and the willingness to create a clear connection to Spirit. Ultimately, the best medicine for building health in our immune system is to remember that human beings are also a part of nature, and that we have the ability to express and receive the awesome healing power of love.

Chapter 10

Respiration and Circulation

RESPIRATION AND CIRCULATION are diverse functions in the body that are both energetically centered by the thymus gland. You'll recall that the thymus gland is linked to the immune system, but it is also at the core of the respiratory and circulatory systems. In fact, the health of these two systems depends on the health of the emotionally sensitive thymus gland.

Respiration and circulation also share a similar connection to the endocrine and nerve system, and share the same purpose of bringing the magical nutrient oxygen, which represents the invisible breath of life, to each of the body's 100 quadrillion cells.

The respiratory system gathers oxygen gas from the air and transfers it to the circulatory system for distribution. The circulatory system pumps oxygen, along with other nutrients in the blood, to the far reaches of the body, and brings back a host of waste products for the body to eliminate.

Many of these waste products are eliminated not through the urine and feces, but by two of the largest organs of elimination, the skin and the lungs. Essentially, human beings eliminate carbon dioxide gas from their lungs into an external environment that contains trees and other green plants. Trees and green plants recycle this toxic CO_2 gas, transforming it back into oxygen to be used as the life breath for all living animals.

Living animals exhale CO_2 gas and breathe in oxygen, while green plants and trees breathe in CO_2 gas and exhale oxygen. This symbiotic relationship that human beings share with trees and green plants is an integral part of our respiration. If the health of trees and green plants becomes jeopardized, so does a major source of oxygen. If our air becomes too polluted it will directly effect our ability to carry oxygen to our cells, which has huge implications on our overall health. As an integral part of our respiration, we must take better care of our external environment.

Respiration also occurs on the cellular level, which means that we are what we assimilate. For instance, if we are able to bring in oxygen and other nutrients to the cell, and move CO_2 and other waste products out, our chances of experiencing vibrant health are vastly improved. If we are not efficient in this process, we will begin to experience dis-ease. The principle of wholeness reflects the understanding that the health of the whole body is represented by the health of the tiny cell.

Another important aspect of respiration is reflected in the very word itself. Whenever we inhale, we breathe in *(in)* the invisible essence of spirit *(spire);* when we exhale, we give back *(ex)* the essence of ourselves. At the very core of our breathing lies our direct physical connection to the invisible realm of Spirit. You might like to spend a few moments thinking about that as you become more conscious of your breathing.

In this chapter we will look at the interdependent nature of respiration and circulation, and I will show you how you can maintain your multidimensional health and well-being in relation to these two vital systems.

The Respiratory System

The lungs are the primary organ of respiration, but the respiratory system also includes the nose, the nasal sinuses, the pharynx, larynx, trachea, bronchial tubes, and the thoracic cavity. The proper function of these ancillary organs is absolutely essential for the lungs to do their job.

The nose, for example, filters, cleans, and warms the air for the lungs. Those persistent nose hairs have an important function. If your nose is constantly stuffed up, the filtering and warming process of respiration is bypassed, and dirt and debris from the air is allowed to pass directly into your lung tissue.

A baby's lungs are perfectly pink, while the lungs of adults tend to be blue in color from a lack of oxygen. The lungs of a smoker are dressed in black.

The four nasal sinuses are paired, air-filled cavities, lined with mucous membranes and located within several bones in the front of our skull. These membranes moisten the air and gather dirt and debris. Sinuses are also designed to lighten the weight of the skull and provide a resonant chamber for the sound of our voices.

Unfortunately, sinus infections are fairly common today, especially in our polluted environment. Chronic sinus infection can be dangerous if allowed to persist, and can seriously effect our vision. Sinus problems can be caused by polluted air, allergic reactions to food, an overwhelming toxic load in the body, and the misalignment of the cranial bones and/or the upper cervical vertebrae. If you are plagued by recurring sinus problems, try the Sinus Drainage Technique included in appendix B. This technique has been used successfully for centuries.

The pharynx, a Greek word for the throat, is a structure that contains passageways for both respiration and digestion, and it contains seven openings that connect our nose, mouth, Eustachian tubes in our ears, voice box, and esophagus. The pharynx begins at the base of the skull and extends to the level of the sixth cervical vertebrae, where it turns into the esophagus. The throat contains a significant number of lymphatic structures that act as the first line of defense for our immune system, and it is an important vocal structure in the formation of sound.

The voice box is a passageway for air that helps us change pure sound into recognizable words. Nine different cartilages allow our vocal cords to open and close in just the right way to produce the wide variety of human sounds for language and expression.

It seems that our Inner Intelligence has put a lot of effort into creating this intricate design in order to give us the ability to express ourselves vocally. Singing, for example, is a powerful form of expression that helps us integrate the functions of our right and left brains. Singing allows us to harmonize our brain while we express our feelings.

The windpipe is the passageway that allows air to move in and out of the lungs. If the epiglottis—the flap of tissue that covers

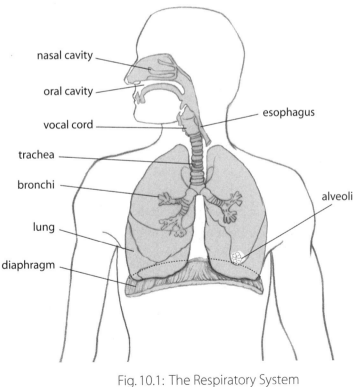

Fig. 10.1: The Respiratory System

our airway when we eat—fails to block the airway, the windpipe can become blocked with food. The Heimlich maneuver forces air through the windpipe by squeezing the chest and lungs. This maneuver is usually quite successful in clearing a blocked airway and can send blocked food sailing across the room.

After six inches or so, the windpipe divides into two branches called bronchi, each of which connect to a lung. The bronchi form a tree-like structure inside our lungs, and allow air to pass in and out of our lung tissue. Bronchitis occurs when these tree-like structures become inflamed or congested. The bronchi terminate into small air sacks called alveoli that look like bunches of grapes on the branches of our tree. A tree of life is present at the core of our body, and resides at the center of our lungs.

The alveoli are composed of elastic tissue and have the ability to expand to many times their original size. They are the site in which oxygen and CO_2 gas are exchanged. Each day the alveoli process some 5,000 gallons of air as they expand and contract over 26,000 times.

The Mechanics of Breathing

Understanding the mechanics of breathing will help you to visualize the correct way to breathe, which allows the maximum amount of oxygen to get to your alveoli. The more oxygen gets to your alveoli, the more oxygen gets to your cells.

The inhalation phase of breathing is only possible due to the difference in pressure inside of our lungs and the atmospheric pressure outside them. A variety of conditions must exist in our external environment, extending for miles into space, to set up just the right conditions for us to breathe.

The inhalation phase of breathing is initiated by the involuntary contraction of the muscles of respiration. This process occurs naturally as the amount of air in our lungs decreases and the difference between the pressure in our lungs and the atmosphere increases. In other words, when we start to run out of air, we inhale automatically.

Inhalation is accomplished by contracting our diaphragm and the muscles between our ribs, which elongates our chest and increases its size and volume.

This change in volume decreases the pressure between the lungs and the chest wall, causing the lungs to expand automatically. This expansion creates a pressure difference between the alveoli of the lungs and the atmospheric pressure of the earth, which allows air, containing just the right amount of oxygen, to rush into our lungs.

Exhalation, on the other hand, demonstrates the exact opposite principle. As our diaphragm and rib muscles relax, the size and volume of our chest decreases, shrinking our lungs. The difference in pressure between the alveoli of our lungs and the atmospheric pressure of the earth forces air out.

Voluntary breathing is also possible in our respiratory system, as we can take a breath whenever we want. This happens when the respiratory centers—located at the base of the brain—are stimulated, and our diaphragm and rib muscles contract. If we wish to hold our breath, we activate the respiratory centers in the cerebral cortex, which gives us control of respiration up to point of putting our life in jeopardy. At that point, the Intelligence of the body takes over and we start breathing again. This same mechanism occurs when fear or emotion blocks our ability to breathe normally, and we pass out.

Other factors that influence our breathing include the levels of carbon dioxide, oxygen, and the pH present in our blood. If the CO_2 levels rise above a certain point in the blood, our respiration centers stimulate us to breathe faster. When CO_2 levels in the blood decrease, our Inner Intelligence slows our breathing down.

A low blood pH, which indicates excessive acidity in the body, triggers an increase in both the rate and depth of our breathing, which is a significant factor for all of us. The breathing techniques presented in this chapter can help your body become more alkaline by decreasing the level of toxins in the blood.

As most people know, hyperventilation occurs when too much oxygen is taken in at one time. Hyperventilation can be corrected by breathing into and out of a small paper bag. Why? Because the controlled breathing environment temporarily reduces the available amount of oxygen and returns your breathing to normal. As a rule, if oxygen levels are either too high or too low in the body, our Inner Intelligence automatically adjusts our breathing to make up for the difference. Our bodies are truly amazing.

The Natural Phenomena of Respiration
Coughing, Sneezing, Yawning, and Hiccupping

Several natural phenomena occur in the respiratory system to keep respiration on track. These include coughing, sneezing, yawning, and hiccupping.

Coughing is an essential mechanism used by the body to clear the airways of obstructions and foreign matter. Our entire respiratory system is extremely sensitive to foreign matter, toxic chemicals, and outside irritants. Whenever an irritant is present, we instinctively take a short breath of air; the epiglottis automatically closes; the vocal cords shut down, trapping air in the lungs; and our abdominal and intercostal muscles forcefully contract. This series of events dramatically increases the air pressure inside the lungs.

Suddenly, the vocal cords and epiglottis open wide, expelling the air at the phenomenal rate of nearly one hundred miles an hour, and usually taking most obstructions or irritants right along with it. The speed of air expelled from a cough rivals that of a hurricane.

If coughing is a regular companion in your life, try to evaluate the cause. Are toxic chemicals, smoke, polluted air, cleaning agents, or foods (such as dairy products or grains) clogging you up? Becoming aware of these factors in your environment may lead you straight to the problem. If you do cough a lot, it is usually a sign from your Inner Intelligence to change something that you are doing. You can locate the irritant through a process of elimination, and remove the irritant or habit from your lifestyle. If your cough persists, consult the appropriate member of your health team.

The purpose of the sneeze reflex is to eliminate foreign matter from the upper respiratory system. Sneezing is initiated by the nasal passages whenever irritants such as smoke, toxic chemicals, dust, pollen, or polluted air are present. Allergic reactions, triggered by food or drink, can also cause us to sneeze. I have a friend who sneezes endlessly immediately after eating a bowl of ice cream.

A similar sequence of events occurs during sneezing and coughing; with sneezing, however, the depression of the uvula occurs, enabling large amounts of air to quickly pass through the nasal passages in order to clear the irritant or foreign matter. In contrast to coughing, sneezing emits air speeds of only fifty to sixty miles per hour! If you sneeze on a regular basis, you would do well to evaluate the possible causes and make the appropriate changes in your lifestyle to remedy the situation.

Yawning is another respiratory phenomenon. Surprisingly enough, yawning improves respiration by ventilating the lungs more deeply. When a yawn occurs, it is usually in response to a drop in the oxygen level of circulating blood, which is frequently caused by alveoli that are not ventilating properly or that are closed off completely. Collapsed alveoli are opened again by the long, deep inspiration initiated by a yawn. Yawning also helps to clear our airways and move stagnant blood more effectively through our blood vessels.

Hiccups are a more mysterious respiratory phenomenon. We know very little about their purpose, though it is presumed that a hiccup is caused by substances in the blood or by local circulatory abnormalities, which cause a spastic contraction of the diaphragm. The vocal cords, which are normally open during inspiration, close during a hiccup. Hiccups can be caused by eating too quickly, consuming too much air with your food, a misalignment of the fourth cervical vertebra, or by abnormal function of the diaphragm, as in a hiatal hernia. The diaphragm, which is the divider between the upper and lower abdomen, is intimately associated with our emotions. If hiccups are a persistent problem for you, eat more slowly, chew your food, and make sure that you have a healthy atmosphere in which to eat your meals.

How Well Do You Breathe?

Now, let's take a look at the two types of respiratory breathing: costal breathing, the kind initiated by the ribs, and abdominal breathing, which is initiated by the diaphragm.

Costal breathing is the shallow breathing that results from the contraction of the muscles around and between the ribs, and associated muscles of the back and neck. Costal breathing moves the chest upward and outward, and is classically the type of breathing that is used by athletes at the end of a race.

Abdominal or diaphragmatic breathing, on the other hand, results from the contraction of the diaphragm and dramatically increases the breathing capacity of our lungs. When the dome-shaped diaphragm contracts, it descends, pushing out the lower abdomen. Abdominal breathing is deep and slow, and occurs naturally when we are asleep.

Both types of breathing are important parts of respiration and are designed to function together. When we are awake, most of us become costal breathers. Stop for a moment—don't change a thing—and check your breathing style. If you are breathing at all (you'd be surprised at how many of us tend to hold our breath), you are probably using a shallow, costal breath. As you continue to check your breath, evaluate the feeling tone associated with this type of breathing.

Now, sit up straight and allow your diaphragm to drop down with your next breath. This is easily accomplished by pushing your belly out, relaxing, and breathing in deeply. Breathe in the abdominal breath, and sense the feeling tone associated with that. What did you find?

Chances are you discovered that you are a costal breather. The trouble with shallow breathing is that it generally shuts down most of our feelings, resulting in a limited feeling experience.

Shutdown Feelings and Shutdown Breathing

I find that when we are isolated in our minds, we use the costal breath. When we are connected to our feelings, we use our diaphragms. This makes sense from a scientific standpoint because a large part of our feeling nerve system lies in our abdomen. When we utilize abdominal breathing, we activate our gut feelings.

These two types of breathing effect the efficiency of our oxygen and carbon dioxide exchange. If we are shallow costal breathers, we may get the oxygen down our windpipe or even into our bronchi, but we are usually not getting enough oxygen to the alveoli of our lungs.

Shallow breathing does not allow for fresh oxygen and CO_2 to effectively exchange in the lungs. It may push old air into the alveoli, but it isn't the air we just breathed in. Costal breathing also doesn't allow for a full expiration to take place, which leaves a large concentration of CO_2 in the lungs, directly effecting acid toxicity levels in the body. If you are a shallow, costal breather, it is time for a conscious change in breathing technique.

If you are not actively using the diaphragm in your breathing process, you may develop digestive problems associated with the presence of a hiatal hernia. As you will recall from chapter 8, the diaphragm is also intimately associated with the digestive system.

Learning how to use a combination of costal and abdominal breathing, as they were designed to be used, is of primary importance to your health. This integrated type of breathing is sometimes called the yogic breath.

HEALTH TIP #1: Integrated Breathing Technique

To begin this technique, you will first need to visualize what you are trying to accomplish. I find it useful to imagine an empty pitcher that I wish to fill with water. When filling the pitcher, the bottom fills first, then the middle, and finally the top. Costal breathing fills only the top portion of the lungs, while abdominal or diaphragmatic breathing fills the bottom and the middle as well. The same visualization can be used for exhalation, only in reverse order. First empty the top of your lungs, then the middle, and finally empty the bottom by contracting or sucking in your lower abdomen.

Now that you have the image of how you want to breathe, sit upright and comfortably in a chair, or in a cross-legged position on the floor. When practicing integrated breathing, it is best to have adequate back support to allow for complete relaxation to occur, which is the key to success.

Begin to integrate your breath on your next inhalation. Focus on pushing your abdomen down and out as you breathe, and allow the breath to rush in on its own. Keep filling the lower portion of the pitcher first. As the abdomen fills with air, you will automatically move on to fill the middle portion of the pitcher, which is in your upper abdomen. The final phase of the integrated breath engages your costal muscles and tops off the upper portion of the lungs with air.

Exhalation simply involves reversing the inhalation process. Remember that inhalation and exhalation are a continuous part of one whole breathing process: one phase moves directly into the other. Try not to hold your breath between the two cycles.

It is also important to remember that inspiration and expiration should be of equal lengths. This becomes especially evident as you slow down your expiration rate. A slow, controlled inspiration and expiration allows your mind to follow the breath much more easily, which naturally brings out both the meditative and relaxing features of the integrated breath.

Empty the top portion of the pitcher first by allowing your intercostal muscles to relax. Move down to the middle portion of your upper abdomen, and finally to the lower abdomen and diaphragm. The exhalation process is completed by pulling your lower abdomen in as you release your breath.

Integrated breathing is much easier to perform than it is to describe in words, as it is the natural way for us to breathe. Check in often with your breathing to get a sense of how well you are integrating this important process into your life. Your body will appreciate the changes, and your cells will appreciate the oxygen.

HEALTH TIP #2: Retention Breathing

After you become familiar with the Integrated Breath Exercise and want to learn more, you may add a retention breath to the very top of the inspiration cycle. In times of emotional upset, when stomach upset or hiatal hernia involvement is suspected, you may want to try retention breathing. You an also use this practice to increase lung capacity or to more deeply access the realm of Spirit before meditation. A retention breath is accomplished by holding the breath and pushing down slightly on the diaphragm with a full inspiration. When you reach a full inspiration, simply add three short, quick in-breaths to completely fill the lungs. Try to hold this expanded breath for ten seconds or more, and then release the breath slowly and steadily. If your air rushes out, you are holding your breath too long.

Use the retention breath after first completing three normal integrated breaths. This cycle of four breaths can be followed by two additional cycles of four breaths. Add one more retention breath at the end to complete the exercise.

HEALTH TIP #3: Improve Your Lung Capacity

You can also increase your lung capacity by using a respiratory spirometer. A spirometer is a device that measures the flow rates and volume of air inspired and expired by your lungs. This device not only measures vital capacity of the lungs, but it can be used to improve capacity as well. A spirometer is often given to patients in a hospital setting to evaluate and improve their lung function. Utilizing a bidirectional spirometer allows for improvement in both inspiration and expiration. Sources for spirometers are listed online, or a simple version can be purchased from a medical supplier.

Indications of respiratory system dysfunction include the following in figure 10.2.

Indications of Respiratory System Dysfunctions
Allergies, sinus infections, persistent coughing or sneezing, pain during respiration or a general decrease in lung capacity.

Fig. 10.2: Indications of Respiratory System Dysfunction

Pneumonia is a condition of bacterial infection in which the alveoli are partially filled with fluid and white blood cells. In pneumonia, the alveoli are inflamed and unable to oxygenate blood effectively.

Bronchitis is the inflammation/infection of the bronchial tubes to the lungs, which results in an oversecretion of mucus by the mucous membranes throughout the respiratory tract. The resultant deep cough is the body's attempt to rid the bronchi of excess mucus. Bronchitis is often the result of irritation to the lungs.

Asthma is a condition that is characterized by labored expiration, caused by intermittent obstructions in the bronchi. Asthmatics can be helped enormously by concentrating on emitting a controlled exhalation, as inspiration usually occurs naturally. In children, asthma is often caused by food allergies, yeast or fungal infections, as well as emotional stress. Asthma in adults is usually triggered by allergies to pollen, foods, yeast or fungal infections, as well as emotional stress. Asthma attacks are most commonly preceded by emotional upset.

HEALTH TIP #4: The Sinus Drainage Exercise

Utilize the following exercise to help drain your sinuses and improve your ability to breathe. The exercise works surprisingly well, even though it focuses on an area of the body that is far removed from your sinuses.

Lying on your stomach, bend your lower legs 90 degrees. Begin to swing your feet from side to side, interchanging leg positions on each swing. Maintain this 90-degree angle throughout the exercise. Move your legs in an orchestrated manner until 25 repetitions are completed on each side. It's amazing how quickly this

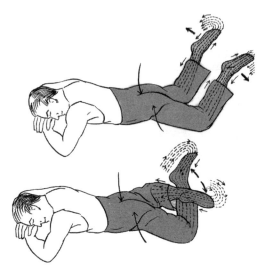

Fig. 10.3: The Sinus Drainage Exercise

exercise can clear your sinuses. An important side note for sinus sufferers: Congested sinuses are often caused by dietary indiscretions, especially the overconsumption of wheat and dairy products.

Respiratory Health Tips Summary

- Integrated Breathing Techniques: Integrated breathing adds a meditative quality by slowing the breath rate. This slower-paced breath should have an equally timed inhalation and exhalation.

- Retention breathing can be practiced on a daily basis to expand lung capacity, give relief for digestive problems, or to relax in times of emotional upset.

- Whole Body Scan: The Integrated Breath Exercise can be added to the Whole Body Scan described in chapter 1 to bring healing to any part of the body. Our breath naturally travels with our awareness and brings healing wherever we send it. Exploring these ramifications is health producing, relaxing, and enlightening.

- Air Filtration: Introduce air filtration into your home or office if the quality of the air you breathe is questionable. In dry climates, the use of a humidifier is also helpful. For more information on air quality and filtration, see appendix A.

- Stimulate Lymphatic Drainage Points: To improve the drainage of lymphatic fluid in the lungs, which helps to enhance respiratory function, stimulate the lymphatic drainage points. Holding the neurovascular holding points (see page 159) associated with the lungs will also assist in enhancing the blood supply to your lungs.

- Organ Trigger Points: Stimulating the trigger points associated with the respiratory system will help stimulate and balance respiratory function.

- Nutrition: Introduce a diet rich in whole foods, especially organic fruits and vegetables. Limit the intake of dairy products, refined carbohydrates, caffeine, and chlorinated water. Drink spring water, filtered water, lemon water, and a

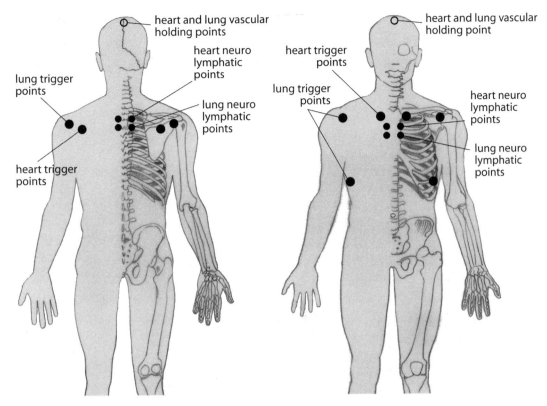

Fig. 10.4: Treatment Point Chart for Lungs and Heart

variety of herbal teas. Use the following herbs to assist respiratory function: osha for supporting the entire respiratory system; mullein for the lungs; plantago for coughing and wheezing; anise for dry cough and bronchial infections; marshmallow for inflamed respiratory membranes; and goldenseal for sinusitis. For persistent sinus problems utilize the ancient sinus-clearing method presented in appendix B.

■ Vitamins and Minerals: Supplement with vitamin A, which promotes the health of mucous membranes; vitamin-C complex, which promotes healing; vitamin F, as flaxseed oil, fish oil, or blackcurrant seed oil, promotes anti-inflammatory activity in the body; and, vitamin-B complex to support overall biochemical function. Supportive minerals include zinc, magnesium, and calcium. Use whole food supplementation for increased absorption and utilization.

■ Whole food supplements: Use antioxidants, immune system enhancers as indicated in chapter 9, and proteolytic enzymes, taken between meals for anti-inflammatory effects. Special formulas for the respiratory system and sources for all supplements are listed in appendix A.

The Circulatory System

The circulatory system is the transit system for the river of blood that integrates all the parts of the body into one living whole organism. The anatomy of circulation includes a pumping mechanism—the heart—and over 100,000 miles of continuous blood vessels, ranging in size from capillaries, which are the width of one red blood cell, to vessels that average several inches in diameter. Blood vessels are also intimately integrated with the lymph, respiratory, immune, and nerve systems.

Lymph fluid, which is similar to the plasma portion of blood, enters the circulatory system by way of two large veins that lie above the heart on either side of the neck. Here, lymph fluid and blood mix together before taking the wild ride through the heart.

Fluid reenters the lymphatic system through millions of tiny lymph vessels that are located throughout the body. The lymph system gathers fluid from the spaces between the tissues. Lymph fluid also contains the waste products of normal cellular activity, fat globules that have been gathered from the small intestine, and an array of white blood cells from the immune system.

The circulatory system carries blood to the lungs for oxygenation, and returns carbon dioxide to the atmosphere via exhalation. Tiny capillaries of the circulatory system gradually form into larger and larger arteries, which deliver newly oxygenated blood to one of the four chambers of the heart. The heart, in turn, circulates this blood out to the cells of the body.

Although the circulatory system is complex, its purpose is rather simple: Circulation gets oxygen and other nutrients to the cells, and moves out waste products.

Blood, the River of Life

Blood is the river of life in the body. It carries beneficial nutrients and harmful waste products to and from our cells. Blood is also the means of transportation for our immune system army, and provides a vehicle for the delivery of hormones from the endocrine system.

Blood is composed of approximately 50 percent plasma and 50 percent blood cells. Blood plasma is over 90 percent water and 10 percent plasma proteins. These plasma proteins include albumin, which helps to control the volume of blood; globulin, which contains important antibodies from the immune system; and two components for blood clotting.

The blood cell portion of blood is composed of red blood cells (RBCs), which are designed to carry oxygen to our cells; white blood cells (WBCs), which are produced by the immune system; and platelets, which are cell fragments important in blood clotting. Red blood cells are produced by the marrow of long bones and live for only about 120 days, after which they are recycled by the spleen, liver, and bone marrow. Up to ten million RBCs are circulated every second in the body.

When looking at a blood test, certain values are assigned to each portion of blood in order to evaluate the condition of the body. A table of the normal values of blood components and possible health-related scenarios are listed in appendix B.

The average woman has about seven pints of blood, and the average male has about ten pints. A newborn infant has only a half a pint of blood, which is the origin of the term "half-pint."

Blood can be separated into different types, which is especially important to know when receiving transfusions. Most blood types contain antibodies to other blood types, which can cause severe reactions. The blood types are type A, which is present in 40 percent of the population; type B, which is present in 10 percent of the population; type AB, which is present in 5 percent of the population; and type O, which is present in 45 percent of the population. As we discovered in chapter 7, these blood types can be helpful in considering biochemical individuality and dietary practices.

The Heart

The heart is a hollow four-chambered muscular organ about the size of a man's fist, and it lies between the lungs in the middle of the chest. Our ten-ounce heart includes several accompanying structures, including the pericardium, which is the sac surrounding the heart. This heart sac is attached to the inside of the sternum and to the diaphragm. This diaphragm attachment is significant to both our breathing and our digestion, and is often symptomatically associated with a hiatal hernia.

The walls of the heart are composed of three layers. The middle layer, called the myocardium, is the part of the heart that receives the nurturing blood supply from the coronary arteries. When too many denatured fats are eaten in the diet, these arteries often become clogged, interfering with the circulation of blood to the heart

The walls of the heart also receive instructions from the nerve system about when to contract or relax. The walls of the heart are actually responsible for pumping blood through the entire body.

The four chambers of the heart include two upper chambers called atria, and two lower chambers called ventricles. The atria, which are named after the central hall of a Roman house, receive blood from various parts of the body, just as the Romans received their guests. The right atrium receives blood from all the tissues of the body except the lungs, while the left atrium only receives life-giving, oxygenated blood from the lungs.

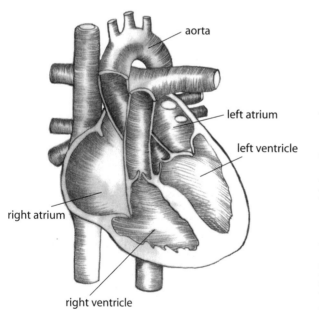

Fig. 10.5: The Heart and Its Chambers

The right atrium pumps blood into the right ventricle below it. The right ventricle then pumps this blood to the lungs for oxygen and CO_2 exchange to take place. The left atrium pumps its blood down to its left ventricle through the largest blood vessel in the body, the aorta. The left ventricle pumps blood out to every part of the body except the lungs.

In short, during a contraction of the heart, the right side of the heart pumps blood to the lungs, and the left side pumps blood to the rest of the body. During the relaxation phase of the heart, the right side of the heart fills with blood from the veins, and the left side fills with oxygenated blood from the lungs.

The heart is both a receiving chamber and a pump. I hope it's clear how intimately the heart and lungs are connected. Half of the heart's activities are dedicated to lung function. Breathing and heart function always go hand in hand.

The heart also has four valves, which regulate the amount of blood passing between chambers. The tricuspid valve regulates the flow of blood between the chambers on the right side of the heart, while the mitral valve regulates blood flow between the chambers on the left side.

Two other valves keep blood from flowing back into the heart once it is pumped out. These are called the semilunar valves, because they are shaped like half moons. These half-moon valves lie between the right ventricle and the pulmonary artery, and the left ventricle and the aorta.

Why so much detail? Because so many of you have been exposed to these terms by your doctors and friends, and it is good to have some basic knowledge of how the heart functions and what these terms actually mean. If and when you are confronted with them, you will have a better reference point to understand the essence of what is happening.

Lub-dub, lub-dub: These are the sounds of a healthy, functioning heart. As the function of the heart becomes altered, so do these telltale sounds.

The sounds of the heart, which you usually don't hear unless there is a problem, are made by the closing of its valves. The lub-sound is the closing of the mitral and tricuspid valves, while the dub-sound is the closing of the two semilunar valves.

After a short pause, the first heart sound is followed by a second heart sound. The resting phase of the heart is determined by an even longer pause between the second sound and the beginning of another first sound. Heart murmurs occur when the valves don't close crisply and cleanly. A murmur is an extra sound that represents a leak in a valve.

The heart is composed of special cardiac muscle that will beat for a lifetime with only the short rest between beats. The heart pumps some four thousand gallons of blood every day, which is amazing considering there are only ten pints in an adult male.

I have worked with the nutritional components of the heart for many years and have found great success in reducing or eliminating heart murmurs with nutritional substances and special formulas, which I list at the end of this chapter. These substances have also been shown to enhance the function of the heart and its related blood vessels.

Timing Is Everything

There is a normal rhythmic cycle of contraction and relaxation in the heart muscle that is a marvel of perfect timing. Each side of the heart contracts at a different rate, which is only possible because of the electrical nature of the heart and its relationship to the nerve system. Valves opens and close, and blood flows at rapid rates in and out of the heart muscle; different chambers fill with blood and eject this life-giving substance out to every part of the body. There are even different sections of the heart that contract at different times. This is the story of life inside the heart, where everything is timed to perfection by an Internal Intelligence that doesn't miss a beat.

The timed sequence of contractions and relaxation in the heart muscle is initiated by specialized nerve-sensitive fibers in the walls of the heart so that every action of the heart can be made with controlled regularity. Electricity sets off the heart's pacemaker to establish a coordinated rhythm that is relentless in generating over thirty-six million beats every year.

The Intelligence of the body regulates heart function through the action of sympathetic nerves that stimulate heart function and utilize the vagus nerve to inhibit heart function. Using the simple tools of stimulation and inhibition, our Inner Intelligence is able to bring about the right balance of contraction and relaxation necessary for every possible circumstance that the body will encounter, from sleeping at high altitudes to extreme exercise.

As human beings, we can become much more aware of the needs of our bodies and learn how to provide it with the raw materials necessary to create health on all levels of our experience. This is especially true for the function of our heart.

Circulation

Circulation in the body refers to the route that blood takes as it leaves the heart pump and makes its way back again. Circulation can be broken down into three smaller units: systemic, which travels throughout the body; pulmonary, which travels to and from the lungs; and portal, which is the circulation involving the liver. The vehicles for transporting blood are the arteries and veins. Arteries go from the largest—the aorta—which is several inches in diameter, to the smallest of capillaries, in which red blood cells have to line up in a single file to get through. Arteries are filled with oxygenated blood, and veins are generally filled with deoxygenated blood.

The systemic circulation carries blood filled with oxygen, nutrients, and waste products throughout the body by way of the aorta, which is largest artery in the body. The aorta, which arches up out of the heart, carries a huge amount of blood and provides a resonant frequency chamber that echoes specific tones throughout the body. Even though they are smaller, the arteries connected to the aorta carry the same tonal frequency.

When capillaries become joined to smaller veins, it indicates that the journey back to the heart has begun. Blood flows back to the heart through a series of veins that get larger and larger until they reach the huge veins that empty blood directly into the heart.

Veins also have little valves that allow for the one-way flow of blood. These valves keep the blood from flowing backward on its journey to the heart. Some of the exercises at the end of this chapter, the inversion exercises in particular, help the body recycle blood back to the heart from distant veins in the arms and legs. This is especially important as we get older and when we stand still for long periods of time.

Varicose veins occur as the result of stagnant blood remaining in the veins. This stagnant blood stimulates the liver to elevate the blood pressure in the legs in order to get the blood to return. Hemorrhoids are also varicose veins that are directly related with liver function.

Obesity increases the possibility of varicose veins. For every additional inch of fat, an additional five hundred miles of blood vessels must be added by the body. The more overweight we are, the more difficult it is to get deoxygenated blood from the extremities back to the heart.

The pulmonary circulation carries blood from the right ventricle of the heart and back to the lungs, where oxygen and CO_2 gas exchange takes place. Oxygenated blood then circulates back to the left atrium for distribution to the body. Pulmonary circulation includes the circulation to some 250 million alveoli sacs, which are directly responsible for exchanging oxygen and CO_2.

The liver is so rich in blood supply, and its functions so important to the body, that it basically has its own blood circulation loop. As a matter of fact, the portal circulation, which is the blood that flows to and from the liver, can contain about 30 percent of our entire blood supply at any one time.

The circulation to the liver actually occurs on the way back to the heart, and most of its circulation is received after passing through the blood vessels of the intestines. In the intestines, the blood collects the nutritional end products from our digestive process, which include sugar, amino acids, and fats. After a meal, the liver cells remove these nutrients, convert them into more usable forms, and slowly release them into the circulation to nourish the body over the next eight to twenty-four hours. The liver also collects unwanted bacteria from the intestines, digests them, and passes them on to the lymph system. Over half of the entire lymphatic system surrounds the liver.

The body needs to increase the blood pressure to the liver in order to circulate some ninety quarts of blood per hour through its vast number of blood vessels. This increase in pressure allows the liver to expand and contract as it extracts nutrients and cleanses the blood.

If the toxic load on the liver becomes too high, the blood in the liver becomes more and more congested, requiring a higher blood pressure to push the blood through the portal circulation. Fibrous tissue in the liver slows down the ability of the liver to filter blood, which marks the beginning of liver disease.

Eating a diet composed of whole foods, utilizing the right kind of fats and oils, and limiting your intake of alcohol, drugs, and toxins usually ensures a higher level of liver function. The structural component for the liver relates to the upper portion of the thoracic spine. To assure that the five hundred different liver functions take place with ease, it is important to keep this area free of structural interference.

Blood Pressure

Currently, high and low blood pressure readings are treated as if they were diseases, when in reality they are symptoms of trouble in circulatory system function. In other words, blood pressure is not the problem; it is the *indicator* of a problem—and a much larger one. This larger problem involves the inefficient function of the heart, and the slow but steady increase in the body's resistance to the pumping of blood through the vascular system.

The pressure exerted against the walls of the blood vessels is called the systemic blood pressure. Blood pressure is usually the highest in the brachial arteries, where it is classically taken, yielding the ideal blood pressure reading of 120/80. The systolic pressure, the first of these numbers, is the blood pressure at the exact time the ventricles of the heart contract. The second number, called the diastolic pressure, is a measure of blood pressure during the resting phase of your heart's beating.

The systolic pressure is dependent on the amount of blood ejected from the ventricle, the elasticity of the blood vessels, and the thickness of the blood. The thicker the blood, the greater the resistance occurs in the blood vessels, and the higher the blood pressure.

The diastolic pressure is dependent on the amount of resistance in the blood vessels and the length of time that the heart rests between beats. The longer the rest, the lower the diastolic pressure. The greater the resistance in the blood vessels, the higher the blood pressure needs to be to pump blood through the vessels.

Blood pressure is subject to vast fluctuations and is influenced by numerous factors. Blood pressure normally rises with exercise, and abnormally rises with mental or emotional stress. Blood pressure is lowered with rest, relaxation, and meditation, and is abnormally lowered by adrenal fatigue.

More specifically, an increase in the systolic blood pressure indicates that your heart is inefficient in its pumping, that the blood vessels are not as elastic as they need to be, or that there is a buildup of bad fats and cholesterol within the arteries. An increase in diastolic blood pressure indicates an increased resistance of the blood vessels, a possible liver involvement such as toxicity, or an increase in resistance in blood flow to the kidneys. Low blood pressure, on the other hand, can indicate that your body doesn't have enough blood or that you are in a state of exhaustion and/or severe adrenal fatigue.

The pulse is present in all arteries of the circulatory system but is more easily felt in the arteries nearer to the surface of the skin. The pulse is an indication of the alternating expansion and contraction of the walls of the arteries as the result of the beating of the heart. The pulse can be easily felt in the wrist and in the carotid artery on the side of the neck.

The pulse can tell us the number of heart beats per minute, the strength of the heart, and even the amount of tension on the arteries. Under the direction of a highly trained physician, close to one hundred different types of pulses can be detected. The pulse pressure is the difference between the systolic pressure and the diastolic pressure. The ideal pulse pressure is 40.

Your pulse rate is an important part of your exercise equation. Finding the ideal heart rate for your specific age and exercise needs will allow you to exercise safely and burn fat instead of your precious sugar reserves. For details on how to find your ideal exercise heart rate, see appendix B.

In some cases, blood pressure regulation with drugs may be necessary, but it is only a temporary solution. If you are experiencing consistently high blood pressure, this is an indication of an overall loss of health. High blood pressure is a signal from your Internal Intelligence that you need to slow down and reduce your physical, mental, and emotional stress levels.

If you experience high blood pressure, please explore the following:

- A change in lifestyle
- The presence of dietary imbalances
- The possible presence of structural misalignments
- Whether it is a time to initiate beneficial habits, such as meditation and breathing exercises
- A monitored exercise program
- A general shift in perspective

Remember, high and low blood pressure are symptoms, not diseases. If you have either one on a regular basis, it is an indication from your Inner Intelligence that something is not quite right.

Indications of Heart-Related Problems

Heart disease is a broad classification that includes the following:

- Stroke—a blockage in the blood supply to the brain
- Angina—chest pain caused by blockages of fat and cholesterol in coronary arteries that supply the heart with oxygen and vital nutrition
- Arrhythmia—problems with the timing of heart related events
- Heart muscle weakness—inefficiency of heart muscle contractions
- Valve problems—leaking of the heart valves, usually accompanied by a buildup of fat, cholesterol, or calcium around the valves, which are all signs of nutritional deficiencies/imbalances
- Lack of oxygen and nutrients to the heart—caused by poor dietary habits and poor circulation
- Increased homocystene levels in the blood—caused by eating too many animal products
- Skin problems—appear when poor circulation is present, and are indicated by poor color, texture, and lack of resiliency of the skin. Blood supply to the skin is often compromised when poor circulation and inadequate heart function are present. A variety of skin conditions can result from increased toxins and a lack of essential nutrients to the skin.
- Swelling of extremities—common when heart function is diminished and leaky valves are present. The heart is unable to overcome increasing resistance in the blood vessels to pump fluid and blood back to the heart. Swelling in the extremities can also occur when fluid leaks directly through unhealthy blood vessels and into the tissues.
- Blood Vessels/Arteriosclerosis—fatty deposits and cholesterol accumulate on the inner walls of blood vessels, causing a narrowing of vessels and a reduction in blood circulation.

Cholesterol is manufactured and recycled by the liver. Seventy-five percent of our brain is actually composed of cholesterol, which is essential for the production of hormones and of bile for the digestive system. Cholesterol is in abundance in the body because it is so necessary for normal body function. LDL, or low-density lipoproteins, are termed bad cholesterol, as they oxidize and build up on the inside of our arteries. When trans-fatty acids build up inside the walls of blood vessels, LDL cholesterol attaches itself to these trans fats, forming plaque, which hardens on the walls of the blood vessels, reducing blood flow and elasticity. HDL, or high density lipoproteins, are the beneficial type of cholesterol created by eating healthy fats and oils.

HEALTH TIP #5: Enhance the Functioning of the Circulatory System

■ Nutrition

Many nutritional experts agree that heart disease is a deficiency disease caused by consuming too many refined foods, especially fats and oils. Deficiencies caused by refining and bleaching our flour, refining and processing our foods, and the denaturing of our fats and oils are part of the cause. Processing destroys essential vitamins, minerals, and synergistic factors present in whole foods.

Foods to eat:
A diet rich in whole foods, whole grains, organic fruits, vegetables and beneficial fats, such as unheated extra virgin olive oil

Brewer's yeast and whole grains that are abundant in B vitamins

Raw, unprocessed wheat germ, which is a rich source of vitamin-E complex

Rice bran syrup, which provides niacin for nerves and reduces triglycerides and LDL cholesterol

Avocados, which are abundant in beneficial fats

Eggs, which have generous amounts of lecithin that counteract dietary cholesterol

Fiber in the form of oat bran, brown rice, and flaxseed meal, which can help lower cholesterol

Avocado and grape seed oils, which have a high smoke point and can be best used for cooking

Foods to avoid:
Fried foods

Excess animal protein

Nonorganic dairy products

Saturated, hydrogenated, and trans fats

Fluoride, chlorine, and other toxic chemicals

Additives and preservatives in foods and drinks

Coffee, cigarettes, and excess alcohol consumption

Cleansing the arteries and veins of your circulatory system is accomplished by eliminating hydrogenated trans fats in your diet and adding essential fatty acid supplementation in the form of flaxseed oil and certified mercury-free fish oils. Both omega-3 and omega-6 fatty acids are important to circulation. Omega-3s have been shown to reduce blood pressure, cholesterol, and triglycerides. Omega-6s, which are found in black currant seed oil, borage oil, and evening primrose oil as GLA, have been shown to reduce plaque inside arteries.

■ Whole Food Supplements

The vitamin B complex includes both the B-complex group (for stimulation) and the G-complex group (for relaxation). Vitamin B6, B12 and folic acid are necessary to reduce circulating homocysteine levels in the blood formed by the consumption of high amounts of animal proteins.

Vitamin-C complex, E2, and heart protomorphogen are special whole food vitamin complexes that help to build a healthy heart muscle.

Chlorophyll is plant blood that helps cleanse, detoxify, and thin the blood that is thickened with toxins and cellular debris. Chlorophyll is found in all green plants, kelp, and seaweed, and is especially rich in magnesium. Chlorophyll can be found in all green food supplements. See appendix A for all whole food supplements and special heart-related formulas.

■ Exercise

Mild inversion exercises are beneficial to the heart and help remove stagnant blood from the extremities. For exercise, you can try the slant board, inversion table, or the yoga swing.

Walking, swimming, and mild aerobic exercise—utilizing a heart monitor to find your ideal heart rate for exercise—are all great for building a healthy heart.

▦ Herbs

Hawthorne berries help to open up blood vessels to the heart and assist in lowering blood pressure.

Cayenne pepper can be a magic tonic for the heart, and is especially effective when combined with hawthorne berries. Take a capsule of cayenne pepper each day with food to improve circulation. Garlic is an excellent blood purifier and has even been found to dissolve blood clots.

▦ Minerals

Organic minerals, organic trace minerals, calcium lactate or citrate, magnesium, chromium, and selenium.

▦ Amino Acids

A whole food source of all the essential and some nonessential amino acids assist the heart by providing the raw materials necessary for repair. All whole food supplements for the heart are listed in appendix A.

▦ Neurolymphatic Reflex and Vascular Holding Points

Stimulating lymphatic reflex points as illustrated will help to improve lymphatic drainage and enhance the function of the heart, circulatory system, and liver. Holding the related vascular holding points will improve the circulation to the heart and improve the function of the circulatory system.

Emotions and the Heart

Emotions are also at the heart of the matter, and it is no coincidence that we address our physical and emotional heart by the same name. Our physical heart usually reflects the state of our emotional heart, and vice versa. If you or someone you know experiences heart problems, chances are that unresolved emotions lie directly below the surface.

When our emotions get bottled up, something in our heart or circulation has got to give. There are exceptions, and genetic problems can explain many heart defects, but heart problems usually don't show up unless emotions are involved.

Science and medicine don't often make the connection between emotions and heart health, because emotions are not easy to explain scientifically. Emotions and Spirit don't fit neatly into the medical model of the world, but our emotional health is at the very core of our health.

Our true feelings and emotions are often kept inside of us, ready to burst out at a moment's notice. When they finally do, we sometimes don't survive the process. It's no coincidence that heart attacks are most likely to occur at 9:00 a.m. on Monday morning while at work. Let's discover creative ways to express our emotions and feelings before our physical bodies pay the price.

Conclusion

Heart disease is the biggest killer of human beings in the United States, causing over 50 percent of the total deaths at a cost of over fifty billion dollars yearly. Yet heart disease is very preventable when all the components of optimal health are addressed.

Diet and nutrition are especially important in maintaining normal heart function, and we will usually be successful in maintaining a healthy heart and circulatory system when we understand what kind of foods the heart needs in order to function at optimal levels, and avoid the foods that interfere with that function. Healthy heart nutrition can be practiced by anyone who has the desire to create health.

Another huge consideration for health involves maintaining normal spinal function in relationship to the heart. This is especially true when we understand the heart's electrical connection and the rhythm of the heart cycle as coordinated by the nerve system. If nerve interference is present in the upper thoracic region of the spine, or anywhere in the cervical spine, the nerve impulses to the heart become compromised. Maintaining a spinal system that is free from spinal misalignments, which is the job of a doctor of chiropractic, is an important component of healthy heart function.

Our state of mind can be a big help or a big hindrance in maintaining a healthy heart. The heart represents a different realm of experience entirely, one that cannot be explained by logic and reason. The stressful interaction of the universal male and female principles also lie at the core of heart disease.

Stress is a condition in which we create a huge strain on our physical hearts. We usually create our own stress by pushing ourselves beyond our limitations, and our cardiovascular system often pays the price.

We create stress in our lives when a gap exists between what we know is the right way to live and how we actually live. If mental stress or strain is present in your life, you owe it to your cardiovascular system to change to a healthier lifestyle. As a matter of fact, your life may depend on it.

If there is a magic potion that produces a healthy heart, Spirit is that ultimate elixir. The essence of Spirit relaxes the heart and opens the mind to possibilities greater than itself. Spirit also provides the perspective in which the heart and the mind are seen as complementary. When we access this perspective in relation to our heart, all things seem to come together with ease. As we've learned, it is our perspective that alters our perception and changes our experience.

Chapter 11

The Mind

INTERESTINGLY ENOUGH, it is often our mind that stands in the way of our quest toward vibrant physical health. The mind continually tries to control what happens to us and to think its way to the next solution. In fact, the way to a healthy body that is vibrantly alive lies in knowing how to work with the mind, how to move beyond it, and how to understand what is beneath it.

It is difficult to write about a such a process, because the process is not about words or thoughts. This chapter was designed to encourage you to release mental control and allow the Innate Mind within you to take over. This is about moving your educated mind out of the way long enough to allow a most incredible experience to take place.

The mind is certainly a powerful tool for creating health and well-being, depending on how we choose to use it. The educated mind tries to figure everything out, answer every question, solve every problem, but without really seeing the larger context of wholeness. Educated mind is associated with the male principle. When a women shares a problem with a man, he quickly tries to solve it. In reality, she just wants someone to talk to about it, to share her feelings, and is not actually seeking a solution. But the educated mind is into finding solutions and solving problems and is more likely to react to a situation than to consciously act.

"I am, therefore I think" is a more accurate summary of our Innate Mind and the connection to the source of our Being. In the presence of our Innate Mind, our educated mind becomes a valuable ally that brings with it an entirely different experience.

How we relate to our minds is similar to the way people walk their dogs. People with a dominant, educated mind let the dog walk them—pulling them in every possible direction. When these people get home from their walk, they are often exhausted. In contrast, people who are present in their Innate Mind are able to control their dog and to instinctively find a different path, perhaps arriving at an exciting new location.

When we create space for our educated mind to move out of the way, our Innate Mind can take over and do the rest.

We can ask the question, "What is guiding me?" Am I being guided by the same power that directs the movement of the planets and stars, or am I the one being dragged around by a leash? Am I led by my own self-directed thinking, or am I guided by a greater vision of wholeness? If you are like most of us, you are only occasionally, and fleetingly, connected to that more expansive sense of yourself. And yet the key to unlocking the extraordinary lies in that connection.

We will take a look at ways to improve the function of the educated mind, and then we will look at moving beyond it entirely. See if this chapter can't help nudge open the doors of your perception into that expanded realm.

The Educated Mind

Our Belief Systems

All of us are guided by belief systems, whether or not we can articulate what they are. Religious beliefs, cultural beliefs, beliefs about our inherent separateness or connectedness to/from one another, even beliefs about health and disease—these core beliefs about the world act as filters that overlay our perception. We may even be aware that we hold these beliefs, but we are often not aware of how these filters keep us from experiencing our own deepest sense of truth and reality, and how they restrict our flow of creativity into the world. Ironically, many of us see these filters in other people, but rarely do we see them in ourselves. If we don't like what we are getting in our world, or how things are working out for us, chances are that our beliefs are involved in setting it up that way. If you allow yourself to acknowledge it, you will see that your world is probably pretty consistent with your worldview.

Our belief systems begin to form in early childhood when we take on the ideas and perspectives of our parents, friends, teachers, and peers. The accuracy of these ideas is rarely the issue, of course. We simply adopt beliefs that in turn help determine our basis of understanding, where we fit in the world, and how we feel about ourselves and other human beings.

Not only are individual filters of perception placed upon us, we also inherit collective filters of perception that are either widely or entirely shared by all humankind.

Discover the hidden beliefs and stuck attitudes that limit your life experience.

At the time of Christopher Columbus, people shared the limited belief that the world was flat. Even though they believed it to be true, it did not make the world flat. Collective beliefs don't always coincide with reality. Contrary to current beliefs, the nature of the table on which you placed this book is mostly space, not solid substance. Similar filters tell us the earth is standing still, when in reality it is moving through space at tremendous speeds. These collective filters still keep human beings from acting as if we are a unified, whole Being.

Our core beliefs are usually kept in place with strong emotional anchors, which can be expansive or limited, inclusive or exclusive. For example, if at our core we believe that we are not enough, guess what? We never will be strong enough, fit enough, slim enough, or pretty enough. To make things worse, we won't ever have enough either. In contrast, when we perceive ourselves as more than enough, we will be enough on all levels of experience.

I occasionally run into people who don't believe in chiropractic. I always shake my head. Their beliefs don't change anything about the nature of chiropractic, which helps millions of people every year. The belief simply keeps nonbelievers from experiencing the benefits of structural balance.

When we know for ourselves that maintaining structural balance beneficially effects our health and well-being, that belief can provide a great benefit, and we can begin to determine for ourselves when we need structural help to maintain that balance. If you find yourself saying, "I don't believe in this or that," stop and reorganize your perceptions. See and feel what is actually going on underneath your beliefs. You may be missing a very important opportunity.

When we release our beliefs and attitudes, and let our higher mind take over, we become part of the solution, not part of the problem.

As a practitioner in the healing arts, I am particularly aware of how our beliefs limit our experience of health. So many patients come to me with terrible fears of illness, bacteria, and disease. They don't realize that the fear itself is fueling their disease and weakening their immune systems. Fear of disease begins to overtake them, and they begin to act out of fear, abandoning the positive nature of their own healing power. The thymus gland negatively reacts to fear, becomes weaker, and allows bacteria and other agents of dis-ease to gain more of an upper hand. Instead of weakening your immune system through your mind, you could be using those same powers to strengthen it.

Positive Thinking

We have all heard of the power of positive thinking, and many people use it all the time. The power of positive thinking supports our every step, while negative thinking continually undermines our progress. Quantum physics has shown us that the way we choose to interact with the world determines the way that the universe/world interacts with us. Sometimes a positive attitude about something can turn the tide in favor of success as we enlist the help of Spirit. Likewise, when we succumb to negativity in our thinking, we shut out the possibility of help and insight from Spirit. The power of positive thinking adds to our health with every breath, while negative thinking detracts from our health.

Be aware of what you say and how you say it, because your body is listening to every word. In fact, your body is so eager to serve you that it will carry out any instructions you give it.

When you say you hate something, your body hardens, constricts, and closes down. But notice how your body softens and your reality expands when you speak of loving something or someone.

We often don't realize the power of our words. They have the ability to create or destroy. A great example of this was shared by Norman Cousins in his book *The Healing Heart.* While pursuing a postdoctoral fellowship with the renowned physician Dr. S. A. Levine, professor of cardiology at Harvard Medical School and head physician at the Peter Bent Brigham Hospital, Cousins encountered a woman who was in the hospital for routine treatment. During a session with interns, Dr. Levine offhandedly mentioned that the woman they were observing had TS (tricuspid stenosis), and then he left the room.

Immediately, the woman's condition started to change for the worse. Her breathing became labored and her lungs congested. When Cousins asked her about the sudden change, the woman said she knew that TS meant "terminal situation." She was convinced that she was going to die. Despite Cousins' insistence that this was not true, the woman's condition continued to worsen, and rapidly degenerated into massive pulmonary edema. Efforts to reach the physician who had cast the fatal spell failed, and the woman died later that day.

This woman believed that her situation was terminal, and her belief created her immediate reality. I often shudder when I hear parents scolding their young children, calling them names and telling them how stupid or bad they are. In due time, these same children will start to believe it. Stories such as these have made me much more aware of what I say and how I say it.

Our choice of words reveals our true feelings and beliefs.

Our words reveal the real feelings in our hearts. It is important to listen to your words as you say them and to become aware of how they affect those around you. Be sensitive to feedback from other people, especially unspoken feedback, and use it to change your choice of words. Avoid using phrases like "I'm dying to see that movie," "These long hours are killing me," or "I hate doing that." Remember that the energy of a waveform becomes a particle when we give it our attention; we are encoding a message to the universe. When we encode this message using negative thoughts and language, the results will reflect it. Conversely, when we send a message encoded in the language of love, the resulting forms reflect that. Be aware of how you are programming the universe.

Intention vs. Chance

To understand the nature of the mind we need to look at the nature of the universe, as they both follow the same universal laws and principles. This is the practical application of the wave and particle discussion I presented earlier. Whatever we create in waveform by our intention shows up in particle form as physical reality.

The blank slate of the universe manifests whatever we create energetically. And what we create is dependent on our intention.

Our words set the stage for creating health and well-being.

The way in which we support ourselves truly lies in our hands. If we use the creation-by-chance method, which allows our unconscious mind to do the bidding, many unknown factors will contribute to the outcome. But if our intentions are clear, what comes back to us is clear. Our intent, or lack thereof, is also responsible for creating our life circumstances.

Combining the right words with the power of feelings sends a strong message to the universe, and it always responds.

🙢 WAVEFORM

It's waveform; it's particle

It seems it's up to me

Creation brings such wonders

In forms we've yet to see

We move to different drummers

Yet the drumbeat is the same

Lub Dub connects us all

It's more than just a game

The breath of life

Breathes us in

No matter what the color

Magic is the norm, you see

Impostors any other

The Present Moment

How do we set a clear intention, and align our hearts and minds, when our minds are so full of chatter? We must be in the present moment. We can endlessly spin ourselves in circles, fretting over the past or worrying about the future, but the limitless expression and creativity of our Innate Mind lives in the present moment. The present moment is the place from which our Inner Intelligence guides us.

It is the curse of human beings to be enslaved by the past or enamored by the future, but to be aware of the vastness of the present moment is our blessing.

Listen to Your Inner Guidance

In this moment, your Inner Intelligence is directing myriad functions that are essential to your body, like expanding and contracting your blood vessels to direct the movement of your blood, or bringing the images of these lines to your brain and changing them into electrical impulses, but your Inner Intelligence is also available to provide guidance for you. Simply be present, with a quiet mind and an open heart, and ask for guidance.

Sit in a quiet place and close your eyes. Just breathe. Feel your beating heart. Be present. This is how you cultivate your inner connection. What is your Inner Intelligence telling you right now?

In this moment, you can receive the guidance, wisdom, and direction of your Inner Intelligence.

Using Your Whole Brain

Our bodies are designed to accommodate consciousness. We are wired for it. Our brain and nerve system have the inherent ability to create new pathways as fast as we can open up to them. Our Inner Intelligence knows when we express the qualities of our Inner Being, and creates the neurology for us to sustain it.

You may be familiar with the terms "left brain" and "right brain." These phrases give us a clue about how our minds work. While the brain is designed to function as an integrated whole, the left brain is linear, logical, rational, and associated with the functions of the male principle and the conscious mind. Our right brain is expansive, nonlinear, spatial, and associated with the feminine principle, the feeling realm, and the subconscious.

Right and left, male and female, spatial and linear, together these halves create a truly dynamic and balanced human being. We are given two distinct, interconnected brains in order for them to work in tandem. You might think of your brain as a house. You can create a living space that is both spatially open and functionally practical, a space that engenders a sense of peace, while at the same time is oriented toward useful space. Your right brain creates the living space while your left brain sizes things up. The two fit together perfectly, and you need them both to produce a great design.

You are similarly designed with the ability to utilize both the male and female aspects of your Being and to express them in a balanced way. If you are a pretty logical, left-brain type (which is often the case), you might try to find some balance by introducing right-brain activities, such as music, movement, or dance. If you tend to be more right-brained, you can find some balance with left-brained activities, such as reading, writing, or doing puzzles. Singing is one of the few brain-balanced activities: it involves making sounds (which is right-brained) and making word progressions (which is left-brained). Singing on a daily basis also helps to balance your heart and mind. In fact, using both sides of your brain brings balance to your whole body.

Mental Patterns

We have already seen how our patterns of movement go hand in hand with the function of our nerve and muscular systems. Now we can see how our mental patterns or mind-sets show up in our physical bodies, and how our physical ailments reflect our mental patterns. This sounds complicated, but it's really very simple. For example, if you shoulder a lot of responsibility in your life, you often develop shoulder problems. Conversely, if your shoulders bother you, consider whether you have been taking on too much responsibility. The accompanying chart shows some of these body-mind relationships. This process is called aspecting. See if you can find meaning and cues in your aches and pains.

Problem Area	Aspect
Head	Unable to maintain connection to source
Neck	Stiffness, stubbornness, unable to see what is around you
Upper back	The presence of physical and emotional burdens
Mid back	Unable to connect with one's source of power
Lower back	Lack of support in one's life
Shoulders	Shouldering too much responsibility
Hips	Blockage of sexuality, lack of movement
Knees	Inflexibility, inability to bend
Ankles/wrists	Lack of intention
Feet	Lack of understanding
Hands	Inability to give (right) or receive (left)
Elbows	Unable to give to one's self
Eyes	Far sighted - inability to see what is in front of you Near sighted - Inability to see the big picture
Stomach	Unable to stomach certain circumstances
Digestion	Inability to digest ideas and feelings
Immunity	Inability to to resist what is not supportive to one's self
Respiration	Unable to give and receive
Heart	Inability to experience emotional health

Fig. 11.1: Aspect Chart

The Conscious and Subconscious Minds

Our minds are incredibly complex. The portion we utilize is only a fraction of the whole. I like to use the image of an arc welder to describe this important connection.

An arc welder has two different electrical charges, positive (+) and negative (−), each attached to a welding rod. Visualize if you will one rod coming from above and one coming from below, as in the accompanying illustration. The nature of the electrical current coming from above is the positive masculine charge, while the current coming from below represents the negative charge of the feminine. The nature of these charges has nothing to do with good or bad, but simply represent the nature of the two separate but equal charges of electrical energy.

As we bring these two separately charged rods closer together, an arc of energy forms between them, emitting a powerful light. In our analogy, this powerful light represents the interaction between our conscious and subconscious. The synthesis of the positively charged and negatively charged aspects of our Being results in a powerful light that is designed to illuminate the way for human beings through the darkness of an unknown world.

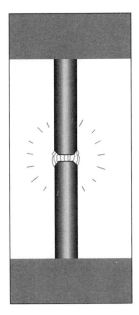

Fig. 11.2: Arc Welder: Conscious & Subconscious Mind

The conscious mind is only aware of what it needs to know right now for the task at hand. It is the thin, top layer of the mind.

Our subconscious mind, on the other hand, records everything we have ever been exposed to, no matter how obscure it may seem. Our subconscious mind records millions of bits of information every second of our lives.

When something or someone in the present moment provides the trigger, pertinent bits of information pop into our conscious minds from our subconscious. The subconscious mind acts as a vibrational hard drive that automatically retrieves associated information and experiences. One of the more important functions of the conscious mind is to act as a guardian for what goes into our subconscious. And we seem willing, at times, to let almost any kind of information and experience into our subconscious minds, which comes back to haunt us.

For example, we can't seem to get enough of scary movies. Unfortunately, that material sits in our subconscious, waiting to be triggered—and we don't get to control when or how it expresses itself.

We can use our conscious minds to screen out experiences by not admitting them into our subconscious in the first place. If you attend a movie that is too strange or scary, get up and leave. If a movie that your child is watching is not fitting for them to see, change it to something else. Our conscious minds are in control of our actions, and as parents we act as guardians for the conscious minds of our children. Be a responsible guardian.

Inner Wisdom

One way of improving the connection to our subconscious is by consciously choosing to do so. Instead of reacting to the distracting events in our external world, we can choose to turn our attention inward and receive the guidance and direction of our Inner Wisdom. When we find that place of stillness within, we can access the wisdom of our Inner Intelligence. This kind of deep thinking allows us to make decisions in a whole new way, guided not by what we *think* we *should* do or be, but by what we *know,* internally, is right and true for us. This simple shift changes everything in our lives.

When stillness is present in our conscious minds, we can access the wisdom of our Inner Intelligence. Once we get the hang of returning to stillness before we take action, life becomes much less stressful. Things happen in a natural flow, which proceeds from the invisible realm into the visible world. Life becomes more creative and much more interesting.

The Innate Mind

Try to become a witness to the many thoughts and ideas that move through your mind. Simply stand aside and let them move through; thoughts only become your own if you lay claim to them. Our Innate Mind simply observes thoughts as they pass by, inspects them, learns from them, and lets them go. This process makes room for clearer thoughts to enter, and, eventually, it creates a place of stillness and peace. After practicing the discipline of observing and letting go of ideas for a period of time, many of the stray and extraneous thoughts begin to thin out and dissipate.

When we begin to dwell in the spaces between our thoughts and ideas, we also find that the content of these thoughts begins to change. The Innate Mind occupies the spaces between our thoughts, between our words, and between our actions. When the educated mind steps aside long enough, when we allow that inner stillness to penetrate the intermittent chatter, we can become the Presence that occupies the stillness. From the depths of that place arises just the right thought for the situation at hand—not a hundred scattered thoughts, but exactly the right one.

It is like what happens when you pick up the right book, open it to the right page, and hear exactly what you wanted to know. We still use our conscious mind to screen incoming thoughts and ideas, but as we become clearer, and dwell in the stillness, our Innate Mind begins to retrieve exactly the right things. Release the need to know, and rely on the Innate Mind to provide the right thoughts at the right time. Learn to be content with the experience of no thoughts.

Take a few moments to be by yourself. Use your breath to quiet your educated mind and to seek the resting place of stillness that lies between your thoughts. Be content when nothing is happening at all. Be fulfilled with no mental activity. Cultivate this experience of emptiness with every breath, and release your untamed thoughts with every sigh.

Fig. 11.3: Educated vs. Innate Mind

Educated Mind	Innate Mind
"I think, therefore I am"	"I am, therefore I think"
Male principle	Female principle
Reacts to situations	Consciously acts
"Dog walks you"	Instinctively finds a new path
Self-directed thinking	Greater vision of wholeness
Overlays perception	Deepest sense of reality
Lives in the past or future	Lives in the present
Guided by distracting events	Guided by stillness
Led by what we think we should do	Led by what we know is right
Prisoner of the mundane	Unlocks the extraordinary

How to Get There

The practices below are designed to exercise your mind and free your spirit, which allows life to be more clear and purposeful.

Visualization and meditation are two practices that have been utilized for centuries to quiet the mind, open the heart, and directly connect the practitioner to their Inner Wisdom.

Here I offer a basic visualization process and a meditation practice that I have taught for a number of years. I know that when I don't begin my day with meditation, things kind of take off haphazardly and the days can be rough. When I do begin with meditation, everything goes much more smoothly and the details of the day just seem to fall into place. I still have all the same things to plan and do, but beginning from a place of stillness makes all the difference. I move from a resting place of stillness to a place of creative action.

In order to enjoy the experience of mental clarity in your life, you need to create the space for it to exist. No space, no clarity. Big space, lots of clarity. You choose.

If you want more peace, joy, ease, health, lightness, and wholeness in your life, my advice is to meditate every day without exception.

I recommend meditating first thing in the morning and, if your life is stressful, again in the evening before bed.

HEALTH TIP #1: Visualization and Meditation Practice

This simple meditation process will provide peace and quiet for your mind, and relaxation for your body. You can complete this meditation in about ten minutes. If time is a particular concern, you might want to set a timer. Just be kind to yourself and pick a timer that isn't too jarring when it rings. Over time, you will probably find yourself wanting about twenty minutes for your morning meditation.

Sit comfortably on the floor in a cross-legged position with good back support, or sit in a comfortable chair. Make sure that you are sitting upright with your spine erect. Place your hands at your sides or in your lap, whichever feels more natural. The more comfortable you are, the less you will be distracted.

Become conscious of your breathing. Think of breathing in peace and tranquility, and breathing out tension.

Your breath will relax your body, slowing down your body's metabolism and encouraging the experience of stillness. Breathing entrains the mind and allows it to find its own natural rhythm.

Using your mind's eye, focus all your attention on what is happening right now in the present moment. Extract your mind from all past events and future possibilities in order to fully participate in the meditation.

■ Meditation Tip

Initially, meditation is like training a dog to stay on the front porch. At first you may need to tie your dog to the porch, but after he gets the idea, and with a little encouragement from you, he will usually stay there all by himself. Like your dog, you may have to tell your mind to stay put on the porch for a while; eventually, however, it will love being there.

As your breathing becomes more steady, and you allow yourself to be with the present moment, focus your awareness and attention very softly on the space between your eyes. This is the location of your third eye, which connects your pituitary and pineal glands. Your soft focus at this location helps to activate your higher consciousness. Maintain this focus as you continue to relax. A soft focus is important here, as you want your awareness to expand to include this important location, not to focus so intently that you exclude everything else. Just let your breath breathe you into a meditative state.

After a good stretch of time with a soft focus of attention resting between your eyes (about ten minutes), take an exhalation breath and let go of everything. See if you can experience an attitude of gratitude throughout your entire Being—gratitude for anything that comes to consciousness, even for your breath itself. Be thankful not just with your mind, but with your body, mind, heart, and spirit

During the meditation, your mind will try to interrupt your peace and quiet with really important thoughts like, "What am I going to wear today?" Simply lead it back to the porch.

Your breathing will usually let you know when your meditation is complete, as you will naturally take a deep, cleansing breath. Consciously enjoy the experience for a few more moments before getting on with your day.

If your life is particularly stressful, meditate again that day, even if only for a few minutes. Make your morning meditation a priority, and you will soon experience the benefits of peace and tranquility. There is always a good excuse not to meditate. In my experience, none of them are ever good enough.

Even in the midst of the confusion and chaos of today's world, an intimate connection with your Innate Mind will bring peace, beauty, and joy into your world, and will help you to cultivate wisdom. Vibrant health and well-being are the blessed side effects of living in the natural flow of life, with your mind open and receptive to the essence of Spirit.

THE INNATE MIND

When I connect with the Innate Mind

Something greater comes upon me

When the Innate Mind becomes my own

All is very well

The wind is suddenly at my back

I know that I am safe

My direction is homeward bound

And I know the way

I've waited my whole life for this

Another world has opened

It's the adventure of a lifetime

And I am thrilled

Chapter 12

Bring in Your Heart

IN HEALTH AND HEALING, we often refer to the body-mind connection with a vague idea that this includes matters of the heart. But so often, it doesn't. In our collective worldview, the heart has been perceived as subordinate to the mind—and part of the (less valuable) feminine realm—and has been omitted from consideration in almost every area of human endeavor, especially science, health, education, and business. Ironically, it is our capacity of heart that leads us to our Inner Intelligence, the place from which radiates our greatest health and vitality.

Why is it that we trust our minds more than our hearts? Perhaps because the mind is more clear cut, with its rational capacities and conclusions. We can always count on the mind to come up with explanations for things, even if we really don't understand them. The heart, on the other hand, is messy and complicated. It appears completely foreign to the mind and relates to an entirely different realm of experience. As such, it also requires a completely new level of sensitivity.

Our heart is literally the energetic center for the body: It has the pineal, pituitary, and thyroid energy centers above it, and the gonadal, adrenal, and pancreatic centers below it. Our heart is right in the middle of the action, where it belongs, blending the higher and lower energies that power the human body.

How do we connect with this vital part of ourselves? How do we return to the path of wholeness? How do we align our minds and hearts, and open the door to the magic of our Inner Being?

First, we can recognize and acknowledge how we have elevated the role of the mind and downplayed the role of the heart in our individual and collective lives. Women are not immune from this either. Having gained greater access to the world of business, women now have the blessing of experiencing more heart disease than men. Why? Because their hearts have become hardened in order to win at the game, and when anyone becomes hard-hearted (as is often the case in business), heart disease can become a natural consequence. Anyone that is incapable of expressing feelings of love, compassion, and forgiveness will more than likely share that same hardened experience in their own lives and in their own bodies.

The heart refers to the most vital organ in the body, and to the realm of emotions and feelings. It is our healthy relationship to this realm that creates physical health and emotional well-being.

In this chapter we will explore the following heart aspects:

The healing power of love

The important distinction between feelings and emotions

The reason why the heart is the energetic center for the entire body

The mysterious function of the limbic system

The effect that sound and feeling tones have on our heart realm

The effect that our feeling realm has on the health of our immune system, respiratory system, circulation, and our physical heart

Techniques for clearing the heart of stuck emotions

The important connection between movement, sound, and breath

Techniques for a heart-centered meditation

How our minds and hearts can work together in the present moment to form an exceptional creative partnership

The Limbic System

Our system of sensory perception is so sensitive that we feel our feelings and emotions with every cell in our physical body. We have the innate ability to feel those feelings by utilizing the circuitry within our nerve system and the biochemical sensitivity inherent in our endocrine system. We feel through the combined effort of every nerve and organ in our body. We are born to feel.

The limbic system, which is a series of brain structures arranged in a circular pattern and located at the heart of our brain, is the center for our feelings and emotions. The limbic system also interfaces with our endocrine system by way of our brain chemistry, which means that any distortion in the delicate chemistry of our brain can cause an associated disturbance in our emotions and feelings. The reverse is also true: Emotional upset can cause a corresponding imbalance in the chemistry of our brain.

Imbalance in our emotional patterns, or brain chemistry, or the presence of structural misalignments (especially in the upper cervical vertebrae and cranial bones) can result in anxiety, depression, and a variety of emotionally based disorders.

Although drugs may be necessary to suppress and control these emotionally-based disorders, many people have had great success with the combination of nutrition, structural alignments, and emotionally based therapies aimed at changing their filters of perception. Suppressing emotions with drugs can only be a temporary solution, but changing our perspective and perception can have lifelong effects.

How can you move out negative emotions to better accommodate the healing power of love in your heart? You accomplish this by opening the channels to your heart.

The Healing Power of Love

Our hearts have an incredible capacity to probe the depths of our Being and to feel what is happening in us and in the world around us. With a little practice, we can sense what is occurring in the feeling realm of others as well. We can accomplish this by tuning into the tonal quality that a person carries in their heart.

Each person carries a predominant tonal quality that represents the sum total of their emotional experiences. It is the resonant frequency of this tone that ultimately determines our experience. These different frequencies explain why we feel good in the presence of some people, while others make us want to get as far away as possible. The tonal qualities speak volumes about who we are and what we are about.

We determine for ourselves what tonal qualities we carry. Unfortunately, it is rarely a conscious choice for many people. We may unconsciously carry the tone of a parent, friend, or loved one, or even remnants of a traumatic emotional experience. Because we are unaware, many of us carry these disruptive tones to the grave. The tones we carry color everything about the way we interact with the world. One of my goals for this chapter is to help you become more aware of your tonal quality and to help you make the kinds of shifts in tonal quality that will result in a greater engagement with and fulfillment in the world.

We can either embrace a tone that represents the perspective of love and joy, or we can embrace the spirit of complaint, anger, and resentment.

Posture of Heart

When we become stuck in an old perspective or posture of heart, it can impose the same limitations on us as our mental belief system. We see the world in a certain way because of our past experiences. If these experiences were hostile in nature, we try to protect ourselves from similar experiences by filtering our perception. Perceptions not only protect us, but they also change our view of the world. Unless we discard them, these filters stay with us forever.

I often use the example of a person wearing a pair of yellow sunglasses: they would swear that the world is yellow, and in a way, they would be right. If a person has had an abusive childhood for instance, they would view the world through that same obscuring filter of abuse. This filter often determines who they are (victim), how they perceive the world (unsafe), and even with whom they choose to be in relationship (perpetrator). In the same way, a posture of heart can keep a past experience in the present and enable a person to live in a limited, yellow world of their own creation.

This same person will no doubt complain that life is unfair, that they never get a break (victim), that the people they are associated with are abusive (perpetrator), and that the world really stinks (unsafe). Again, they would be right, but they are the ones who set up the parameters for their experience. They continue to write the script, audition the actors, and sit in the director's chair calling, "Lights, Camera, Reaction."

Our Inner Intelligence needs the constant input from our feeling realm to round out our human experience. Feelings open the heart to the intuitive influences of Spirit. But if the heart is occupied, or tied up in emotional reactions, there is no available space for the creative action of Spirit to move. There is no room in the inn, and Spirit passes us by. When open space is available in our hearts, we have the opportunity to receive the influence of Spirit in the present moment.

When our hearts are open, we begin to receive the qualities and characteristics of our Inner Being, and we begin to generate spiritual substance. As we become accustomed to creating this open space, spiritual substance begins to penetrate every level of our experience.

This same process is true of the mind. When the stillness of the mind is present and space is available to accommodate the nature of our Inner Being, the mind also generates its own spiritual substance.

When our mind and heart are in agreement, they begin to generate a collective substance that attracts new forms into our lives and brings a new level of experience.

This experience is exponential in nature, and joins the magnetic energy of the endocrine system (heart) with the intensified electrical energy of the nerve system (mind), and results in a body filled with vitality. This is the essential multidimensional experience of vibrant health.

When the fine line of separation between heart and mind begins to dissipate, and we begin to receive the awareness generated by the perspective of wholeness, a new level of conscious understanding opens to us. On the physical level, this translates into an improvement in the function of our endocrine system and an increase in the capacity of our nerve system as new pathways are created to accommodate the experience.

Feelings and Emotions

Many of us confuse feeling with emotion. I suggest that feelings are an essential part of the experience of human beings, but emotions are not. Let me explain. Feelings can be described as the quality of awareness that is present in our heart realm. This realm is designed to accommodate feelings written in the language of love.

Pure feelings of love are designed to fill our hearts. Although our feelings may include love for another person, the love of which I speak is the love between Great Spirit and human beings.

There is nothing on earth like this love. It is based on the experience of communing with our Inner Being and is centered in nonattachment.

As we let the feeling of love move through us in every dimension of our lives, we become unattached and free—free from the emotions that bind us, and free in the love that liberates us from an earthbound experience.

As it moves through us, the powerful force of love removes anything that stands in its way. The love of Great Spirit also creates its counterpart in the world of form by manifesting the perfect circumstances, events, and people in our lives.

Love brings out the best in human beings, and it provides healing for our bodies and souls.

Love creates additional space for the experience of Spirit. In the process, it expands our perspective and sharpens our perception. Love not only dissipates our experience of separation, which is ultimately the cause of all dis-ease, but it institutes a new experience of integration. This experience of integration fills us with the ways of Spirit and connects us with our true life purpose.

Carrying the feeling of love in our heart refreshes and revitalizes our life. This life-changing experience is reflected in our state of multidimensional health, our overall attitude, and the quality of our relationship with others. As an added bonus, this elevated experience of love also connects us to the principle of abundance. When we fully participate in the balanced expression of love and truth, we will also experience abundance in the outer world of form.

The power of love moving through our feeling realm creates an experience that is beyond our wildest imagination, as love is truly the creative gift of Spirit.

The power of love creates a feeling tone that resonates throughout our hearts, minds, and bodies, shaking loose anything that is not of the same quality and resonance.

Emotions, on the other hand, are a completely different story. The word "e-motion" represents energy in motion, and I'm sure we have all had the powerful experience of energy moving out of our heart realm. Emotions are powerful, and I believe they occur when the energy of feelings become attached to judgments from the mind.

The mind tries to explain and classify feelings in order to understand them and, in the process, creates a variety of emotions that become stuck in our heart realm and lodged in our bodies. When the mind judges a feeling as being either good or bad, it attaches that judgment to a free-flowing feeling, creating a more dense and sluggish emotion, often stopping it dead in the tracks of our heart.

It is really impossible for the mind to understand the feeling realm, as thoughts and feelings are two distinctly different animals.

This is not to say that one is better than the other, just uniquely different. The functions of mind and heart have a relationship to each other that is revealed when they share the same common denominator, which is Spirit. When the mind and heart don't share a common perspective, chaos and confusion usually prevail. When mind and heart realize that they are both important parts of the wholeness of Being, they begin to consciously complement each other in amazing and unique ways.

When emotions are present, it is usually evidence that we have become stuck in a perspective of the past. This perspective creates congestion in our heart and confusion in our mind, takes us out of the flow of the present moment and away from the creative perspective of wholeness. As emotions start to take up space in our heart realm, the powerful flow of love from spirit is often reduced to a trickle and the life-force in our body starts to shut down.

When we are angry, for instance, our heart is filled with the uncontrollable power of emotion, which can completely take over our identity. Instead of being aligned with our Inner Being, we are stuck with the identity and perspective of anger. We can rightfully feel anger, but it doesn't need to take over who we are.

In my opinion, this is the state in which most human beings currently find themselves: shut off from the free flow of love, and tossed around by the tumultuous tides of emotion. As our faithful servant, the body follows along, experiencing a relatively low level of function and manifesting a variety of symptoms and diseases related to this limited state of consciousness.

Instead of being the crowning glory of creation, we often find ourselves disconnected from the source of all life.

Your Feeling Tone

I have mentioned how tone plays an important role in the expression of our feelings and emotions, but that tone also relates to the frequency of the sounds that come out of our mouths. Some people are meek and barely emit a peep, while others hardly ever stop emitting sounds. Some people are confident, while other have been beaten down by their life experiences. These few examples represent a small portion of the multitude of feeling tones that fill the spectrum of human experience.

The tone we carry with us not only triggers responses from other people, but it triggers major responses inside of our own bodies.

The tonal quality that we carry with us is the major contributing factor to our health. Our systems, organs, tissues, and cells are so sensitive to this tone that they alter their function to comply with it.

We all take notice when someone uses a harsh tone of voice. This harsh tone is not only present in their voice, but resonates throughout their whole being. This feeling tone is usually evidence of an inner pool of stuck emotion that sends the same feeling tone into the world. It is this tone that actually attracts our future experiences.

If we utilize the full extent of our sensory equipment, we can usually determine if the nature of the tone a person carries is needy, greedy, angry, aggressive, aloof, or violent. Our sensory system, which includes our whole body awareness, can even detect feeling tones at a distance. When we are attuned to our Inner Intelligence, we can sense almost immediately what is headed our way and the appropriate action we need to take.

All human beings carry feeling tones. While our tone changes throughout the day, the underlying feeling tone usually remains the same. This feeling tone activates our body to function at a certain vibrational level, creates our overall life perspective, and attracts to us the people and circumstances that best suit this tone. Our feeling tone is a reflection of our true state of consciousness.

We all wonder why some people have it so easy, while others seem to run into one major obstacle after another. It could be bad luck, but I am suggesting that we actually create our own luck. We create our own circumstances through who we choose to be and the tone we choose to carry.

Of course, most of us don't choose our tone consciously. Chances are we learned it from someone else, beginning with our parents. They, in turn, most likely took their tone from their parents, added in their own successful or unsuccessful emotional experiences, and passed that new tone down to us. If our parents experienced a perspective of wholeness, they would likely have passed the beneficial results of that experience on to us. If they had an experience based on separation and disconnection, they would also pass down the results of that experience.

We receive their tone, adding in our own successful or failed experiences. We then plant the seeds of that collective experience, and pass them on to our children. This process is the recipe of tonal genetics and can determine the quality of experience for entire families.

Many times the tone that we carry is determined by an experience from which we have not been able to recover. For example, someone who has been abused carries the tone of abuse, which often attracts even more abuse. If we are unable to recover from a past event, we still carry that perspective and the accompanying tone with us, attracting more of the same. For a person to move on, they must choose not to continue in the same tonal pattern. They must clear out the stuck emotions and fill this reclaimed heart space with new experiences.

The Feeling Tone of Health

At any moment, we can assume the nature of our Inner Being, the place within us that was never abused, is always whole and complete, and always offers us the opportunity to embrace only love, regardless of our past or present circumstances. When we unite with the nature of our Inner Being, and let go of our past emotional experiences, we become whole and complete.

This may prove to be more difficult than it sounds, but it can be accomplished in this very instant. I have found that when people agonize over traumatic experiences for decades, they often anchor the problem even deeper into their identity. We become stuck with the perspective and the tone of a victim.

Tone is a powerful thing. It either paves the way for creative action and success, or it continually throws a monkey wrench into the works.

I'm sure we all know people with whom it is difficult to work and for whom nothing ever goes smoothly. They are always interfering with the natural rhythm of whatever they are involved in. And, as a result, they travel a very rocky road.

If we are honest with ourselves, sometimes we can observe how the tone we carry creates an attitude that interferes with the free flow of our own life. On these days, nothing seems to go smoothly. We don't realize that we can change that tone before it turns into a major problem, and we can carry the healing power of love instead. We may need to clear the air in order to make that change possible, but the process can be rather simple.

For example, check out the tone you carry in your workplace. Change the tone related to your work, and you will find that the experience of work changes along with it.

You may also find that you love to be around the healing tone or vibration of a certain person. Without either of you even knowing it, this person may be helping you to sound a new tone, one that helps you heal old emotional wounds. As you continue to sound this tone with your teacher/friend, you are really learning to sound that new tone for yourself. Eventually, you may even be able to offer this new healing tone to someone else.

Human beings can help each other by tuning each other to a higher level of function or frequency. Unfortunately, we can also tune each other down by assuming the tonal frequencies of a lower emotional state. In my service as a health care provider, many people come to me because of the tone I carry. I realized years ago that although people come for a physical tune-up, many of them were unconsciously needing to sound a healing tone with me as well. I realized that this was the real tune-up, and it made me much more aware of the tone that I carry, especially when I am working with others.

It became important for me to carry a tone of love and compassion, and to share it with those who came to see me, which was as helpful for me as it was for them. On days when I wasn't feeling physically well myself, whatever was bothering me usually disappeared within a few short hours of carrying a healing tone with my patients.

Human beings are extremely sensitive to electromagnetic frequency waves that are generated by the universe and by other human beings. This is why we are so beneficially effected by being in nature. Once we release the negative tone that we have been carrying, nature simply retunes our human instrument.

Clearing Your Heart Realm

How do you reclaim your stuck energy and embrace the connection with your Inner Being? First of all, you can recognize that stuck emotions are most likely present in your heart realm. This acknowledgment begins a process of purification in which you start to detach yourself from your emotions. After all, you are not your emotions. The first step is to realize that fact.

HEALTH TIP #1: Move Stuck Emotions

▪ Recognize Stuck Emotions

Emotional situations are usually present in your life for a good reason, and they provide you with the opportunity to clean up your emotional act. Try to observe them in yourself and see if you can identify who and what triggers them for you. Recognition is always the first step. Resisting, denying, blaming, or resenting the emotions only allows them to work more powerfully against you. When you recognize and observe your emotions, you are loudly proclaiming that you are not your emotions.

When you can observe your emotional imbalances, you can realize that you are the Being behind them. This recognition creates space between you and your emotions. You can stop feeding, maintaining, and caring for your unresolved emotions, and release them from your heart realm.

▪ Use Your Breath

Regardless of how you choose to move stuck energy, include the power of your breath (outlined in chapter 10) as an integral part of the clearing process. Bring your awareness to your breath, as it will reconnect you with your Inner Being. Anytime your vision and perspective become obscured by judgments or emotions, a few minutes of conscious breathing will usually create enough space in your heart and stillness in your mind for something new to occur. As you breathe, feel the energy course through your body, mind, and heart. Visualize your breath moving out the stuck energy. If the emotions are intense, intensify your breath. If emotions come up while breathing, release them with a strong exhale. Without judgment, express any associated sounds that come along with them.

▪ Move Stuck Energy

The emotional clearing techniques presented later in the chapter are effective in moving the stuck energy of emotions out of your heart, and in creating space for the healing power of love to take their place. Each of these techniques utilizes a combination of breath, sound, and movement as an integral part of the process.

The stuck energy of emotions will move out of the heart realm when you express the amount and intensity of energy that currently holds them in place. Powerful emotional experiences need powerful emotional releases. When this occurs, you can reclaim the space that these emotions have occupied.

Moving out stuck emotions can be as simple as recognizing when stuck emotions are present and taking responsibility for releasing them. Be sure to release your emotions by yourself or with a trained therapist. Do not direct them toward another person.

To release emotions, you can begin by lying on the floor in a comfortable position. Using your breath, create a strong breathing pattern. Your breathing can start out slow and deep, but it may need to build to the point where it can trigger stored emotions. Continue to build your breath until it completely fills your attention. The point will come when your breathing will release an emotional charge. At this point, use sounds to express the emotions in a strong and powerful release. You may find that movement, such as rocking, helps to make the emotional release more complete. Continue with your breathing, sound, and movement pattern until the emotional charge has dissipated. The process of emotional release is like letting a huge wave of energy pass through you. Let the wave move.

When the emotional charge has been released, new space is created in your heart realm. This internal work is as valuable as anything you can ever do for your health. The emotional release is often followed by a period of quiet and calm, which is the perfect opportunity for the healing power of love to fill your heart space.

▪ Fill this Cleared Heart Space with Love

Whenever any new heart space is created, the space should be filled as soon as possible with spiritual substance in order to reclaim it as your own.

In essence, you are reclaiming a part of yourself that has been tied up in past emotional experiences. It takes persistence to nurture and care for this fragile space and not refill it with similar emotions.

The heart-centered meditation on page 365 is a great way to fill this space. Step by step, reclaim another piece of your wholeness and fill it with the energy of love. Remove your identity from past events and move it into the present moment.

Emotional Clearing Techniques

There are many emotional release techniques that are effective in moving stuck emotions from your heart realm. In my experience, choosing to embrace the spirit of love and shifting to the perspective of wholeness is the most simple and effective technique. Occasionally, it is necessary to release deep-seated emotions, which can be done in a quiet space by yourself or in the presence of a trained facilitator or therapist. Taking responsibility for moving stuck emotional energy is essential for the success of this activity.

A wide variety of movements can help release emotions. Hitting a stack of pillows, batting a bed with a plastic bat, or stomping up and down like children during a tantrum may be necessary to release resurfacing emotions. This process must always be done in an appropriate, safe, private space with no interruptions. Movements such as rocking, shaking, or vibrating can help prime the pump for emotional release to occur quickly.

Have you ever noticed that children usually don't have much trouble releasing emotions? They just let them go in the moment. They will cry, yell, jump up and down, or throw a tantrum in order to release emotional energy. A moment later, they are back to laughing and singing. We can certainly learn a lot about emotions from our children.

I'm not suggesting that you throw a tantrum in front of your mother, or your boss for that matter. But observing how children express their emotions, and borrowing a few of their techniques, may prove to be very enlightening. Most children don't build up emotional blockages early in their lives because they constantly release them.

When our feelings begin to shut down, so do our breathing and movement patterns.

This pattern is clearly expressed by the autistic child who rocks back and forth in an effort to move stuck emotional energy. Movement patterns reflect the overall function of our body, mind, and emotional realm. Most of the time, we will be successful in moving and releasing stuck emotional energy by using a combination of movement, breath, and sound. When these three components are used individually, or creatively combined in a clear and focused way, the results can be transformational.

When we are clear about the intent of our actions, we can use almost any activity to help clear out emotional debris. The point of this entire activity is to reclaim emotional heart space and fill it with feelings of love and peace. This can also be accomplished through meditation, contemplation, prayer, breathing, singing in the shower or car, sounding or toning a particular note, chanting, yoga, integrated movement, dancing, walking, running, bicycling, playing tennis, or through almost any active physical activity.

Just for Fun

Here is a fun exercise that will physically demonstrate the process I have just described. Perhaps it will help clarify the overall picture. Place a clear glass or plastic container in your kitchen sink and fill it with a few inches of dry dirt from your yard or potting soil. Do not use big rocks or clumps of grass. Your mind may try to talk you out of this simple exercise, as it most likely will when you try to move your stuck emotions.

Fill the glass with water and note how cloudy and murky the water becomes from the dirt. In my experience, this resembles the state of one's heart realm when filled with stuck emotions. Try to get a clear impression of your relationships with others as you perceive them through such a muddle.

Now, let a steady stream of water flow from the tap and into the glass; let it overflow into the sink and run down the drain. The steady stream represents the spirit of love flowing into your heart realm. Let the water continue to flow into the glass.

Looking into the sink, you will see dirty water everywhere. Let the image go, and focus your energy on the endless stream of clear water from the tap. Note that the glass is not so filled with dirt anymore, but has begun to clear. The key to this process is to let the water continue to flow.

This is especially true when dealing with emotions. Let your breath and sound continue to flow. Feel the creative movement, and focus not on the dirt but on the clear flow of love from your Inner Being. As incomplete emotions depart down the drain, and the spirit of love continues to flow freely into your heart realm, you will create more space in your heart realm. Let this newly cleared space be filled with the joy and clarity of your Inner Self.

Soon enough, the water will be clear. Realize that even though you are responsible for your emotions, they are not you. When sufficient water has moved through the glass, the water will be clear enough to drink. Toast to your health and drink this elixir of life.

Toning

The use of sound is essential for attaining the depth of feeling necessary to complete the clearing process. At first, almost any sound will do. But as you refine the process, you will realize that certain tones and intensity of sounds are directly linked to your stuck emotions. Looking a little further, you can even detect specific areas of your body to which these emotions are connected. Let the sound reverberate through those areas of your body.

HEALTH TIP #2: Sounding the Tone

Let a tone sound from the depth of your feeling realm. Sound connected to your breath will move the logjam of emotions from your heart. Primitive sounds work really well, as emotions and feelings are directly related to your primal self.

Connect with your Inner Intelligence, as it will help you locate just the right tone, sound, note, and intensity associated with a particular emotional pattern. Be assured that you will likely have more than one emotional pattern. The sounding technique at the end of this chapter provides ample means of exploring the further use of sound. Eventually, you can create your own sounding or toning techniques.

Singing and toning are also great ways to move energy through your body on a regular basis. Singing by yourself or with others is a wonderful way to maintain a clear heart space. As they say, sing your heart out.

As you sound out the tones of your own song, stuck emotions will move out right along with them. If your voice is weak, cracks, or is shut down, this is a huge clue as to the location of the right note. The art of toning is to locate just the right tone, the one that resonates with your heart strings, and to sound it out as clearly as possible with all of your heart, not necessarily with all your might. Toning helps to establish your connection with Spirit, and it speaks the language of your Inner Self.

The seven notes of the musical scale are directly associated with the seven energy/endocrine centers of the body. Beginning at the base of the spine, the gonadal center is associated with the note C, the adrenals with D, the pancreas with E, the thymus with F, the thyroid with G, the pituitary with A, and the pineal gland with the note B.

When these notes are sounded, they will actually help to strengthen a weakened endocrine organ. For instance, if a thyroid weakness is present, sounding G on the musical scale will strengthen the thyroid gland, at least temporarily, and its associated teres minor muscle. This opens up myriad possibilities for healing, as specific healing tones are associated with specific areas of the body.

The thymus gland is the endocrine connection to our heart center, and is located at the core of the endocrine system. For that reason, the thymus gland and the immune system are usually the first areas of the body to show the ill effects of imbalanced emotions. Whenever we hold on to negative emotions, we can create an associated weakness in our thymus gland, which can in turn create weakness in our immune, cardiovascular, circulatory, and/or respiratory systems.

There are various techniques that use muscle testing to sort out emotional imbalances and to reveal the associated belief system. Resources for these connections are listed in appendix A. Sounding out our associated heart tone with feeling will go a long way in creating a new level of function in the body, as well as a new pattern of behavior.

Breathing

Breathing seems so simple and natural, but in reality it is something that very few people know how to do correctly. Most of us use only a fraction of our breathing capacity, which is often reflected in our level of health and well-being. Our inability to breathe is symbolic of the limited amount of inspiration we usually have in our lives.

Fully breathe in the breath of life, and fully breathe out a new level of experience.

HEALTH TIP #3: The Walking Breath

The Walking Breath is a simple technique that helps open up the breath and improves your physical and emotional health. This technique adds movement and sound to the art of breathing.

During each of your next seven steps, partially inhale until you reach full inhalation on the seventh step. Maintain a full breath for another step, and then slowly exhale over the course of the next seven steps. Maintain a full exhalation for one more step, and then begin the inhalation process again. Continue this breathing for several minutes.

Breathe the Walking Breath in a very slow and controlled manner while walking with focused intention. After you feel comfortable with the breath, sound can be added to help move stuck energy in the form of emotion.

Care should be taken to enlist your Inner Intelligence to guide you. Always use caution when exploring forceful breathing techniques, as hyperventilation can happen quickly.

Hyperventilation can be easily avoided by controlling the speed and intensity of both your inhalation and exhalation. With breathing, slow and steady wins the race. If hyperventilation feels imminent, slowly breathe in and out of a medium-size paper bag. This technique reduces the amount of oxygen that you inhale and will soon reduce the effects of hyperventilating.

HEALTH TIP #4: Heart-Centered Breathing

Breathing in and out of your heart center is another effective tool for clearing the heart of emotional clutter, and it can quickly change your perspective and your perception.

Sit comfortably with your eyes closed, and focus your attention on breathing in and out through your heart center, which is located in the middle of your chest. Allow your inhalation to carry peace into your heart. Release any chaos, ill feelings, or tension with your exhalation. As you breathe in, visualize the breath coming from every direction. Breath comes from the front of your body, the back, and the sides. As you become aware of this, you can eventually draw your breath from a 360-degree circle that surrounds your heart center.

Focus your intention to bring in feelings of love and peace with your inhale, and to release everything else with your exhale. Continue for several minutes, using a slow, steady, controlled breath until you experience a level of peace and tranquility. Pay particular attention to achieving an equal duration in both inhalation and exhalation, as this creates balance within your respiratory system and within in your ability to give and receive.

When the exercise is complete, spend a few moments appreciating the benefits of the experience and allow it to penetrate your heart center. Repeat the Heart-Centered Breathing technique as needed throughout the day to improve your level of peace, tranquility, and awareness. It is important to consciously choose the experience of peace and tranquility over anything else, especially if you are still prone to episodes of emotional upset.

There is no life without the breath. Breathing is the key to bringing the inspiration of Spirit into your body and into your life. According to Chinese medicine, chi, or life energy, enters the body through the lung meridian and connects us to the present moment.

Movement

Physical movement is another common way that people move stuck energy from their heart realms, and it can include almost any type of aerobic movement, including running, swimming, basketball, tennis, or soccer. If intense emotions are stuck in your heart realm, they will eventually come out during your play.

We may play enraged basketball, angry tennis, or even violent hockey. This is often seen in the professional ranks of organized sports. Emotional reactions from angry athletes often play an important role in their exceptional accomplishments, which makes it a very scary business.

Of all the aerobic-type exercises running, or playing an individual sport is often your best bet. Aerobic exercise intensifies our breath, which by itself can move emotions. Remember, the purpose of moving emotions is not to pin them on somebody else, but to create space in our heart realm for new experience. It is always important to take responsibility for resolving your own unfinished emotional business.

Other great possibilities for moving out the stuck energy of emotions include yoga postures, yogic breathing, hand-drumming, weight lifting (which can really push out emotions quickly), the energy exercises included in chapter 4, and dance, which is probably the best of the lot.

Unless you live in a remote area, you can usually find a variety of movement classes somewhere near your home, or you can work along with a video. A list of movement videos associated with moving stuck energy is included in appendix B. Your own free-form movement allows you to develop your own movement style, which can be utilized to trigger emotional release. Create your own way to move, breathe, and sound out your emotions. This process should be an integral part of any multidimensional health care program.

The sweet tone of Spirit that has been present in the background all along has been obscured by the raucous tone of our unresolved emotions.

When emotional blockages are cleared, and clear feelings begin to flow freely through your heart realm, there is less internal noise to obscure the underlying music of life.

This sweet tone, which is music to the ears of your body, mind, and heart, is the ultimate source of multidimensional health and well-being. Consciously receiving this tone into your life brings along with it the pleasant side effects of joy, happiness, and abundance.

As we express the qualities of our inner nature, we soon realize that we are the Being underneath our thoughts and feelings. We have thoughts and feelings, but we are not our thoughts or feelings. Feelings come to be experienced or expressed, and thoughts come to be acted upon or not.

HEALTH TIP #5: The Sounding Technique

This is a simple method for locating the areas of blocked energy in your body, using sound as a diagnostic tool. This exercise is best done standing, as it allows the diaphragm to move easily and your breath to be more effective in vibrating sounds throughout your body. This process can be done alone, but is much more fun when others are included. You don't need to be a good singer to perform this technique.

First, do some warm-up stretches and the Twisting Exercise from chapter 4. This will free up any kinks in your spine that may interfere with the process.

Stand with your eyes closed, and inhale from the tip of your toes to the top of your head using the Integrated Breathing Technique outlined in chapter 10 (page 311). Let your breath fill your entire body with life force, release the breath from the top of the head to the tip of the toes, and forcefully exhale while sounding the tone "Ah." Repeat this warm-up breath three times with the addition of sound.

You are now ready for the Sounding Technique. After you take in another full breath, begin to sound your lowest note, and quickly move up the tone scale until you reach your highest note. This is done quickly, in one breath, as the purpose is to explore the full range of your voice. Then, taking another breath, move from the high note back down to the lowest. Repeat this exercise several times until you get it right. Sound out your voice loud and clear.

In the process of sounding, you will discover an area within the range of your voice that is much weaker than the rest, where your voice may crack, break, or produce a sound that is discordant or sketchy. You may even find that you completely skip over several notes on the way up or down this sliding scale. Unless you are trying to hide the results, you can easily find specific areas of need.

Narrow your sound scale down to the most obvious area of need, and zero in on your most difficult note. This is the tone or note that your voice has the most difficulty expressing.

This also represents an area in your body in which you are unable to sound out a clear tone. In essence, this area represents a blind spot in your expression, your awareness, your perception, and your voice.

What can you do with this information? Continue to sound out this specific note as best you can, even though the sound is still unclear.

Try to locate the specific area of your body in which this sound resonates the most. This area is usually located in the chain of endocrine organs along the midline of your body. The associated area will correspond with the specific energy center related to the note. First, feel the note throughout your entire body, and then focus your total awareness on the related area.

Continue to sound out this tone. If you have a piano or other instrument, try to locate the exact note. This is the specific tone for you to sound out when you meditate, tone, chant, or sing. For now, it is also the area of your body to integrate when you consciously sound and breathe. Even a soft tone will send a clear new frequency of awareness throughout your body.

After a short time, perform the Sounding Technique again. You may notice another area in the sound spectrum that may now need your attention, or you may still need to focus on the original area. Don't be in a hurry to change the tone or to "fix" anything. Just let the tone sound, and let the rest of the process take care of itself.

Try to bring this new tone into your awareness and expression, and notice any changes that it may bring. Consciously integrate this new tone into your body, mind, and heart. Above all, have fun with the process.

It is important to recognize that this is a process of reclaiming a part of yourself.

HEALTH TIP #6: The Heart-Centered Meditation

First, let's do a warm-up.

In a comfortably seated position, begin to breathe in a natural and relaxed manner. Focus your inner awareness and intention on following your breath and on allowing feelings of ease and relaxation to penetrate your body, mind, and heart. With daily practice, you will spend less and less time training your conditioned mind to sit and stay, and more time experiencing peace and tranquility.

As you enter your inner realm, notice how quickly your breath changes. Notice how the possibility exists for your breath to breathe you. Allow the breath to be slowly inhaled up the front of your body until it reaches the crown of your head. Pause here for a moment, and then slowly exhale your breath down the back of your body until it reaches the tip of your coccyx at the base of your spine. Pause here for a moment, until the next inhalation begins the slow and steady journey up to the crown of your head. After several breaths, relax and let go of all instructions.

The heart center acts as a hub in balancing the energy from the other centers. If the heart is open and clear, the other centers tend to be open and clear. If the heart is congested with stuck emotions, the other centers will also become functionally impaired. Our heart center is the core of our experience as human beings, and the Heart-Centered Meditation emphasizes this fact.

Now, draw the next inhalation up from the base of your spine and down from the crown of your head, both at the same time. The breaths will meet in your heart center. Feel the energies as they mix together. Exhale from your heart center in a 360-degree circle that extends in all directions, just as you did during the Heart-Centered Breathing Exercise in health tip #4. Allow these two aspects of your breath to meet in your heart center, mix together, and fill your whole body with love, peace, and tranquility.

This breathing meditation integrates the two polarities of life, the feminine from the earth, and the masculine from the heavens, and joins together the yin and the yang aspects of your Being.

Your mind will be busy orchestrating the mechanics of this breathing technique, so remember to be the Presence behind the activity.

Incorporate a soft focus into the mechanics of the meditation. Focus on the details, but softly. After several complete cycles of breathing, let go of everything and experience an attitude of gratitude in your open heart. Be thankful with all of your heart.

🙂 EMBRACE ONLY LOVE

Identify with Love

And the Universe fills your sails

Embrace only Love

And the course that leads to your island paradise

Is laid out before you

Listen to the wind as it guides you

As your inner voice trims your sails

And reveals which stars to head for

On your journey home

Steady as she goes!

Chapter 13

Being Spirit

AS YOU CONTINUE to open your heart and quiet your mind, the realm of Spirit opens. This invisible realm is the most significant aspect in any model of health. Unequivocally, there is no real health without it. Spirit is the wellspring of life, the all that is, the quintessential essence of all creation, the one unifying force that aligns everyone and everything on planet Earth. It is the one consistent thread that unites all human beings—beyond race, color, country, or ethnicity—into one unified whole, one universe, which is beyond the mind and the heart. From this higher perspective, all human beings are one people.

Many of us get very confused about the whole topic of Spirit. We may have learned early on, through our religious traditions, to rely on others for our spiritual insight and experience. We may feel alienated by religious rules and rituals that seem to rob us of personal power. Although ancient customs and rituals can aid us in making a personal connection, it is our personal rituals and efforts that create an intimate connection with Spirit, which is unique for each person.

The experience of Spirit is like eating an ice cream cone: our direct participation is required to really enjoy the taste. Others can describe it, categorize it, or organize it for us, but in order to really know the nature of Spirit, we must taste it for ourselves.

Our perspective expands because of our unique connection with our higher Self, which happens when we create space for it in our lives.

Many people have a hard time dealing with invisible realms and often embrace the attitude that they can't believe it unless they can see it. This is especially true from the perspective of the scientific mind, which tries to use logic and reason to interpret reality. Unfortunately, the nature of the heart and Spirit lie beyond the ability of the mind to comprehend.

For us to directly tap into this realm, our minds and hearts need to relinquish control. When our minds and hearts stop contending with each other, and realize that they are truly complementary, our view of the world and our perspective of life will change dramatically.

When our minds and hearts surrender to the higher perspective and vision of Spirit, they speak with one voice.

From this higher perspective, the mind and heart are already complements, as seen in the yin-yang symbol. The male aspect of mind is the yang energy, and the female aspect of heart is yin in nature. Both are present throughout our bodies and the universe.

To achieve a larger perspective on the unique states of body, mind, and heart, we can take a look at the nature of water, which also manifests as three different states. On the gross level of physical form, water can be experienced as ice. Even though science has taught us that huge amounts of space exist between solid particles, we can compare our physical body to solid ice.

The state between solid ice and flowing water can be compared to the realm of the mind. Crystallized structures and conceptualized thoughts are integrated by the mind into a unique system of concepts and beliefs. Mind and body are intimately connected, and share a cause-and-effect relationship (body-mind), which often allows our mental powers to quickly manifest into form. With focused intention, the mind seems to exercise control over physical reality and can temporarily manipulate the realm of effects.

The more fluidity that is present in our mental concepts and beliefs, the more flexible and expansive our mind becomes. The more we allow thoughts and beliefs to flow freely through the mind without attaching who we are to them, the more available our minds become to accommodate the greatness of Spirit. The more fluid our minds, the more possible is the connection and merger with the next level of experience, the realm of the heart.

Water also exists in a fluid state that differs from crystalline structures and solid ice. Water flows from the clouds, forms rivers and streams, and ultimately becomes part of the vastness of our oceans. The fluid state of water represents the fluid state of our feeling realm.

Add heat, and the nature of water changes dramatically and becomes steam at the next level of experience, which directly relates to the realm of Spirit. Steam, which includes the evaporation of water, rises up from the earth to form clouds that return as rain in an endless cycle of renewal. Steam returns to earth as liquid, just as the essence of Spirit can pass through the fluid, open, heart realm of human beings.

In order for human beings to touch the realm of Spirit, a fundamental shift in perspective needs to occur.

When we are centered in our body and the gross level of physical form, we will primarily concern ourselves with external events and appearances, such as how we look, what shape our body is in, and how can we get more things to satisfy our desires. When our experience is centered at the level of physical form, most of our life force is consumed with getting more.

When we are too identified with our thoughts, we can become consumed by mental chatter. Our minds will always find problems to solve, and we become centered in our small self. On the other hand, a mind that is tempered by a higher perspective holds endless possibilities and illuminates the world.

As our hearts provide a direct link to our Inner Being, a heart cluttered with unresolved emotions stands as a roadblock to the gift of higher consciousness. In contrast, an open heart that yields to these higher impulses is a powerful force for change in the world.

As who we are becomes more conscious, our hearts continue to open, and our minds begins to illuminate and enliven our world and our bodies. This shift in identity is about making the essential shift from our small self to our large Self. Multi-dimensional health and well-being is a natural outgrowth of a life centered in the large Self.

Here, we no longer live in fear of disease. Instead, we understand the causes of true health, and we see the possibilities for striving in that direction. Making this essential shift in consciousness requires a flexible mind and an uncluttered heart, and a willingness to surrender to something higher than ourselves.

Our Inner Being patiently waits for this shift in consciousness to occur.

The Heart of the X

The following illustration represents the natural connection that exists between human beings and Spirit. This important connection is initiated and strengthened when spiritual substance (represented by steam) is generated by human beings in their daily living. Steam then forms into clouds, which rain down blessings on human beings.

When we are centered in an attitude of getting instead of giving, it not only keeps us away from Spirit, but it separates us from our gifts as well. The following drawing illustrates our true relationship to Spirit. As you can see, this requires a willing body, a peaceful mind, and an open heart, combined in an attitude of giving or surrender. In this posture, we breathe in the feminine essence from the earth, up through our feet, into our hearts, and out through our fingertips. As we surrender in this posture, the spiritual substance of connection rises up to fill our hearts with love and our minds with truth. This connection revitalizes our physical body. When we surrender ourselves to Spirit, we set ourselves up to receive blessings. The physical posture illustrated here embodies this principle.

The heart of the X, the place where the two lines cross, represents the heart center of human beings. This is the place where heaven and earth meet, the place where Spirit and matter join together in the human heart. X marks the spot for the true dwelling place of consciousness in human beings, where the duality of heaven and the earth join together in one living Being. This is where the mind and heart come together, and where the human joins Being.

Try the X posture and see firsthand how easily Spirit can flow through you.

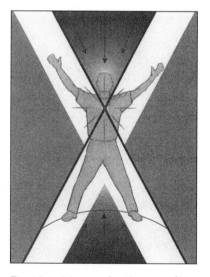

Fig. 13.1: Man at the Center of X

Stand with your arms and legs wide apart, forming the shape of an hourglass as illustrated, and fully extend your arms to the sky. As you fully extend your giving nature between the earth and the sky, the essence of Spirit enters the body, just as sand enters the base of an hourglass.

Hold this posture for a minute or two until this important connection is made, which can happen rather quickly. If it doesn't cause you any pain or discomfort in your neck, extend your head, face the sky, and close your eyes. To release the posture, lower your head back to center first, and then come back to a normal standing position. Feel the essence of Spirit coursing through your body.

Breathe energy in from the earth through your body, and out through your fingertips in the direction of the sky. As you exhale, receive the blessing of Spirit through your body, mind, and heart, and release it into the earth.

When our minds and hearts come together at the center of the X, the world of opposites merges into a world of wholeness.

From this new perspective, we perceive a world that is interdependent and interconnected.

There is no separation or competition between our minds and hearts, and no separation between Spirit and matter.

Energy and Matter Are One

When our minds and hearts agree to embrace a higher perspective, we can all simply live together at the center of the X. Remember Einstein's famous equation, $E=mc^2$? At the center of the X, "E" always equals mc^2, as energy and matter are one. This is more than metaphor. The body actually creates energy as electricity and manifests a corresponding magnetic field.

Electricity and magnetism can be measured by scientific instruments, and they are constantly generated from our heart, our brain, and each of our 100 quadrillion cells.

Surprisingly, our heart generates over one hundred times more electricity than our brains, and it has a magnetic field that is five thousand times stronger.

In contrast, the electromagnetic field of the earth is about one million times stronger than that of the human heart.

The electricity produced by the human body flows through established energy pathways in the nerve system and through energy pathways where there are no nerves. Energy flows through our tissues and cells in an energy bath that nurtures and heals our body.

Our entire body is electromagnetic in nature and represents the electrical nature of the male principle and the magnetic field of the feminine.

Bones are crystalline in nature and, along with tendons, connective tissue, and fascia, are specifically designed to conduct electricity in the body. Our cells generate electricity to communicate with each other, our bodies create electricity as a precursor to movement, and our brains generate electricity that can be measured as brain waves.

When we are in a meditative state, the production of theta and delta brain waves (associated with creativity, dreaming, and deep sleep) increases, along with the coherency of our brain wave patterns. This coherent energy pattern indicates an overall alignment of energy, which acts to renew and recharge our minds and enliven our bodies.

In the heart, feelings of love and compassion have also been shown to enhance our energy field, while feelings of anger and hatred create energetic interference. The nature of the emotions we embrace effect the quality of both the electrical energy produced by the heart and the resulting magnetic field that accompanies it.

Whichever mental state we embrace, whatever feeling or emotion we give into, whatever spirit we embrace as our own produces a corresponding electromagnetic state that is immediately shared with every tissue, organ, and cell in our body.

The nature of the subtle electromagnetic energy field that circulates and surrounds our human body is the underlying cause of both our health and dis-ease. When we intentionally connect to Spirit, our electromagnetic energy field connects our body to the same subtle energy fields that power the living universe.

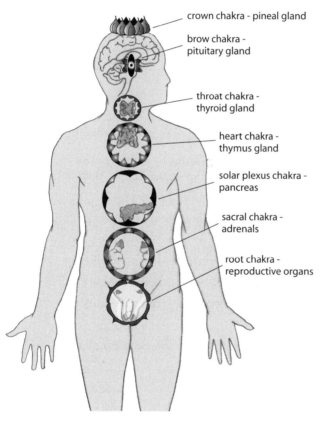

crown chakra - pineal gland

brow chakra -
pituitary gland

throat chakra -
thyroid gland

heart chakra -
thymus gland

solar plexus chakra -
pancreas

sacral chakra -
adrenals

root chakra -
reproductive organs

Fig. 13.2: Chakra Energy Centers/Endocrine Organs

Energy Centers of the Body

Spirit is energy, and the human body is all about circulating energy patterns. As a matter of fact, there are seven major energy centers aligned with our physical body that have Spirit at their source. These interconnected energy centers, called chakras, extend along the midline on both the front and back of the body. These energy centers directly correspond to specific endocrine organs.

It is no accident that our energy centers power our endocrine glands. If Spirit and matter are one, our energy centers and our endocrine organs are also one.

A connected nerve system plexus is also aligned with each energy center and corresponding endocrine organ. This major convergence of nerves functions together with one purpose, much like the solar plexus, which is the nerve center for our digestive system and an integral part of our feeling realm.

Each invisible energy center vibrates at a certain frequency pattern, which refers to the number of oscillations per second of an electromagnetic wave. The frequency of each chakra energy center is consistent with both the accompanying endocrine organ and nerve system plexus. The correlations continue to include a corresponding color, which is a vibrational frequency of light; a corresponding sound, which is represented by a specific tone for each energy center; a corresponding attitude, or associated mind-set; and a corresponding feeling tone.

Each energy center contributes to an elaborate energy field that flows throughout the human body, forming established energy pathways. Acupuncture meridians also represent the flow of energy in the body that are associated with these energy centers. Dr. Randolf Stone's version of energy flow in the body, as well as the energy flow of acupuncture meridians, are shown in the accompanying illustrations.

Corresponding Vibrational Frequencies

Energy flows of various kinds surround the human body and contribute to an energy field similar to a simple magnet and to the vast energy field that surrounds the earth.

These energy fields have been documented to exist in all living things.

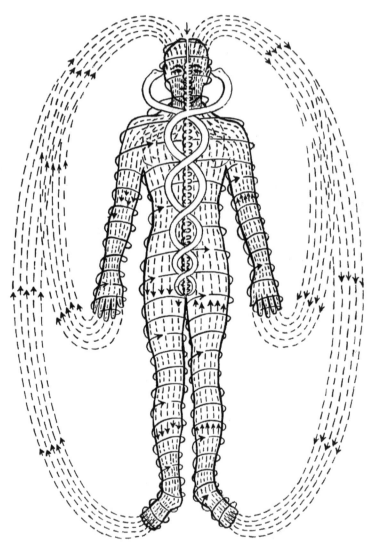

Fig. 13.3: Energy Flow Illustration

Chakra	Endo	Plexus	Attitude	Feeling	Color	Tone	Mineral	Vitamin	Element
Crown	Pineal	Cerebral	Wholeness Cortex	Joy	White	B	Light	Light	Light
Brow	Pituitary	Hypo-	Wisdom thalamus	Peace	Indigo	A	Manganese	E	Intent
Throat	Thyroid	Cervical	Courage	Hope	Blue	G	Iodine	A/B	Ether
Solar	Pancreas Plexus	Solar	Assurance	Confidence	Yellow	E	Chromium	B	Fire
Sacral	Adrenals	Sacral	Clarity	Tranquility	Orange	D	Potassium	C	Water
Coccygeal	Gonads	Coccyx	Creativity	Trust	Red	C	Magnesium	F	Earth

Fig. 13.4: Corresponding Frequency Chart

More and more subtle energy fields continue to be discovered in relationship to the earth and in relation to the human body. It is also suspected that energy fields connect all human beings together in an expanded matrix of super-refined energy, which in turn connects all of humanity into one unified, living Being.

Because of these energy pathways it is possible to tap into the energy field of another person and participate in hands-on healing. When the consciousness and intent of the healer and the healed are aligned, powerful changes can occur in these subtle energy fields, causing dramatic changes in the physical body.

Healing occurs when two or more people come into agreement within an energy field, which points to the healing axiom that subtle energy fields control the gross elements of physical form.

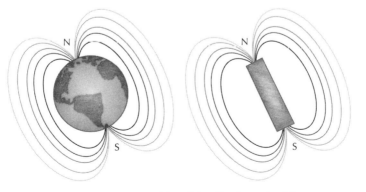

Fig. 13.5: Magnetic Fields of the Earth and a Magnet

Aligning Your Energy Centers

The Corresponding Frequency Chart displays the vibrational relationships that exist between energy centers, endocrine organs, nerve centers, notes on the musical scale, colors, attitudes and feelings, and essential nutrients and elements.

Just as subtle energy precedes gross physical form, the health of our subtle body predetermines the health of our physical one.

Subtle energy is a difficult topic for many human beings, as most people cannot see it and therefore doubt its existence. But through the technology of Kirlian photography, we have been able to photograph the subtle energy fields that surround the human body, as well as those that exist around trees and plants. The phantom leaf effect in Kirlian photography is an amazing condition in which the energy imprint of a leaf still persists energetically even after the leaf is removed. This same phantom effect is also true for human beings who experience pain in a limb after it has been removed.

Some people do have the ability to perceive subtle energy fields, and with practice, anyone can get a glimpse of this subtle reality. It is often possible to see the energy field surrounding the head of someone who is speaking, for instance, especially when they are standing against a light-colored wall with just the right lighting. This energy field of the body, or aura, is like the halo depicted in a painting of a religious icon. In reality, all human beings have an aura. When looking for a human aura, it is helpful to look a little off to one side, as seeing energy requires a different use of our vision. The more spiritual substance a person generates, the greater the intensity of their energy field.

Positive and Negative Attitudes and Emotions

Below is a list of positive and negative attitudes, feelings, and emotions. When we embrace these negative attitudes and emotions, we usually disconnect ourselves from the expansive perspective and guidance of our higher Self.

Fig. 13.6: Attitudes and Emotions Chart

Energy Center	Positive Attitude	Negative Attitude	Positive Feeling	Negative Feeling
Pineal	Wholeness	Separation	Joy	Sorrow
Pituitary	Wisdom	Short-sightedness	Peace	Frustration
Throat	Courage	Discourage-ment	Hope	Despair
Heart	Forgiveness	Blame	Love	Resentment
Solar Plexus	Assurance	Indecision	Confidence	Guilt
Adrenal	Clarity	Confusion	Tranquility	Anxiety
Gonadal	Creativity	Survival	Trust	Fear

Destructive attitudes and emotions reduce the effectiveness of our mental and emotional capacities and reduce the flow of life energy to our physical body.

Rising Spiritual Substance

When the light of universal Self enhances our vision, it expands our perspective and our experience. The light of Spirit illuminates our mind, brings love into our heart, and increases the level of health and vitality in our body.

Our spiritual substance rises up from our first energy center, enters the second energy center, and, as we embrace Spirit in our lives and consciously open up to the next level, we continue up the energy ladder.

Along with this rising energy, we experience a corresponding rising awareness, which includes our attitudes and feelings. The accompanying chart offers a perspective on the positive attitudes and feelings connected with each energy center and endocrine organ system. As we let this life-giving energy rise up our developmental ladder, our awareness will also continue to climb, and we will experience the side effects of these positive attitudes and feelings. If we allow negative emotions to get in our way, we can easily become stuck at its level.

If we exprcience recurring negative feelings or attitudes that are associated with a particular energy center, such as resentment or blame, look to the energy center to resolve the issue. Use sound, color, and movement to help open the pathways to that particular center.

HEALTH TIP #1: Sound Healing

Sound healing is a powerful tool for a human organism that has its foundations in the realm of vibration. The resonant system of sound, presented in chapter 1, shows how sound vibrations are transmitted to every part of our physical body.

Whatever tonal frequency we embrace, whatever sounds we express, whatever music we listen to, those tonal frequencies resonate through every cell, tissue, organ, and structure in our body. Sound vibrations vibrate our physical structures and actually change their cellular patterns.

Sound Awareness

We can become more aware of the sounds we express, what it is that we say, and the tone or context in which we say it. Our underlying tone is the essential part of our communication that lies behind the words.

We can pay attention to the type of music that we listen to, as music enters into our multidimensional core. Music has either a beneficial or detrimental effect on our health and well-being. Studies have shown that heavy metal, rap, and a host of other musical genres actually weaken our physical body, whereas classical music and soft rock strengthen it. If health is your priority, listen to what your body is saying about the nature of your music.

You can often advance your own health and well-being through sound. Experiment with the effects of sound by sounding the same notes that correspond to a specific energy center or endocrine organ in which you suspect problems. Use a piano or tuning fork as a guide to find just the right note. You will feel it. Trust me.

You can even create a sounding meditation in which you tone or sing each related note on the endocrine scale. Spend a minute sounding out each specific tone while you focus on the location of that energy center.

Color Your World

Vibrational healing includes many different techniques, with color healing ranking as one of the most powerful. Light, which is the core foundation of the human organism, comprises the essence of color healing. Color has a powerful effect on every system, organ, tissue, and cell in our body. Correlating colors to the organs of the endocrine system is of particular value.

The colors listed on the Vibrational Frequency Chart demonstrate the interrelationship of color to the endocrine organs and the chakra energy centers. These interrelationships represent extremely powerful pathways that can be utilized to create physical healing.

Many of us already use color therapy on a daily basis without even being conscious of it. Open your closet and take a look. If you are like most people, one color predominates. The dominant colors of the clothes you like to wear indicate the connection with the endocrine organ and chakra energy center to which you are most attuned. Depending on your current state of health, this color can also indicate the energy center and organ that needs your help.

Whether you realize it or not, the color of your car, the color that you paint your house, the colors you use to decorate your home indicate areas in which you naturally use the principles of color healing.

The way you dress each day usually reflects the colors you need to improve your current state of mind. It is no accident or coincidence that you choose the colors that your body needs the most.

Wearing colored glasses that correspond to the colors of the energy centers offers another way of introducing color therapy into your life. In my practice, my patients use a set of glasses for short periods of time to stimulate corresponding energy centers, endocrine organs, and related nerve system structures. Many people use colored sunglasses inadvertently as color therapy. The correct color glasses will make you feel better, give you more energy, and make you feel more alert. The proverbial rose-colored glasses often reduce stress and make you feel more at ease.

However, just as the right colored glasses will help to strengthen you, the wrong colored ones will make you weaker. You may discover that you have been wearing the sunglasses that are draining you of energy. It can be very enlightening to play around with color and become conscious of how your body responds to it.

HEALTH TIP #2: Color Healing

Check the right color for your own healing by utilizing the self-test on page 276 in chapter 9. This test can be used for myriad questions involving health and healing, and can be used to determine the appropriate color glasses as well as the specific color support that your body needs at this time.

Lighting is also an important aspect of color therapy. Natural light contains a full spectrum of color that contributes to our multidimensional health. An incomplete spectrum of light, which is the kind found in most types of lighting, can weaken the body, tire the mind, and frazzle the emotions. Bad lighting is depressing and drains your body of its vitality. Research has shown that children who attend school under fluorescent lights are more prone to have behavioral problems. Make sure that the lighting at your work place and at home supports your health and is of the full-spectrum variety.

HEALTH TIP #3: Check Your Breathing Patterns

Your breathing patterns can also be used as a tool to communicate with your Inner Intelligence. First, evaluate how deeply you are breathing at the moment and the level of ease with which you can take a breath. This will establish a normal baseline for your breathing. Now, try on a pair of colored sunglasses or ask your Inner Intelligence a question. Wait a moment or two for the body to respond, and then check again for the depth and ease of your breathing. It is amazing how significantly your breath can change in just a few moments. A positive response brings a deepening and sense of ease to your breath, while negative responses yield a more shallow breath with a bit more difficulty.

Anything that is beneficial to your health and well-being will expand your breathing capacity and increase the ease of breathing. Anything that is not beneficial to your health and well-being will contract your breathing, making it more shallow and difficult.

This breathing technique can be applied to a host of different multidimensional life situations. Just notice what happens to the body when it is exposed to different possibilities of experience. These changes in your breathing pattern will tell you exactly what you need to know in the present moment. Muscle self-testing can also be used for the same purpose.

HEALTH TIP #4: Affirm Your Health

The use of affirmations is another beneficial method of strengthening your energy centers and endocrine organs. Certain affirmations are associated with particular energy centers and act as a useful tool to change behavior, attitudes, and emotions when practiced on a daily basis. Affirmations need to be repeated several times in succession, several times throughout the day, in order to entrain your mind and heart to the possibility of having a different experience. The following affirmations relate to specific energy centers and endocrine organs. You can also create your own affirmations for specific needs and circumstances. Discover your purpose and intent, and create an affirmation that supports it. For example, if you want to improve your health, create an affirmation that you can use when you are tempted to eat junk food, such as "I eat the food that supports my health and well-being." Or, if you wish to work at a job that supports your beliefs and aids humanity, you could say, "I will create a job that supports the increase of consciousness in the world." Affirmations are more powerful then you can imagine when you mean them and send them off with the power of your feelings. Use them throughout the day to support your continued growth and movement.

Fig. 13.7: Energy Centers and Affirmations Chart

Energy Center	Affirmations
Pineal	I am whole and complete within myself.
	Joy, Beauty, and Harmony surround me and those in my world.
Pituitary	The Wisdom of Spirit guides my thoughts and feelings.
	I embrace the Peace and Harmony of Spirit in this moment.
Throat	I am Courageous in my expression of the truth.
	Living in a world that is guided by Spirit brings Hope for humanity.
Heart	I Forgive myself and others for all past wrong doings.
	I give myself the Love that I deserve.
	I breathe the Love of Spirit into my open heart.
Solar Plexus	I build Confidence in knowing the Will of Spirit.
	I am Assured that the light of Spirit guides my life.
Sacral	I experience Tranquility of mind as I surrender to my higher Self.
	I experience Peace on earth and extend good will to all men and women.
Gonadal	I Trust Spirit to bring Health and vitality to my body.
	I feel the Creative power of Spirit in every aspect of my life.

Pathway of the Ancients

Generating spiritual substance is the single most important factor in creating multidimensional health and spiritual awareness. This all-important connection to Spirit is strengthened or weakened in each moment, depending on what we choose to express. Embracing the positive attitudes and feelings that characterize our higher Self increases our spiritual substance, while expressing negative attitudes and emotions makes our connection with Spirit more distant.

Many of us have had the unfortunate experience of seeing this principle up close and personal. Whenever our emotions get the best of us, or whenever we embrace negative attitudes in relationship to ourselves or others, we dissipate our spiritual substance, making our connection to Spirit more tentative. This is not to say that we should avoid expressing our feelings and emotions, but we should avoid directing them toward ourselves or others.

A word of caution: Above all else, protect your spiritual substance, as it is your passport to the guidance, protection, and insight of Spirit.

Without this substance, we are devoid of the perspective and awareness that makes our life work easily and allows health to naturally manifest in our lives.

As surely as we can find ways to dissipate our spiritual substance, Spirit always gives us another opportunity to allow our energy to rise up and reestablish this precious connection. This rising up of energy is nothing new, as human beings have been aware of it for centuries. The process is represented by the ancient symbol of the caduceus, or the staff of Hermes. Hermes was a Greek god (called Mercury in the Roman tradition), the son of Jupiter and Maia. Mercury is the messenger with wings on his feet. He invented the lyre, which he traded to Apollo for the caduceus. The caduceus is a staff around which are two intertwined serpents, representing the male and female energies in the human body—separate yet entwined, rising up around a central staff.

The central staff in the accompanying illustration represents our spine, with the male and female energy ascending from both sides of the sacrum and surrounding the seven chakra energy centers.

The masculine and feminine energy of our life-force arise out of the sacrum, or sacred bone, entwine around each living energy center, and end in the pair of wings at the top of the staff. The wings represent the Presence of our higher Self.

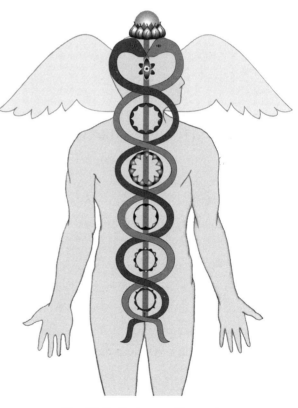

Fig. 13.8: Caduceus Illustration

Ideally, all seven energy centers of the body are embraced in the balance of male and female energies. These integrating energies unify the mind and heart, unite our left brain and right brain, and integrate the masculine and feminine energies that are present throughout our body.

The male and female energies represent the opposites of expansion and contraction, positive and negative electrical charges, electricity and magnetism, inspiration and expiration, the lub and dub of our heartbeat, and the union of the visible earth and the invisible heaven. These seemingly separate energies are the principle forces that unite human beings in the experience of wholeness.

As the serpents symbolize the union of the ascending male and female energies, the central staff of the spinal cord represents the pathway of energy from above descending into our bodies. This important connection manifests when our energy rises through the ascending chakra energy centers, and returns back to us in the form of a new perspective and a new level of awareness.

The energy pathways suggested by the caduceus bring with them an understanding of how energy moves as it brings health and healing to our body, mind, and heart.

HEALTH TIP #5: The Caduceus Meditation

One way that we can consciously integrate the role of the masculine and feminine energies into our lives is by performing this simple meditation.

1. Sit up straight and tall using a straight-back chair, or sit with your legs folded beneath you. Be sure that your spine is in proper alignment with gravity, as this allows your body to conduct energy through the spine more effectively.

2. With an inspiration breath, visualize the dual energies rising up out of your sacrum, one on either side, and surrounding each energy center as your breath rises. Initially, you may only be able to encompass one or two energy centers with one inspiration breath, but with time and practice, this will change. Use the illustration of the caduceus to visualize the process.

Initially, bring these dual energies up into your heart center. Eventually your inspiration will lead you all the way to the crown of your head. You need not worry about crossing the energies, so concentrate more on feeling each center being bathed in the balanced energy of the masculine and feminine.

As you bring your awareness up through each energy center, you may notice different feelings associated with particular energy/endocrine centers. Your breath may move more easily through some, while others may take more time and effort. After the meditation, you may wish to familiarize yourself with the attitudes and emotions associated with the more difficult ones.

When your breath moves the twin energies up to the top of your head, simply let go of your breath, and let it descend the central core of your spine back into your sacrum, through your legs and feet, and into the earth. Let the energies move up with your inhalation and descend back down with your exhalation. Let the energies move and circulate. Direct the caduceus meditation for several minutes, and then release all instruction, letting your mind rest in meditation for 10–20 minutes.

When the meditation is complete, you most likely will recognize the following truths:

You are more connected with your source.

Love is abundant in your heart and your mind is peaceful.

There is increased awareness and activity in each energy center.

Your body is supercharged with life-force energy.

The world within you and the world around you have shifted dramatically.

Your awareness has changed, and who you are is noticing this awareness.

Perform the meditation on a regular basis to integrate your energy centers, your endocrine system, and your masculine and feminine energies with the essence of universal Spirit.

The "I Am" of Spirit

As you become more familiar with the chakra energy centers, you may notice that you feel more attracted to the qualities of one particular center.

Your language, your desires or passions, your interests, and the way you spend your time and energy usually indicate the energy center with which you identify the most.

There is no reason to judge the energy center, as all energy centers are equally important in the overall scheme of things. As you let your perspective ascend to your crown, it will activate all of your energy centers and bring with it the awareness of the "I Am."

All of us have the opportunity to be centered in the "I Am" identity in the present moment, and to let that identity fill our body, mind, and heart. When most human beings use the "I Am," it is in relationship to the external world. I am smart, good-looking, fat, short, angry, etc. Even the perspective of "I am healthy or happy" shows a connection to a somewhat limited perspective. "I Am" simply is, and needs no qualifier to explain it.

If we find ourselves more aligned with the three lower chakras, which are centered in our small self, we become overly identified with what we want or need. The worldview or vision from these lower chakras is also limited, as is the amount of spiritual substance we have generated. The amount of spiritual substance generated is directly associated with our perspective and our perception of the outside world.

As we rise up in our level of growth and development, we begin to embrace a higher level of awareness, and our vision expands as we gain altitude. The more light we generate in the form of spiritual substance, the higher up the totem pole we rise, and the better vantage point we have from which to see the world. As we continue to generate spiritual substance, our identity naturally elevates to our heart center, the gateway to the realm of Spirit.

Our open heart provides an open door to the upper energy centers and marks the transition from an external to an internal perspective. Our open heart transforms the world of human nature into a world blessed by the divine.

Each energy center represents a particular perspective, contains a corresponding perception, and produces a related experience.

Our Seven Multidimensional Energy Centers

The first energy center relates to the physical body, the second to the lower aspects of the mind or ego, the third to the power of will, the fourth to an open heart, the fifth center relates to the expression of life-force, the sixth center relates to the higher elements of truth, and the seventh center relates to the full spectrum of love and light. The seven energy centers can be seen as stages of development into which we have the full capacity to grow, and they represent expanding states of consciousness.

But how do we build spiritual substance? By consciously choosing to do so in every moment.

HEALTH TIP #6: Restore a Sense of the Sacred

▦ Physical

You can build spiritual substance in your physical body by embracing the perspectives presented throughout this book and by following the structural and biochemical guidelines. Become aware of what is going on in your body.

▦ Mental

Allow your mind to stop acting as if it were God. In order for the mind to be a point of illumination, it must first yield to the inner essence of your Being and allow a complementary relationship to exist between your mind and heart. Here, masculine and feminine energies consciously come together as one.

Until your mind and heart become aligned, sharing a higher perspective becomes as limited as the opportunity to build your health and well-being. A cooperative mind and heart brings understanding and insight into your life and into the lives of others.

When humility is present in the mind, the physical body becomes charged with vitality.

When love fills the human heart, and humility is present in the mind, the physical body becomes charged with vitality.

▦ Emotional

Allow your heart to become open to a connection with your Source, and clear out emotional blocks that occupy your heart space.

Learn how to clear your heart of emotional debris (chapter 12), and create space for the powerful feelings that originate from your higher Self.

Shift your orientation from one of reacting to external events to one of acting from internal guidance.

Practice bringing love into your heart for the benefit of yourself and others.

■ Spiritual

Create space for something higher in your life. This can be done by practicing meditation or prayer first thing in the morning and, if possible, the last thing each evening, regardless of your life circumstances.

Meditation acts like a generator for producing spiritual substance.

The right form of prayer generates spiritual substance, especially when it is not self-centered in its approach.

Recognize that you are an integral part of Spirit. Instead of perceiving Spirit or higher Self as something separate from you, shift your perspective and end the false distinctions. Separation is the cause of all suffering. Use affirmations to remind yourself that all healing originates from this valuable connection, and be aware of the spirit that you consistently express in your relationships.

Be present in your integrity. Living with integrity rapidly builds spiritual substance and health. As you build your integrity and do your very best to bring it into every aspect of your life, you bring change to both your external and internal worlds.

Consistently build spiritual substance by connecting with the essence of Spirit, in your own way, everyday. Yielding or surrendering yourself to this essence creates the necessary polarity for co-creation, which is the most powerful experience available to human beings.

Nurture the rising feminine energy in yourself and in your world. The creative aspect of the feminine, which is present in us all, grows more powerful in the world each day and holds the solution to many of the problems of mankind. Align yourself with this incredible rising power, and you create a direct pathway to Spirit. Once you get in touch with your own feminine energies, you can consciously begin to blend the power of the feminine with your enlightened masculine. The symbol of yin and yang acts as a model for these two complementary energies. Whenever you bring the energy of earth and heaven (the divine feminine and masculine) together in yourself, the power of Spirit rushes to be in their midst.

Restore the sense of the sacred. Let sacredness spread from your heart realm into all of your relationships, through to your family, out to your tribe and clan, and toward all of humanity. When a sense of the sacred is present in our bodies, minds, and hearts, the powerful essence of love will expand into the earth.

Another practical way of creating spiritual substance is to create a sacred space or altar in your home. An altar is the symbol of your intent to include something higher in your life. It should be created in a private space, away from public view.

An altar is a place where you meditate, pray, put your intentions out to the universe, and generate the substance necessary to heal yourself and others. An altar can consist of a small, simple space or an elaborate one, depending upon your purpose and accommodations. On it you can place the sacred things that represent what is most important to you.

An altar represents a part of yourself that you make consciously available to Spirit. Whatever it is that you value, whatever you hold to be important, whatever you hold to be sacred and true can be represented on your altar. You can burn incense as an offering, or light candles, which symbolize the increase of light in your world. Perhaps you will place statues or figurines on your altar, which can represent the integration of the principles of the female and male. Or you might choose to include pictures of those you love and cherish. Whatever you hold sacred in your life can be honored and reinforced on your altar.

The altar also represents your purpose, intention, and plan to co-create your multidimensional health and well-being. It provides a focal point for implementing changes in your life, which can alter both your direction and your experience.

Use spoken affirmations at your altar to empower your intent. You enliven your affirmations with your spiritual substance and send them on their way with the power of your feelings. Affirmations put your energy in motion.

You want to create meaningful affirmations that engender the power of your Inner Being. Use these affirmations to generate richness and power in your life, as they are often precursors to success. There is no right or wrong way in any of these matters, as whatever level of sacredness and purpose you wish to create in your life is totally up to you.

You can create your own rituals and attach your own importance to any event. You can pray by yourself, affirm with another or with a group. Relationships are usually strengthened and empowered by a sense of sacredness, especially when you begin each day together at your altar. The Bible affirms this theme in a lovely sentence: "Whenever two or more gather in my name, there I am in the midst of them." Ultimately, your altar will help you create a better world for yourself and others.

Creating the Reality of Wholeness

As we become more conscious of what we create with our substance, we can begin to create a better world for ourselves and others. We can begin to withdraw from a world that is based on the principles of fragmentation and separation, and move into a world that has its basis in wholeness.

We can begin to change our worldview from one of exclusiveness to one of inclusiveness. We can choose to live in a world of complementation, not competition. We can move out of the world of my, me, and mine, and into a world where each person contributes an important part to the whole, which is much greater than the parts alone could ever be.

When the higher power of Spirit becomes a partner, we find that the energies of mind and heart are entwined in a powerful dance of life in which the "I Am" is present in their midst. As equal partners, the divine male and female energies combine together into the perfect combination of creativity and action. Together, these energies elevate you into a new realm.

When we embrace a perspective of wholeness, we open up to something greater than ourselves. In essence, we willingly surrender to the will of something higher, which brings in return the side effects of health and happiness. When the mind yields to the Source of its power, it receives wisdom in return, and when our hearts surrender to this same Source, we become filled with the creative power of love. In this state of wholeness, we can truly be in the place of the "I Am," where wonder and beauty and abundant health reside.

Conclusion

The three phases in the process of creating multidimensional health can be described by following the three Rs: reclaim, renew, and restore.

Reclaim

First, you must reclaim your true identity, which requires a shift from your small self to your large Self. In the process, you reclaim your birthright and illustrious heritage, which is based in the value of Spirit.

You can also reclaim your sense of the sacred, establish a new benchmark for your integrity, and begin to reclaim your sense of humility and innocence. From the vantage point of your higher Self, innocence is present in someone who brings a fresh impression to the world, where all things are made new.

Consciously reclaim your health, happiness, and well-being. Under the guidance and direction of Spirit, you can align your life with your highest intentions.

Renew

The second step in the process of creating multidimensional health and well-being is based on the principle of renewal. Renew your commitment and connection with your Source on a daily basis, which is best accomplished in the morning and the evening.

Renew your connection with your rising feminine energy, both inside and outside of yourself. The feminine principle, which has been largely disregarded in the external world, actually provides the basis for the right action of the enlightened masculine. For heaven and earth to be one in your own experience, acknowledge, protect, and embrace the divine feminine as the natural starting point for every creative action.

Once you renew your connection to the sacred feminine, you can begin to resurrect the consciousness of the enlightened male. This creative process is true for both men and women. The power of the divine feminine always proceeds the action of the enlightened masculine.

Using these fundamental truths, you can renew your commitment to create health in your body, peace in your mind, and love in your heart.

Restore

Revitalize your body, mind, and heart by using the restorative principles and practices presented in this chapter. Let your Inner Intelligence teach you how to become more aware of the stumbling blocks in your life that keep you from experiencing multidimensional health. Begin to see through the veil of your own experience, and restore your ability to re-create your health.

As you continue in the process of aligning yourself with the Source of your Being, use the light generated from additional spiritual substance to perceive the truth for yourself. Restore your spiritual connection, be conscious of your actions, and be responsible for their consequences. Restore the balance in your life in as many areas as possible, and, above all, restore your health by doing things that produce health.

This formula begins in being, continues with renewing, and ends by doing.

Conclusion

THROUGHOUT *Health Is Simple* I have stressed the importance of creating multidimensional awareness, which will lead us to the experience of vibrant physical health, and mental and emotional well-being.

The physical body is truly a miracle to behold, and we learn more about it and the cosmos every year. It is our faithful servant, serving up the physical counterpart of what we create in our lives on a daily basis. The state of our physical body, for the most part, reflects our mental, emotional, and spiritual state of awareness.

Throughout this text I have provided an abundance of tools on both the structural and biochemical levels, which can support and increase your physical health.

These tools help to create structural alignment through posture, movement, and exercise. As a chiropractor I am acutely aware of the importance that attaining and maintaining structural alignment has on the function of the central nerve system. Chiropractic provides an amazing vision of health that is unparalleled in the health care field today. I highly recommend seeking out chiropractic assistance to help maintain a state of balance in your structural health.

Cranial work, which uses your body's own internal rhythm to align the structures of skull and sacrum, is also an important tool in achieving structural balance. The subtle energies that reside within the physical body respond amazingly well to the gentle touch of a qualified cranial sacral practitioner.

All of us at one time or another need the help of healing practitioners. When you listen to your Inner Wisdom, it will let you know when that time has arrived. Let your Inner Wisdom guide you in finding the right practitioners to assist you. Let your Inner Wisdom guide you in all things!

I have stressed the biochemical importance of the endocrine system, and how it functions as the key to the organ systems in the body. Endocrine organs literally control all biochemical functions.

In order to experience vibrant physical health, you must discover your own biochemical weaknesses and the appropriate means to strengthen them. Many of the tools I have presented throughout these pages will be sufficient for most of you. Those who have more serious health problems will likely need the assistance of a holistically oriented chiropractor or other health professional who perceives the benefit of a multidimensional approach to health.

I have also included a host of self-help tools to assist you in balancing your biochemical health. These include a variety of reflex points that will help you determine and strengthen areas of weakness in your body. These points will help to confirm areas of need and assist your body in your healing process.

Obviously, nutrition plays a huge part in balancing biochemistry in the body. I have included several diet and cleansing possibilities in chapters 7 and 8. Use your intuition and awareness to determine which course of action is right for you at any one particular time. Implement a particular strategy, and then listen for the feedback from the Intelligence of your body. Your Inner Intelligence will always let you know exactly what it thinks about your actions.

In order to express ourselves in the mental realm, we all have created a system of beliefs that reflect our current worldview. Try to be as flexible and unattached to these beliefs as possible, and allow them to change as you do. As you become more aware of their limitations, you can let an expanded truth replace an old belief. As we remain humble and thankful for what we already have, and who we are in the present moment, we can make great strides in expanding our view of the world.

Aligning your perspective with the principles that are already guiding the universe will expand your mind beyond the small view held by the small self. This mental shift from small, self-centered self to the large Self, guided by universal Spirit, can be absolutely life-changing.

What we carry in our hearts is also a vital component in creating health. If our hearts are filled with the remnants of failed emotional experiences, we will have no room for anything magnificent to occur.

As we clear out incomplete emotions that still manage to color our experience, and allow our hearts to be filled instead with feelings of love and joy, we will make the essential shift in our feeling realm that brings with it the side effects of health. This process in itself is the best thing you can ever do for your health and well-being. Forgive old emotional debts and replace them with an attitude of gratitude for the things that you have now, and for everything that brought you to this point of change in your life. Remember: Whatever we focus our attention on, expands. Do you want to carry the frustration and unhappiness of past events with you for the rest of your life, or do you want to take advantage of the fresh start that is being offered to you in this present moment?

Throughout the text I have shared my current understanding of the realm of Spirit. Hopefully, it will provide some insight and understanding. Until we realize that we create our own reality, Spirit will have very little practical value. Embrace this power and responsibility with all your heart as you continue to build spiritual substance, and you will perceive more and more of the true nature of reality.

I have also emphasized the tremendous healing effects that movement, breath, sound, and light have on our multidimensional being. Take advantage of these powerful tools in your daily life. Movement is a sign of life. Keep finding new and creative ways to move your body, as movement clears out the cobwebs of your mind and stuck emotional energy from your body.

Whenever you become stuck in an old perspective, movement provides a level of healing that can be exponential in nature. Use your Internal Wisdom to introduce creative combinations of these essential healing elements into your life on a regular basis. Remember to include breath, sound, and light.

Movement creates new nerve system pathways in your body. The power of your breath quiets your mind. Using sound vibrates emotional tones that retune your heart strings, and the power of light activates the entire spectrum of your life energy.

Use these elements of nature to reset and retune your human instrument to the resonant frequency of life. Use the tools of movement, breath, sound, and light to bring the spirit of health more tangibly into your life. These elements of nature will energize your body, enlighten your mind, and enrich your heart. These are the tools of Spirit that connect human beings to the power of their sacred heritage.

Finally, remember that you are the one who orchestrates your own health care program by aligning yourself with the wisdom of your Inner Intelligence. This Intelligence is of the same basic nature as the universe, which acts upon the energy, intentions, feelings, and beliefs that you set in motion. A friend of mine once counseled me by saying, "If you don't like what your getting, check out what you are giving."

Become aware of the raw materials that you are providing the Universe to create your life. Become aware of the effect that your beliefs, intentions, emotions, and the spirit have on your current experience. Realize that you are in charge of what you are sending out into the world, and what it is that will return. Even though your physical body may have some limitations, your Inner Intelligence has none.

You have the ability to create a multidimensional level of awareness that brings a multidimensional level of health and well-being. Become aware that your Inner Intelligence *is* Spirit working through you, and that you can bring peace and harmony to your own world. You have the ability to co-create a vibrantly healthy world for yourself and for those around you. When you completely surrender yourself to the wisdom of your Inner Being, you literally become the cause of your own health.

Resources for Treatments and Products

Appendix A Resources for Chapter 3

Resources for Finding a Chiropractor

International Chiropractic Association:
www.chiropractic.org or 800-423-4690

Applied Kinesiology: www.icak.com (click on
"Find an AK Doctor")

American Chiropractic Association:
www.amerchiro.org or 703-276-8800

National Board of Chiropractic Examiners:
www.nbce.org

For local information, search online for specific
chiropractic state associations. For example: Colorado Chiropractic Association

Benefit from word of mouth. Ask people you
know who are currently receiving the benefits of
chiropractic care about their doctor(s).

Resources for Finding Osteopathic Cranial Practitioners

The Cranial Academy:
www.cranialacademy.com (click on
"Practitioners")

Recommended Nutritional Supplements and Suppliers

Note: Do not take B vitamins after noon.

Standard Process Labs: Visit www.standard-process.com for information about products and
how to order from a health professional near you.
There are also several other web sites that offer
Standard Process products. Try searching "Standard Process Labs" for other ordering options.

Vitamin, Mineral & EFA Supplements:
Catalyn/1–3x day, Organically Bound
Minerals/1–3x day, Allorganic Trace Minerals/1–3x day

Cataplex B/2–3x day, Cataplex G/1–3x day

Cataplex C, Cataplex ACP/3, 3x day

Tuna Omega-3/2–4 per day

RNA Supplements:
Ribonucleic Acid (RNA)/1–3x day, Ginkgo
Synergy/2–2x day

Biotics Research Corp.: Visit www.bioticsresearch.com for product and professional contact
information. For other ordering options, search
for "Biotics Research Corp."

Vitamin, Mineral & EFA Supplements:
Bio-Multi Plus/1–2x day, Multi-Mins/1–2, 3x
day

Bio B 100/2–2x day, Bio BBB-G/2 3x day, Bio
GGG-B/ 2–3x day

Optimal EFAs capsules/1–3 3x day

RNA Supplements:
Nuclezyme-Forte/1–3x day

Nutri West: Visit www.nutriwest.com for product
and professional contact information. Search
"Nutri West" for other ordering options.

EFA Supplements:
Complete Omega-3 Essentials/2–4 per day
Complete Children's DHA/EPA/ 2–4
capsules per day

RNA Supplements:
Total Brain/1–2x day, RNA-DNA Plus/1–2,
3x day

New Chapter, Inc.: A good source for multiple
vitamin/mineral combination formulas. Go to
www.newchapter.com for product and ordering
information. You can also search "New Chapter
Vitamins" for other ordering options or find them
in your local health food store.

Vitamin & Mineral Supplements:
Unbounded Energy Multiple
vitamin/mineral/3 per day
Coenzyme B Food Complex/2 per day
C Food Complex/1 per day

The Synergy Company: Visit www.synergy-co.com for ordering and information, or call 800-723-0277.

Slant Boards

Slant boards can be found online at www.juicing .com/slant1.htm.

Appendix A Resources for Chapter 4
Sources for Lumbar Sitting Cushions

Improvements:
wwwimprovementscatalog.com
Type in "Ortho wedge Seat Cushion"
or call 800-642-2112.
Brookstone: www.brookstone.com or call
866-576-7337 and ask about Ergonomic
Seat Cushions.

Feldenkrais Resources

For books, audio, and video products and practitioners west of the Mississippi:
www.feldenkraisresources.com or
800-765-1907
For classes, workshops, and practitioners east of the Mississippi: Feldenkrais Institute of New York:
feldenkraisinstitute.com or 212-727-1014

Sticky Mat Distributors

Hugger Mugger: huggermugger.com or 800-473-4888; Yoga Tapas Mats in a variety of colors
Gaiam Living Arts: www.gaiammindbody.com
(click on "Yoga Tools") or 877-989-6321

Appendix A Resources for Chapter 5

Note: Please see *Appendix A Resources for Chapter 3* for supplier and ordering information for products from Standard Process, Biotics, Nutri West, New Chapter, and Synergy.

Nutritional Products That Help to Balance pH

Standard Process Labs: SP Green Food/2–3x
day; SP Cleanse/5–3x day w/meals for
short term; Cruciferous Complete/2, 2x
day; Chlorophyll Complex/2–3x day
Biotics Research Inc.: Chlorella Caps/5–8
capsules per day
The Synergy Company: Pure Synergy/1 TBS
day
New Chapter Inc.: Broccolive/1 per day

Nutri West: Total Veggie/1–2, 3x day
GreensPlus: Greens Plus Superfood/2–3 tsp
day; greensplus.com
Premier Research Labs: pH Powder,
Quantum/ as directed; www.prlabs.com
or 800-325-7734

Sources for Whole Food Vitamin/Mineral Formulas

Standard Process Labs: Catalyn/1–3x day;
SP Complete powder/2 TBS per day;
Cyrofood/4 tablets per meal/powder/
2 TBS per day
New Chapter Inc.: Every Man II/2–3x day;
Every Woman II/2–3x day; Only One/
1 per day
Biotics Research Inc.: Bio Multi Plus/2–3x
day for 30 days/then 1–2x day thereafter
Nutri West: Core Level Health Reserve/
1–2x day

Breakfast Drink Recipe

The breakfast drink includes a low potency, full spectrum, whole foods multiple vitamin and mineral powder; high quality bone meal powder for healthy bones, teeth, ligaments, and tendons; high quality mineral whey protein powder; an essential amino acid powder; nutrition for healthy arteries and veins; a source of whole food B-complex vitamins; vitamin E complex; kefir culture, a great source of pH-balancing chlorophyll; fiber; essential fatty acids such as flax seed oil; and the benefits of fresh fruit, all rolled into one simple drink. I include all of the fixings here, which you may wish to modify according to your needs.

In a blender, mix the following ingredients:
Fresh and/or frozen fruit, such as a banana,
blueberries, etc.
Fruit juice: 8 oz. of dilute non-citrus juice as a
base, or purified water
SP Complete: a full spectrum multiple
vitamin/mineral, available from Standard
Process Labs
Calcifood Powder: bone meal, available from
Standard Process Labs

Capra Mineral Whey: available from Bernard Jensen Intl. (other whey products are much less desirable)

Amino Charge: amino acid powder available from Life Force International

Lecithin granules: Assist in emulsifying fats, available at health food stores

Nutritional yeast: natural source of B vitamins, available at health food stores

Unprocessed raw wheat germ: source of vitamin E complex, available at health food stores

Green food supplement: spirulina, available at health food stores (recommended: Pure Synergy, available from the Synergy Company at www.synergy-co.com)

Flax seed meal: Bob's is best and available at health food stores

Flaxseed oil: Barlean's is best and is available at health food stores

Wheat germ oil: helpful when spinal problems return; it needs to be refrigerated and is available at health food stores

Rice bran syrup: excellent source of B vitamins; try Rice Bran Complex from Bernard Jensen Intl.

A handful of raw almonds: available at health food stores

Products Available From: The Synergy Company (www.synergy–co.com; 800-723-0277), Bernard Jensen International (www.bernardjensen.org; 760-471-9989), Life Force International (www.life-force–intl.com; 800-531-4877)

Connective Tissue/Joint and Muscle Nutritional Formulas

Standard Process Labs: Calcifood Wafers/2–3x day/powder/1 TBS per day, a source of high-quality veal bone; Biost/1–3x day, a natural source of manganese; Ligaplex I/2–3x day, contains essential nutrients for ligament health; Glucosamine Synergy/1–3x day, a complete joint complex

Biotics Research: BioMusculoskeletal Pak/1 pak per day; ChondroSamine S/1–2, 3x day-joint formulation; Osteo B Plus/2–3x day, bone support; Amino Acid Quick Sorb/20 drops 1–2x day, an amino acid formula

Nutri West: Total Joint Support/1–2, 3x day

Dr. David Williams.com: Joint Advantage/as directed; Joint Advantage Gold/as directed. Call 888-887-8262 or visit http://www.drdavidwilliams.com to order.

Generic Orthotics/ Inserts

Birkenstock inserts: The only generic insert with metatarsal arch support. Order from Birkenstock Express at www.birkenstockexpress.com (click on "insoles").

Blue Footbed for Casual Shoes: Call 800-451-1459 or buy them at your local shoe store. Available in narrow and wide, European sizes.

Superfeet Premium Insoles: superfeet.com; Insoles come in a variety of footbeds. See the website for details or visit your local shoe store.

Montrail Footbeds: www.backcountry.com. Purchase online or visit your local shoe store. Helpful Hint: Don't heat insoles in oven before use and they will last longer.

Red Wing Custom Footbeds: See your local shoe store for details.

Sole Custom Footbeds: www2.yoursole.com. Order online or at your local shoe store.

Helpful Hint: Don't heat insoles in oven before use and they will last longer.

Trigger Point Treatment

The Stick is available from Intracell Technology at 120 Interstate North Parkway East Suite 424 Atlanta, Ga 30339. Email them at stickdoc@intracell.net or researchstudies@intracell.net, or call 800-554-1501 or 770-850-1126.

The Ma Roller: Available online at
www.themaroller.com or call 800-830-5949.

B12 Folic Acid Resources:

Standard Process Labs: Folic Acid B12/ 1–2,
3x day

Biotics Research: Folic Acid 800/ 1–3x day

Three-way Foot and Ankle Exercise

Thera-Ciser ™: From Foot Levelers, Inc. at
www.footlevelers.com. Standard is ideal
for variable resistance, Light for upper
extremity injuries and arthritic joints, and
Heavy for lower extremities and strength
training. Order at:
www.greatchiro.com/theraciser.html

Thera-Band System of Progressive Exercise:
Available at www.optp.com or 888-819-
0121. Click on "resistive exercise products"
and choose the desired strength.

Cho-Pat Original Knee Strap: From Cho-
pat.com. Order from Cho-Pat, Inc. P.O.
Box 293Hainesport, NJ 08036 or call 800-
221-1601 or 609-261-1336.

Kinesthetic or Balance Boards

OPTP: A variety available at optp.com or
877-989-6321.

Gaiam/Living Arts: Balance boards available
at www.gaiammindbody.com or
800-367-7393.

Hugger Mugger: Balance board available at
huggermugger.com or 800-473-4888.

Massage Body Roller for Hip Roller Exercise

Gaiam/Living Arts: Gaiam Pilates Body
Roller available at
www.gaiammindbody.com or
800-367-7393.

OPTP: Standard Foam Roller or OPTP Axis
Roller available at optp.com or
877-989-6321.

Hugger Mugger: Pilates Foam Roller
available at huggermugger.com or
800-473-4888.

Fitness Balls

Gaiam/Living Arts: A variety of fitness balls
are available at www.gaiammindbody.com
or 800-367-7393.

OPTP: A variety of fitness balls and
instructional booklets are available at
optp.com or 877-989-6321.

Hugger Mugger: Fitness balls are available at
huggermugger.com or 800-473-4888.

Anti-inflammatory Nutrition

Standard Process Labs: Tuna Omega 3
Oil/2–3 2x day; Source of mercury free fish
oil

Biotics Research: Optimal EFAs/3–3x day

Nutri West: Complete Omega-3
Essentials/2–2x day

Anti-inflammatory Proteolytic Enzymes

Take 4–6 capsules between meals/two hours
removed from food, 2–3 times per day to
reduce the effects of inflammation.

Nutri West: Pro-Infla-zyme

Biotics Research: Intenzyme Forte

Appendix A Resources for Chapter 6

**Note: Please see *Appendix A Resources for Chapter 3* for
supplier and ordering information for products from
Standard Process, Biotics, Nutri West, New Chapter, and
Synergy.**

Sources for Pineal Gland Nutritional Supplements

Standard Process: Ginkgo Synergy/2–3x day,
Folic acid B12/ 2–3x day, Neuroplex/1–3x
day

Biotics Research: Cytozyme PT/HPT/1–3x
day, Cytozyme B/1–3x day

Nutri West: Pineal-Lyph/1–3x day

EMF Protective Devices

There are numerous options available on the
Internet. Below are some of the many possibilities. Q-Link seems to lead the pack.

- qlinkxzone.com
- www.fastfengshui.com/products_emf.htm

- www.blockemf.com
- www.emfdefense.com

Sources for Pituitary Gland Nutritional Supplements

Standard Process: Ginkgo Synergy/2–3x day, Pituitrophin/1–3x day, Cataplex E/2–3x day

Biotics Research: Cytozyme PT/HPT/1–3x day, Cytozyme B/1–3x day

Nutri West: Pit-Lyph-Anterior/1–2x day, Pit-Lyph-Whole/1–2x day; both are contraindicated during pregnancy

Sources for Thyroid Gland Nutritional Supplements

Standard Process: Iodomere/1–3x day, Thytrophin PMG/1–3x day (protomor phagen)

Biotics Research: Thyrostim/1–3x day, Liquid Iodine/20 drops/day

Nutri West: THY #8 tincture/15 drops/2x day

Sources for Thymus Gland Nutritional Supplements

Standard Process: Thymex/2–3x day, Thymus PMG/1–3x day

Biotics Research: Bio-Immunozyme Forte/2–3x day, Cytozyme THY

Nutri West: Total Multimune/1–3x day

New Chapter Inc.: Host Defense Extract/15 drops 2x day

Green Drink Support For Thymus Gland

Standard Process: Sp Green Food/2–3x day

The Synergy Company: Pure Synergy/1 TBS day

Nutri West: Total Green/1 TBS day

New Chapter Inc.: Broccolive Plus/1–2x day between meals

Sources for Pancreas Nutritional Supplements

Standard Process: Cataplex GTF/2–2x day (blood sugar regulation), Lactic Acid Yeast/2–3x day (carbohydrate intolerance)

Biotics Research: Bio-Glycozyme Forte/2–3x day between meals, Cytozyme-Pan/1–3x day. (Both are for carbohydrate intolerance.)

Nutri West: Pan-Lyph Chelate/1–3x day (blood sugar regulation)

Sources for Anti-inflammatory Nutritional Formulas

Standard Process: Tuna Omega-3 Oil/3–6 perles/day

Nutri West: Pro Inflazyme/4, 3x day (between meals)

Biotics Research: Intenzyme Forte (3–3x day between meals)

Sources for Nutritional Supplements for the Adrenal Glands

Standard Process: Drenamin/2–3x day, DrenatrophinPMG/2–3x day

Biotics Research: Cytozyme AD/2–3x day, ADHS/1@breakfast, 1@ lunch

Nutri West: DSF Formula/1–3x day, Ad #1/15 drops 3x day

Weed Botanicals: Adaptogen/15 drops 3x day

New Chapter Inc.: Stress Support Multi/1–3x day

Sources for Reproductive System Nutritional Support

Standard Process: Ovex/1–3x day, Wheat germ Oil Perles/1–3x day

Biotics Research: Equi-Fem/2–3x day, B-Vital 1–2x day (male)

Nutri West: Total Male/1–3x day, Total Female/1–3x day

Weed Botanical Co.: Fem Balance #1/15 drops 3x day, Male Virility/15 drops 3x day, Menopause/15 drops 3x day

Weed Botanical Co.: Call 800-878-1001 for product information and to order.

Appendix A Resources for Chapter 7

Note: Please see *Appendix A Resources for Chapter 3* for supplier and ordering information for products from Standard Process, Biotics, Nutri West, New Chapter, and Synergy.

pH Test Strips

Simply Hydroponics: Offers pH Hydrion test strips and paper at www.simplyhydroponics.com or 727–531–5355.

Products to Elevate the pH of Water

Miracle Works liquid alkaline water additive/Infinite Health Solution—High pH, oxygenated immune support, pH stabilization, detoxification. Infinitehealth@miracle-wrks.com www.Miracle-wrks.com (970) 382-8949

Eco Tech Co, Ltd.: Offers water ionizers to manually control the pH of your water. They can be great alkalizers. The JP 109 Orion/Alphion model is recommended. Visit www.royalwater.com/main.htm for more information or email royal@royalwater.com.

CWR Environmental Protection Products, Inc.: I recommend a CWR Crown Water Filter Series Imperial Ceramic under counter filter, plus a fluoride filter for fluoridated water. More information available at www.cwrenviro.com or 1-800-444-3563.

Extreme Health USA: Offers bottled Micro-Clustered Hexagonal Water. Available at www.ExtremeHealthUSA.com or 800-800-1285.

pH Normalizing Foot Bath/Ion Generator

A Major Difference, Inc.: Offers Ion Cleanse-Ionic Detoxification Foot Bath. Available at http://www.amajordifference.com or 877-315-8638.

Bio Cleanse: Offers Ionic Detoxification Foot Bath. Available at www.biocleanse .info/store or 931-592-7002.

Nutritional Products to Help Balance pH

Standard Process Labs: SP Green Food/2 3x day, Cruciferous Complete/2 2x day, Chlorophyll Complex/2, 3x day

Biotics Research Inc.: NitroGreens/as directed, Chlorella Caps/5–8 day

New Chapter Inc.: Broccolive Plus/1 day, Chlorella Regularis/2, 3x day with meals

Nutri West: Total Veggie/1–2, 3x day

GreensPlus: Greens Plus Superfood/1 TBS day. Available at greensplus.com.

Premier Research Labs: pH Powder, Quantum/as directed. Available at www.prlabs.com or 800-325-7734.

Green Foods Supplements

Standard Process:SP Green Food/2 3x day,

Nutri West: Total Veggie/1–2, 3x day, Total Green/1 TBS day

New Chapter Inc.: Broccolive Plus/1 day, Chlorella Regularis/2 3x day with meals

Premier Research Labs: pH Powder, Quantum/as directed. Available at www.prlabs.com or 800-325-7734.

GreensPlus: Greens Plus Superfood/1 TBS day. Available at www.greenplus.com.

Biotics Research Inc.: NitroGreens/as directed, Chlorella Caps/5–8 day

The Synergy Company: Pure Synergy/1 TBS day. Available at www.synergy–co.com or call 800-723-0277.

Barley Greens: Premium Plus/1 Tbl day. Available at www.barleygreen.com.au or health food stores.

Vegetable Broth Seasonings for 11 Day Diet

Bernard Jensen's Seasoning: Vegetable broth seasonings available at www.bernardjensen.org (click on "products" and "vitamins & nutritional supplements")

Vegex: Can be purchased at most health food stores, or ordered online at http://www.ceaemployment.com/vegex.html

Blender Drink Recipe: See *Appendix A Resources for Chapter 5* for details.

Appendix A Resources for Chapter 8

Note: Please see *Appendix A Resources for Chapter 3* for supplier and ordering information for products from

Standard Process, Biotics, Nutri West, New Chapter, and Synergy.

Hiatal-hernia-related Nutrients

Standard Process: Chlorophyll Complex/2–3x day(cleanses and heals GI tract), Zypan/2–3, 3x day(full spectrum digestive enzyme with HCL)

Biotics Research: Gastrazyme/2–3 3x day just before meals (take until gastric inflammation is resolved then move to a hydrochloric acid supplement), L Glutamine Powder/1–3 tsp day (gastric inflammation), Hydrozyme/2–4 tablets taken in the middle of meal (hydrochloric acid supplement), Bio HPF/2–3x day just before meals (H-pylori formula)

Enzymes & Pancreatic Digestives for Small Intestine

Standard Process: Lactic Acid Yeast/1–3x day (facilitates carbohydrate metabolism), Multizyme/2–3x day (pancreatic enzymes), Zypan/2–3x day with meal (hydrochloric acid plus pancreatic enzymes)

Biotics Research: IPS-Intestinal Permeability Support/2–3 2x day 1 hour before meals (repairs intestinal mucosa), Bio 6 Plus/3–3x day just before meals (pancreas support)

Supplements for Gall Bladder Support

Standard Process: Cholacol/2–3 with meals (provides bile salts), A-F Betafood/2–4 between meals to open bile ducts, Choline/1–2 per meal helps to metabolize fats.

Biotics Research: Beta Plus/2–3 with meals (provides bile salts and bile duct support; vary dosage of bile salts to prevent biliary dependence)

Gall Bladder Cleanse Supplements

Standard Process: Disodium Phosphate/use as directed in cleanse, Phosfood Liquid/use as directed in cleanse

Supplements that Support Correction of Iliocecal Valve

Standard Process: Chlorophyll Complex/2–3x day, Spanish Black Radish/2–3x day, Zymex/2–3x day (maintains healthy intestinal environment), Magnesium Lactate/4–5 at bedtime, Calcium Lactate/3–4, 2x day with meals

Biotics Research: Chlorocaps/1–3x day, Colon Plus/1 tsp of powder or 3–5 capsules per day just before meals, Bio CMP/2–3x day (provides calcium, magnesium and phosphorus)

Nutritional Supplements for Large Intestine

Standard Process: Zymex/2–3x day, Lactic Acid Yeast/1–3x day, Lact-Enz/2–3x day (digestive enzymes plus friendly bacteria)

Biotics Research: BioDophilus/3–3x day before meals (for fungus/yeast problems also take ADP (extract of oregano) and see sections on yeast and fungus in chapter 9)

Metagenics: Ultra Flora Plus/2 3x day; available at metagenics.com or 800-692-9400

Nutri West: Total Probiotics/1–3x day

Probiotic Suppliers

Metagenics: Ultra Flora Plus/1–3x day (dairy and nondairy bifidus formula, capsules, or powder); available at metagenics.com or 800-692-9400

Standard Process: Lact-Enz/2–3x day (digestive enzymes plus friendly bacteria)

Nutri West: Total Probiotics/1–3x day

Biotics Research: Biodophilus-FOS/2–4 capsules 3x day or 1/2–1 tsp powder 1–2x day just before meals

Buying Power: Living Earth /1–2, 3x day (Soil Based Organisms or SBOs). Available at http://www.veromaxhealth.com or 800-577-1826.

Kefir Recipe (Information and Sources for Kefir Starter Grains)

Body Ecology: www.kefir.net (great information and starter culture)

Dom's Kefir-making site: http://users.sa.-chariot.net.au/~dna/Makekefir.html

Health Food Stores: Kefir starter grains may be available at your local health food store

Large Intestine Supplements

Standard Process: Zymex/2–3x day (restores balance in large intestine), Lact-Enz/2–3x day (helps absorption of important nutrients), Cataplex A C/2–3x day (promotes healing)

Health food stores: Aloe Vera juice/1oz. 2x day

Probiotics: See above information.

Sources of Essential Fatty Acids (for Sun Protection)

Standard Process Labs: Tuna Omega 3 Oil/2–3 2x day (source of mercury-free fish oil)

Biotics Research Inc.: Optimal EFA's/3–3x day

Nutri West: Complete Omega-3 Essentials/2–3x day

Pharminex: Marine Omega/2–3x day; available at pharmanex.com (click on "Pharmanex Nutritionals") or 801-345-9800

Enzymes & Supplements for Intestines

Standard Process: Zypan/2–3, 3x day (full spectrum digestive enzyme with HCL), Lactic Acid Yeast/1–3x day (facilitates carbohydrate metabolism), Multizyme/2–3x day (pancreatic enzymes), Spanish Black Radish/2–3x day, Zymex/2–3x day (maintains healthy intestinal environment for ileocecal valve), Lact-Enz/2–3x day (digestive enzymes plus friendly bacteria), Tuna Omega 3 Oil/2–3 2x day (mercury-free fish oil)

Biotics Research: Gastrazyme/2–3 3x day just before meals (take until gastric inflammation is resolved then move to a hydrochloric acid supplement), L Glutamine Powder/1–3 tsp day (gastric inflammation), Hydrozyme/2–4 tablets taken in the middle of meal (hydrochloric acid supplement),

Bio HPF/2–3x day just before meals (H-pylori bacteria formula), IPS-Intestinal Permeability Support/2–3 2x day 1 hour before meals (repairs intestinal mucosa), Bio 6 Plus/3–3x day just before meals (pancreas support), Chlorocaps/1–3x day, Colon Plus/1 tsp of powder or 3–5 capsules day just before meals, BioDophilus/3–3x day before meals

Metagenics: Ultra Flora Plus/1–3x day (dairy and nondairy bifidus formula) capsules or powder; available at metagenics.com or 800-692-9400

Nutri West: Total Probiotics/1–3x day

Buying Power: Living Earth /1–2, 3x day (Soil Based Organisms or SBOs); available at http://www.veromaxhealth.com or 800-577-1826

Sources of Healthy Sunscreen

News Target: www.newstarget.com/001264.html (informative sunscreen/skin cancer article)

Borlind Boutique: store.borlind.com (sunscreen products)

Alba Botanicals: www.albabotanica.com

Kate's Caring Gifts: www.katescaringgifts.com (click on "Green Screen")

Lilou Organics: www.lilou-organics.com (Aubry Organic sunscreen)

Appendix A Resources for Chapter 9

Note: Please see *Appendix A Resources for Chapter 3* for supplier and ordering information for products from Standard Process, Biotics, Nutri West, New Chapter, and Synergy.

List of Protomorphagens (PMG)

Standard Process
- Cardiotrophin PMG—Heart
- Dermatrophin PMG—Skin
- Drenatrophin PMG—Adrenals
- Hepatrophin PMG—Liver
- Hypothalamus PMG—Hypothalamus Gland

- Mammary PMG—Breast Tissue
- Myotrophin PMG—Muscle Tissue
- Neurotrophin PMG—Nerve Tissue
- Oculotrophin PMG—Eyes
- Orchic PMG—Testes
- Ostrophin PMG—Bone Tissue
- Ovatraphin PMG—Ovaries
- Pancreatrophin PMG—Pancreas
- Parotid PMG—Parotid Gland
- Pituitrophin PMG—Pituitary
- Pneumotrophin PMG—Lungs
- Prostate PMG—Prostate Gland
- Renatrophin PMG—Kidneys
- Spleen PMG—Spleen
- Thymus PMG—Thymus Gland
- Thytrophin PMG—Thyroid
- Utrophin PMG—Uterus

Lymphatic Strengthening Nutritional Formulas

Weed Botanicals: Lymphatic Formula / 30 drops 2x day

Hummingbird Herbals: Lymph Mover / 40 drops 4X day

Nutritional Formulas for Thymus and Spleen

Standard Process: Thymex / 2–3x day, Spleen PMG / 1–3x day

Biotics Research: Cytozyme THY / 1–2, 3x day, Cytozyme SP / 1–2, 3x day

General Immune System Strengthening Formulas

Standard Process: Immuplex 1–2, 3x day (broad spectrum), Thymex / 2–3x day (thymus specific support), Congaplex 2–3, 3x day (short-term immune support), Cataplex AC / 2–3x day

Biotics Research: Bio-Immunozyme Forte / 1–2, 3x day (broad spectrum), IAG powder / 1–2tsp, 2–3x day (chronic immune), Immuno G / 2–3x day (colostrum for reduced IgA)

Nutri West: Total Multi Immune / 1–2, 3x day

Sources for Immune System Nutritional Support

Spirulina: Available at health food stores

Pure Synergy: Available from the Synergy Company

Mushroom Formulas (Immune system support): Fungi Perfecti Stamets 7 / 1–2, 3x day, Biotics Shiitake Mushroom formula / 1–2, 3x day

Blue Green Algae: SimplexityAlpha Sun / 2–2x day, Omega Sun / 2–2x day

Green Drink Recipe: See Appendix B page 422

Essential Fatty Acids: Pharminex Marine Omega / 2–2x day, Standard Process Tuna Omega 3 / 2 2x day, Nutri West Complete Omega 3 Essentials / 2 per day

Flaxseed Oil: Barlean's Liquid (available at health food stores), Standard Process Linum B6 perles / 1–2, 3x day

Flaxseed Meal: Bob's Flaxseed Meal (available at health food stores)

Rice Bran Syrup: Bernard Jensen Intl. / 1 TBS day (available at health food stores)

Wheat Germ Oil: Standard ProcessWheat Germ Oil Perles / 1–2, 3x day, (available at health food stores, refrigerated in small quantities)

Wheat Germ (raw): (available at health food stores)

Whole Food Multiple Vitamins: Standard Process Catalyn / 1–3x day, New Chapter Every Woman II / 2–3x day, New Chapter Every Man II / 2–3x day, New Chapter Vit C Complex, Standard Process Cataplex C / 3–3x day, Standard Process Cataplex ACP / 3–3x day, New Chapter C Food Complex / 1 per day

Chlorophyll: source of oil soluble vitamins, ADEK Standard Process Chlorophyll Complex / 2–3x day

Digestive Enzymes: Standard Process Zypan / 2–3x day mid-meal, Biotics Research Hydrozyme / 2 or more mid-meal,

Biotics Research Betaine Plus HP/1–2, 3x day mid-meal (high potency)

Trace Minerals: Standard Process All-Organic Trace Minerals/3 per day, Standard Process Trace Minerals B12/2 per day, Biotics Research Multi-Mins/1–2, 3x day

Natural Anti-bacterial Supplements

Morinda Supreme: Morinda Supreme/1 scoop 3x day

Biotics Research: ADP(Oregano Oil Extract tablets)/5 3x day for 1 week/3–3x day for 4 weeks all taken just before meals, Ultra Olive Leaf (Olive Leaf Extract)/1–3x day just before meals

North American Herb & Spice Co: Oreganol (Oil of Oregano)/take as directed on label; available at 800-243-5242 and select health food stores

Gaia Herbs: Echinacea Golderseal Supreme Tincture (available at health food stores)

Weed Botanical Co.: Inf-Fighter/30 drops 2–3x day

Probiotic Suppliers

Metagenics: Ultra Flora Plus/1–3x day (dairy and nondairy bifidus formula, capsules or powder)

Standard Process: Lact-Enz/2–3x day (digestive enzymes plus friendly bacteria)

Nutri West: Total Probiotics/1–3x day

Biotics Research: Biodophilus-FOS/2–4 capsules 3x day or 1/2–1 tsp powder 1–2x day just before meals

Buying Power: Living Earth /1–2, 3x day (Soil Based Organisms or SBOs). Available at http://www.veromaxhealth.com or 800-577-1826

Anti-Viral Preparations

Morinda Supreme: Morinda Supreme/ 1 scoop 3x day, available at www.morindasupreme.com or 800-922-1744

Standard Process: Garlic/1–2 3x day

Biotics Research: Ultra Vir-X/3–2x day (not during pregnancy or lactation), ADP (Oregano Oil Extract tablets)/5 3x day for 1 week/3–3x day for 4 weeks all taken just before meals

North American Herb & Spice Co.: Oil of Oregano Oreganol/take as directed on label, available at 800-243-5242 or in select health food stores

Biotics Research: Olive Leaf Extract Ultra Olive Leaf/1–3x day just before meals, (olive leaf extracts may be available at health food stores as well)

Gaia Herbs: Echanacia Golderseal Supreme Tincture, (available at health food stores)

Weed Botanical Co.: Vira-Pel/30 drops 2–3x day

Anti-Fungal Preparations

Pure Essence Labs: Candex/Taken as directed (available at health food stores)

Weed Botanical Co.: Fungalytic Formula/30 drops 2–3x day

Morinda Supreme: Morinda Supreme/1 scoop 3x day

Biotics Research: ADP (Oregano Oil Extract tablets)/5 3x day for 1 week/3–3x day for 4 weeks all taken just before meals

Nutri West: Total Yst Redux/1–3x day

Effective Laboratories for Parasite Testing

Parasitology Center Inc.: parasitetesting.com; Dr. Omar Amin, omaramin@aol.com, 480-767-2522; tests can be ordered from the PCI Package Shop at 866-547-2522.

Doctor's Data: doctorsdata.com; a variety of tests are available (blood, hair, stool analysis, toxic metals, water etc.)

Genova Diagnostics (formally Great Smokies Lab): comprehensive stool analysis

Anti-Parasite Preparations

Morinda Supreme: Morinda Supreme/1 scoop 3x day

Biotics Research: Dysbiocide/2 2x day (not recommended during pregnancy/lactation), Parasite Comp/1 tsp 2x day

Standard Process: Zymex II/2–2x day between meals

Weed Botanicals: Vermifuge/30 drops 3x day for 4 weeks

Healing Nutrition Following Parasite Treatment

Standard Process: Zymex/2–3x day: restores balance in large intestine

Standard Process: Cataplex A C/2–3x day: promotes healing

Health food stores: Aloe Vera juice/1 oz–2x day

Probiotics: See Appendix A Resources for Chapter 8

Water-filtering Products

CWR Environmental Protection Products, Inc.: Information at www.cwrenviro.com or 800-444-3563. I recommend a CWR Imperial ceramic under-counter filter, plus a fluoride filter (for fluoridated water). Contact CWR for pricing. Whole house filtration, shower filters and air purification systems also available.

Rainshow'r: shower and bathtub filtration; available at www.rainshowermfg.com or 800-243-8775.

Micro Clustered Hexagonal Water: Helps to hydrate the cell; available from Extreme Health USA, www.extremehealthusa.com or 800-800-1285.

Air Filtration Suppliers

CWR Environmental Protection Products, Inc.: Product information at www.cwrenviro.com or 800-444-3563

Allergy Buyers Club: Air purifiers available at allergybuyersclubshopping.com or 888-236-7231 (also a source for shower filters/water filters)

Web Stores America: www.air-purifiers-america.com

Gaiam: Products available at www.gaiam.com (click on "Natural Home") include the PlasmaWave Air Purifier, UV Air Purifier, Healthmate HEPA Air Filter/Junior

Whole Food Phytonutrient Products

Standard Process: Cruciferous complete/2 per day, Phytolyn/2 per day

Nutri West: Total Veggie/2 per day

New Chapter: Broccolive/1 per day

Sources of Antioxidant Products

Standard Process: Catplex E/2–3x day, Cataplex C/ 3–3x day, Tuna Omega 3 Oil/2–2x day

Biotics Research: Bioprotect/1–2 3x day, Dismuzyme Plus/2–3x day between meals, Co Q-Zyme 30/1–2 3x day, Optimal EFAs/2–4 3x day, Bio-C Plus 1000/1–2 3x day

Nutri West: Total Veggie/ 2 per day, Total Protect/1–2 2x day, Total Green/1 TBS day, Total Alpha Lipoic Acid/2–2x day, Complete Omega-3 Essentials/2–4 per day

Extreme Health USA: Goji Berry and Goji Pomegranate concentrates (add 2–3 TBS of concentrate to water to make juice), Organically Grown Green Tea, (all three products high in antioxidants)

Weed Botanicals: Antioxidant Herbal Formula/30 drops 2–3x day

Nutrients for Toxic Metal Poisoning

Marco Pharma International: Wild Bear Garlic/ 1 tsp 2–3x day, Bio Reu-Rella/3–3x day, Cilantro Tablets/1–3 tablets 2–3x day, dissolve slowly under tongue

Biotics Research: Porphyra-Zyme/4–3x day between meals, Chlorella Caps/5–8 caps day

Standard Process: Cruciferous Complete/2 per day, Phytolyn/ 2 per day, Allorganic Trace Minerals/2–2x day, Cataplex C/ 3–3x day

Extreme Health USA: Detox Heavy Metals Plus take as indicated on web site. Vegetarian formula.

Health food stores: Spirulina/2 capsules 3x day, Ascorbic Acid/ 1–3 Grams per day

Immune System Builders

Standard Process: Immuplex 1–2 3x day (broad spectrum), Thymex/2 3x day (thymus specific support), Congaplex 2–3 3x day (short-term immune support), Cataplex AC/ 2–3x day

Biotics Research: Bio-Immunozyme Forte/1–2 3x day (broad spectrum), IAG powder/1–2tsp 2–3x day (chronic immune), Immuno G/2 3x day (colostrum for reduced IgA)

Nutri West: Total Multi Immune/1–2 3x day

Dust Mite Solutions

Allergy Buyers Club: information and solutions available at www.allergybuyersclub.com.

Allergies

Standard Process: Antronex/5–3x day for active symptoms (natural anti-histamine), Catalyn/1–3x day (multi-vitamin/mineral supplement) Organic minerals/1–3x day, Allorganic Trace Minerals/1–3x day, Tuna Omega-3/2–3 2x day (source of EFA's)

Biotics Research: Histoplex/ 2–4 capsules 2x day between meals (natural anti-histamine), Bio-AE Mulsion Forte/6 drops 2x day taken with Bio-Immunozyme Forte/1–3x day, COQ-Zyme 30/1–2 3x day(antioxidant)

Sources for Whole Food Nutrition

Standard Process Labs
New Chapter Whole Foods

Suppliers

Note: Please see *Appendix A Resources for Chapter 3* **for supplier and ordering information for products from Standard Process, Biotics, Nutri West, New Chapter, and Synergy.**

Extreme Health USA: www.extremehealthusa.com or 800-800-1285; see web site for nutritional products, information and protocols

Morinda Supreme: www.morindasupreme.com or 800-922-1744

Bernard Jensen International: www.bernardjensen.org or 760-471-9989

Life Force International: www.lifeforce–intl.com or 800-531-4877

Gaia Herbs: gaiaherbs.com or 800-831-7780

Pharmanex: pharmanex.com (click on "Pharmanex Nutritionals" and "Marine Omega") or 801-345-9800

Metagenics: metagenics.com or 800-692-9400

Pure Essence Labs: Candexor pureessencelabs.com or 888-254-8000

Buying Power: Living Earth available at www.veromaxhealth.com or 800-577-1826

Fungi Perfecti: www.fungi.com or 800-780-9126

North American Herb & Spice Co.: Oil of Oregano Oreganol/take as directed on label; available at 800 243-5242 or in select health food stores

Hummingbird Herbals: www.hummingbirdherbals.com or 970-259-8965

Simplexity: (formally Cell Tech) simplexityhealth.com or 800-800-1300

Marco Pharma: www.marcopharma.net or 541-677-8300

CWR Environmental Protection Products Inc.: air and water filters available at www.cwrenviro.com or 800-444-3563

Weed Botanical Co.: 800-878-1001

Appendix A Resources for Chapter 10

Note: Please see *Appendix A Resources for Chapter 3* for supplier and ordering information for products from Standard Process, Biotics, Nutri West, New Chapter, and Synergy. See Appendix A Resources for Chapter 9 for supplier and ordering information for products from other vendors.

Air Filtration Suppliers

CWR Environmental Protection Products Inc.: Product information at www.cwrenviro.com or 800-444-3563.

Allergy Buyers Club: Air purifiers available at allergybuyersclubshopping.com or 888-236-7231 (also a source for shower filters / water filters).

Web Stores America: www.air-purifiers-america.com

Gaiam: products available at www.gaiam.com (click on "natural home"); PlasmaWave Air Purifier, UV Air Purifier, Healthmate HEPA Air Filter / Junior

Nutritional Formulas for the Respiratory System

Standard Process: Thymex / 2–3x day (short-term immune system support), Pneuma-trophin / 1 3x day

Biotics Research: ADP / 5 3x day for 1 wk then 3–3x day for 4 weeks before meals (Oil of Oregano tablets), Bio Immunozyme Forte / 3–3x day acute 1–3x day chronic (immune system support), Bio-Mega 3 / 2–3x day (systemic inflammation)

Nutri West: Pro Infla-Zyme / 3 3x day between meals (inflammation)

Gaia Herbs: Echinacea Goldenseal Supreme / 40 drops 3x day in water, Osha Supreme / 30 drops 3x day in 2 oz warm water

Weed Botanicals: Lung Health / 30–40 drops 3x day in 2 oz water

Heart-related Nutritional Formulas

Standard Process: Cardio Plus / 2 3x day, Cataplex B / 2 3x day, Cataplex G / 1 3x day, Cataplex E / 2 3x day, OPC Synergy / 1–3x day

Biotics Research: Bio Cardio Pak / 1 pack daily, VasculoSirt / 4 2x day to improve heart and vascular health, reduce blood pressure and cholesterol and to slow the effects of aging

Nutri West: Total Heart / 1–3x day

Extreme Health: Oral Chelation, am and pm bottle. See web site for information and protocol. www.extremehealthusa.com or 800-800-1285

Weed Botanicals: CV-Tension Plus / 30–40 drops 3x day in 2 oz water

High Blood Pressure Nutrition

Note: Use all 3 products

Standard Process: OPC Synergy / 1–3x day, Garlic Capsules / 1–2x day

Biotics: Aqueous Magnesium / 3 tsp at bedtime, mix with pear or tangerine juice to offset disagreeable taste. For optimal dosage, slowly increase dosage every 2 days until loose stools are reached, and then back off 1 dose.

Low Blood Pressure Nutrition

Standard Process: Drenamin / 3–3x day, Cataplex B / 1 or 2 tabs 3x day
OR
Biotics: ADB-5 Plus / 2 tabs @breakfast, 1@ lunch, Bio 3 B-G / 2–3 tabs 3x day; reduce refined carbohydrate intake

Heart-related Whole Food Supplements

Standard Process: Catalyn / 3–3x day (multiple vitamin), Cataplex B / 2 3x day, Cataplex G / 1 3x day, Cataplex E2 2–3x day, Cardio-Plus 2, 3x day

New Chapter: E & Selenium Food Complex / 1 per day between meals, Coenzyme B Food Complex / 2 per day

Suppliers

Standard Process Labs: Visit www.standard-process.com for information about products and how to order from a health professional near you. There are also several other web sites that offer Standard Process products. Try searching "Standard Process Labs" for other ordering options.

Biotics Research Corp.: Visit www.bioticsresearch.com for product and professional contact information. For other ordering options, search for "Biotics Research Corp."

Nutri West: Visit www.nutriwest.com for product and professional contact information. Search "Nutri West" for other ordering options.

New Chapter, Inc.: A good source for multiple vitamin/mineral combination formulas. Go to http://new-chapter.com/new-chapter.com for product and ordering information or call 800 543-7279. You can also search "New Chapter Vitamins" for other ordering options or find them in your local health food store.

Extreme Health USA: www.extremehealthusa.com or 800-800-1285; see web site for nutritional products, information and protocols

Gaia Herbs: gaiaherbs.com, 800-831-7780

Weed Botanical Co.: 800-878-1001

Appendix A Chapter 12

Dr. John Diamond's Workshop on Releasing Emotions: For books, lecture series, and workshop schedule, visit www.drjohndiamond.com, or call 914-533-2408.

The Mozart Effect, Resource Center: Don Campbell, author of *The Mozart Effect* utilizes a variety of sounding techniques, recordings, books, and resources to educate people on the healing power of sound and music. See www.mozarteffect.com for workshop information, or call 800 427-7680.

Resources for Specific Assessments

Appendix B Resources for Chapter 3
A Systems View of the Body

This expanded viewpoint demonstrates how the systems of the body are both interconnected and interdependent. When we embrace a systems view of the body, we see all the systems as being connected together in a single grand scheme.

In essence, the health of the body depends upon the health of these integrated systems. The health of the body's systems depends on the health of its organs. The health of its organs depends on the health of its tissues, and the health of its tissues depends on the health of its cells. The health of the body's cells is dependent upon the nature of the electromagnetic life force of that travel through the body.

A systems view of the body provides a vantage point in which everything in the body is seen as working together in perfect harmony. If one system is out of balance, the entire body feels the effects, as nothing is ever isolated or separate. When health is present, our whole being is engaged in both creating the cause and feeling the effects.

The accompanying systems view illustration is a limited two-dimensional representation of a multidimensional reality. All the spokes on the systems wheel converge at the center, which is the place where they interact with each other, and receive direction from our Inner Intelligence.

Adjacent spokes have special relationships, such as the nerve and endocrine systems, which share many special functions and can be referred to as the neuroendocrine system. The musculoskeletal system also functions as one system. The only reason to truly separate any of these systems is for the purpose of study and understanding. In essence, all systems are a part of one

whole and help to create our internally balanced living environment.

Integrating these vital systems back together is one of the purposes of this text. The separation of these systems, along with the idea that our bodies, minds, hearts and spirits are separate, has lead us to experience the state of dis-ease.

When we embrace the perspective and guidance provided by our Inner Intelligence, we experience the viewpoint from the center of the circle. From here, we can see and understand how our bodies work. We become aware of specific problems as they arise, recognize which systems are involved, and follow the guidelines and direction provided by our internal intelligence as to the solution. Some great solutions are presented in each chapter.

The human body is amazingly complex, yet there exists within it a profound level of simplicity. One of my teachers once described the human body as being "simply intricate and intricately simple," which sums it all up in my mind.

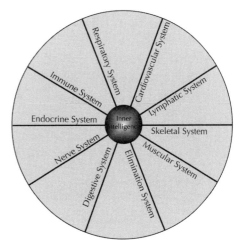

Fig. B3.1: The Systems Wheel

Appendix B Resources for Chapter 4

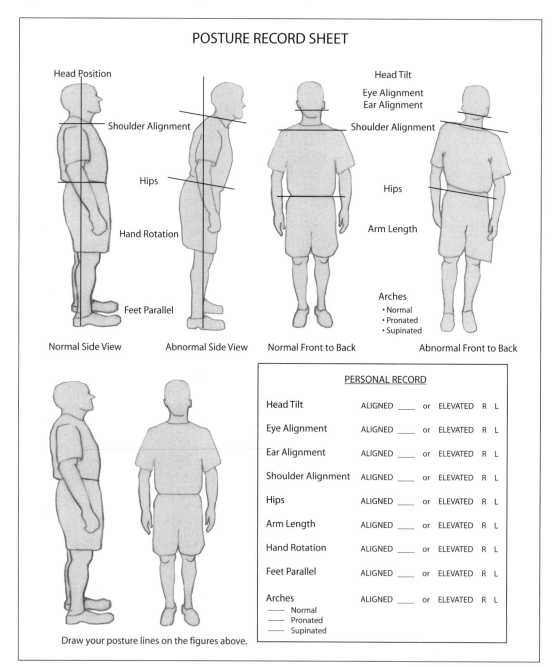

Fig. B4.1: Posture Record Sheet

tibetan eye chart

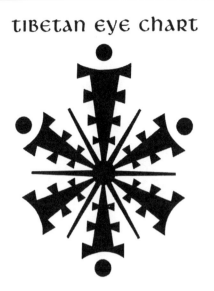

For generations the people of Tibet have used natural methods to correct visual weaknesses and improve their eyesight. Chief among the methods employed has been the use of certain exercises which have proved useful over long periods of time. The figure in this chart was designed by Tibetan Lama Monks to give the necessary corrective exercises and stimulation to the muscles and nerves of the optical system.

A few minutes daily practice, morning and evening, will bring immediate effects, and if maintained over a period of months, most definite improvement should result.

How to use the chart

- Place the chart on a wall with the center spot in line with your nose when your head is level. Now, standing erect and close to the wall, touch the center spot on the chart with the tip of your nose.
- With your head still, move your eyes clockwise around the outer edges of each arm of the figure, including the black spots, until the starting point is reached.
- Repeat the movement in a counterclockwise direction.
- Blink and relax your eyes after each cycle, then do a half minute of palming (palms of each hand over each open eye) when finished.
- Repeat as desired, being careful to avoid strain.

Fig. B4.2: Tibetan Eye Chart

Appendix B Resources for Chapter 5

Alkaline and Acid Food Lists

ALKALINE Foods

apples
apricots (fresh)
artichokes
asparagus
beans (snap)
berries
broccoli
cabbage (red, white, savoy, Chinese)
cauliflower
celery
cherries (sweet, sour)
chicory
coconut (fresh, meat & milk)
coffee substitutes
corn (fresh, sweet)
eggplant
garlic
gooseberries
grapefruit
grapes
kelp
kiwi
leeks
lemons & lemon peel
lettuce
limes
melons
milk (raw)
onions
oranges
papayas
peaches (fresh)
pear (fresh)
peppers (green & red)
potatoes
radishes
raisins
rhubarb
tomatoes
turnips
watercress
yeast
yogurt

HIGHLY ALKALINE Foods

almonds
avocadoes
bananas (ripe)
beans (fresh green, lima)
beets
blackberries
carrots
chives
endive
okra
peaches (dried)
persimmons
plums
pomegranates
raspberries
squash
spinach

VERY HIGHLY ALKALINE Foods

beans (dried lima, string)
bean sprouts
dandelion greens
dates
figs (esp. black)
mangoes
onions
parsley
prunes
raisins
spinach (raw)
Swiss chard
tubers
watermelon

NEUTRAL Foods

Fats:
animal fat
butter
cream
margarine

Oils:
almond
avocado
coconut
cottonseed
linseed
olive
safflower
sesame
soy
sunflower

ACID Foods

beans (garbanzo, kidney, navy, white)
beef
Brussels sprouts
cashews
coconut (dried)
coffee
egg yolk
fish
fowl (chicken, turkey)
fruit (dried)
game
ketchup
mayonnaise
milk products (pasteurized)
molasses
mushrooms
mustard
mutton
pecans
pork
poultry
rhubarb
vinegar

HIGHLY ACID Foods

alcohol
artificial sweeteners
barley
beer

blueberries
bread
buckwheat
caffeine
chocolate
cranberries
custard
honey
ice cream
lentils
millet
oatmeal
pasta
peanuts
potatoes (sweet)
rice
rye grain
soft drinks
sugar
tobacco
walnuts
wheat
wine

Tools of the Trade

1. Fitness Balls

Many of the range of motion exercises offered in chapter 5 can be effectively performed on a fitness or gymnastic ball. Using the principle of the clock, rotation around the cone of motion is simple, effective and fun. The ball actually aids in rotational movements, especially for the trunk and pelvis. Explore the range of motion exercises with the ball, and create new exercises on your own.

Fitness balls come in a variety of sizes, and are measured in centimeters. Use the proper size ball for your height. I recommend a 55 cm ball for those from five feet five inches to five feet nine in height and a 65 cm one for those from six feet to six feet four. If you are smaller or larger, check with the distributor for your proper size.

Fitness Balls are also extremely effective for mobilizing the vertebrae in the mid and lower back areas. Lying on your back with your head sup-

ported by your hands or by the ball, slightly roll forward and backwards, and from side to side. Using the Fitness Ball while on your stomach, is helpful for the lower back, and can be used for massaging your internal organs as well. Locate *Appendix A Resources for Chapter 5* for distributor contacts and a short booklet on how to use a fitness ball.

2. Theracisers

A theraciser is a simple device, a combination of elastic tubing and Velcro strapping, that allows for a variety of exercises to be performed in the extremities. Theracisers are extremely helpful for exercising the feet, shoulders, knees, elbows, wrists and hands.

A theraciser can be inserted into a closed door, or around the leg of a sturdy piece of furniture. It is a great tool for providing resistance for exercise, without a lot of expensive equipment. It is also great when traveling, as the theraciser is compact and lightweight. For more information on theracisers, look to *Appendix A Resources for Chapter 5*.

3. Kinesthetic Boards

K boards are of great assistance in improving balance, and for exercising the large stabilizer muscles of the feet, ankles and knees. Standing on a K Board will let you know right away if your weight is balanced on the foundation of your feet. The idea is to keep the board from bottoming out on the floor. If difficulty is encountered, begin on a rug and progress to a hard non-slippery surface.

Whenever foot, ankle or knee problems exist, the muscles of the feet are usually weak. Within a short time, the K board usually makes a big change in these important stabilizing muscles. For further instructions and resources, see *Appendix A Resources for Chapter 5*.

4. The Ma Roller

The Ma Roller is not for the faint of heart or for those long in the tooth. It is a hard wooden roller that can be effectively used to stimulate the association points that run up and down both sides of the spine. Using the Ma Roller on a bed works best, its effect is not so intense on a soft surface. Begin at the lower back and slowly move the

Appendix B Resources for Chapter 6

1. Take your temperature, in your armpit, first thing in the morning, before you get out of bed. If you are using a glass thermometer (not digital) leave it under your arm for 10 minutes.
2. Record the temperature on the chart below.

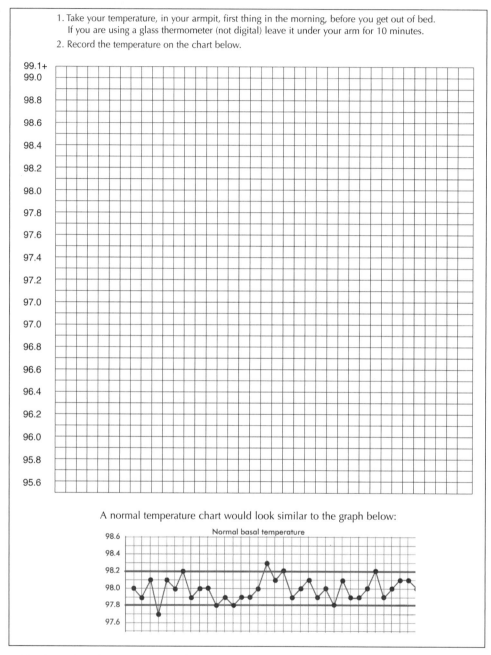

A normal temperature chart would look similar to the graph below:

Fig. B6.1: Basal Temperature Chart

roller up the spine. Pause for a moment or two at each tender spot. More in depth instructions are included with the roller. The Ma Roller is an excellent means to stimulate your organs, and work our some of the kinks in your spine. See *Appendix A Resources for Chapter 5* for more information on the Ma Roller.

5. The Stick

The stick is an excellent way to work trigger points on yourself or on a friend. As the name suggests, each end of the stick is held in each hand, while plastic sleeves roll over your muscles looking for trigger points. The Stick is designed to release trigger points quickly and effectively. See *Appendix A Resources for Chapter 5* for more information on The Stick.

6. Sitting Cushion

For those who spend a lot of time sitting, the Sitting Cushion is a must. The hole in the back of the cushion and the tapered shape allow for the right relationship to occur between your sitting bones, your sacrum and your spine. The Sitting Cushion is excellent for your home, work and especially your car.

Appendix B Resources for Chapter 7
Smoke Points of Oils (sorted by temperature)

200s
225 F:
Canola oil, unrefined
Flaxseed oil, unrefined
Safflower oil, unrefined
Sunflower oil, unrefined

300s
320 F:
Corn oil, unrefined
High-Oleic sunflower oil, unrefined
Olive oil, unrefined
Peanut oil, unrefined
Safflower oil, semi-refined
Soy oil, unrefined
Walnut oil, unrefined
325 F:
Shortening, emulsified vegetable
330 F:
Hemp seed oil
350 F:
Butter
Canola oil, semi-refined

Coconut oil
Sesame oil, unrefined
Soy oil, semi-refined
356–370 F:
Vegetable shortening
361–401 F:
Lard
375 F:
Olive oil
389 F:
Macadamia nut oil

400s
400 F:
Canola oil, refined
Walnut oil, semi-refined
406 F:
Olive oil, extra virgin
410 F:
Corn oil
Sesame oil
420 F:
Cottonseed oil
Grapeseed oil
Olive oil, Virgin
430 F:
Almond oil
Hazelnut oil
435 F:
Canola oil

438 F:
Olive oil, Light
440 F:
Peanut oil
Sunflower oil
450 F:
Corn oil, refined
High-oleic sunflower oil, refined
Peanut oil, refined
Safflower oil, refined
Sesame oil, semi-refined
Soy oil, refined
Sunflower oil, semi-refined
460 F:
Olive pomace oil
468 F:
Olive oil, extra light (best choice for cooking)
485 F:
Grapeseed oil
495 F:
Soybean oil

500s
510 F:
Safflower oil
520 F:
Avocado oil, refined

Glycemic Index and Glycemic Load

The Glycemic Index and Glycemic Load values of 750 additional foods can be found at www.-mendosa.com/gilists.htm.

How to Take an Enema

You will need the following equipment to take an enema:

1. an enema bag purchased from your local drug store, preferably with a two-quart capacity
2. a natural lubricant
3. a large towel
4. a strong clothes hanger

Complete the following steps:

1. Prepare the enema bag, making sure that it is clean and retains water.
2. Shut the hose clamp that comes with the enema bag. The clamp should be placed about 10–12 inches from the nozzle end of the tube, and be easily accessible while you are lying on the floor.
3. Fill the enema bag with lukewarm to slightly cool filtered water.
4. Hold the enema bag upright from its hook and open the clamp to release any air trapped in the hose. Do this over the sink or toilet.
5. Hang the enema bag from the doorknob, or secure it from something in the bathroom that is about the same height. The key word here is secure, as a full enema bag is heavy.
6. Lie flat on your BACK on the towel.
7. Lubricate and gently insert the end of the speculum into your anus.
8. Relax.
9. Open the clamp and release about one cup of water from the bag, and then close the clamp.
10. Massage your colon in a counterclockwise direction, as indicated in the accompanying illustration.
11. Let another cup of water into your colon, close the clamp, and slowly massage your abdomen. The massage will allow you to make the most out of the enema.
12. Fill your colon with yet another cup of water, close the clamp, and massage your abdomen.

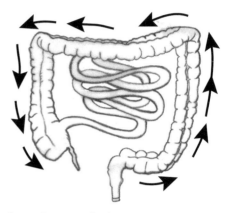

Fig. B7.1: Counterclockwise Colon

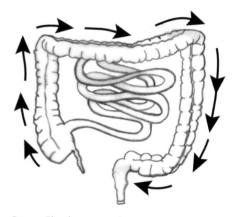

Fig. B7.2: Clockwise Colon

Somewhere about this time, you will begin to feel the pressure of the water inside your colon. When you do, turn on your LEFT side. Make sure that you secure the speculum as you turn on your side, so that the speculum stays inserted.

When you are settled on your LEFT side, let in another cup of water and massage your colon in a counterclockwise direction.

Continue to let in water a cup or so at a time, opening and closing the clamp, and massaging your abdomen. When you are beginning to feel the internal pressure build again, turn on to your RIGHT side. This lets the water move further up the colon.

13. Continue to let in water a cup at a time, followed by the abdominal massage. Continue this process until you have let in all the water, or until you feel that you are too full to let in any more.

14. Breathe, relax, and continue to massage your abdomen.

Remove the speculum and hook it on to the hanger with the clamp securely closed.

15. Breathe, relax, and turn from your RIGHT side onto your BACK. Massage your abdomen again.

16. Try to hold the water inside for at least 5 minutes. Continue to massage your abdomen.

17. When you are ready, sit on toilet, massage your abdomen in a clockwise direction this time, and release the water and toxic fecal matter.

When you are complete, rinse out your enema bag and wash the speculum with detergent.

If you can, take another enema within a day or two. If extreme discomfort or pain should result, which is extremely rare, discontinue use and visit your health professional.

Enemas are uncomfortable, yet productive in cleansing the colon of excess waste material. You may remember that the average colon contains about ten pounds of excess waste material.

Appendix B Resources for Chapter 8
Food Categories

Foods High in Carbohydrates (listed in order from highest carbs to lowest carbs)

  Grains:
  Barley
  Rice
  Spaghetti
  Bagel
  Oatmeal
  Cold breakfast cereal
  Muffins
  Breads
  Vegetables:
  Beans (kidney, lima, navy)

  Potatoes
  Corn
  Artichokes
  Peas
  Carrots
  Fruits:
  Dried Figs
  Grapefruit Juice
  Bananas
  Cherries
  Dates
  Apricots
  Pineapples
  Raspberries
  Plums
  Dairy:
  Dried nonfat milk
  Yogurt
  Nuts:
  Chestnuts
  Cashews

Foods High in Fats

  Cheese
  Pork
  Avocados
  Almonds
  Macadamia Nuts
  Peanuts
  Hazelnuts
  Butter
  Oils
  Salad dressing
  Cream cheese
  Olives (black or green)

Foods High in Protein

  Soy flour
  Lobster
  Crab
  Fish
  Ground beef
  Fried chicken breast
  Ground Turkey
  Tofu

Broccoli
Skim milk
Soybeans
Duck

Low Carbohydrate Foods
Cranberries
Strawberries
Turnips
Bacon
Duck
Beets
Rhubarb
Greens
Leeks
Mushrooms
Pumpkin
Olives
Tomatoes
Coconuts
Walnuts

Simple vs. Complex Carbohydrates
Simple carbohydrates
white sugar
white flour
white rice
white corn grits
honey
barley malt
peas
maple syrup
milk sugar
fruits
fruit juices
Complex carbohydrates
whole grains
whole wheat and oats
brown rice
whole grain pasta
corn
peas
lentils
beans
potatoes

- Carbohydrates are broken down by the body into sugars.
- Too many refined carbohydrates can stress adrenal glands and lead to exhaustion.
- Too many refined carbohydrates and not enough protein can cause live damage.
- Excess refined carbohydrate intake effects protein utilization.

Excess refined carbohydrates can lead to:
Unstable blood sugar levels
High or low blood sugar levels
Cardio-vascular dis-ease
Weight gain
Bloating
Fatigue
Food cravings

Sample Food Combining Menus
A **Protein Breakfast** consists of protein, fats, acid liquids and low carbohydrate vegetables.
Good combinations:
- Eggs, fish, poultry, bacon or ham (occasionally)
- Citrus juices, buttermilk, butter
- Coffee or herbal tea, black, or with cream, but not milk, sugar or sweeteners

Avoid:
- Toast, bagels, breads, grains, sweets, Danish, potatoes, cereals, or dairy products

A **Carbohydrate Breakfast** consists primarily of carbohydrates.
Good combinations:
- Whole fruits
- Whole grain cereals with organic milk but no cream
- Toast and breads with jam but no butter
- Tea or coffee with sugar or honey if needed, but not cream

Avoid:
- Citrus juices, protein and fats

A **Protein Lunch** consists of protein, fats, acid liquids and low carbohydrate vegetables.
Good combinations:
- Meat, fish, poultry and eggs
- Low carbohydrate vegetables

- Soup or broth
- A vegetable salad
- Oil and vinegar, French or Russian dressing
- Cheese or low carbohydrate fruit for dessert

Avoid:
- High-carbohydrate foods and sweets

A **Carbohydrate Lunch** consists primarily of carbohydrates.

Good combinations:
- Soup or broth (not cream-based)
- Vegetables, beans, potatoes
- Vegetable salad with a little Russian dressing or fruit salad
- Bread or crackers, but no butter
- Sweet desserts, low fat ice cream or ices, but no cream

Avoid:
- Protein, fats, oils, cheese, and acidic liquids

A **Protein Dinner** consists of protein, fats, acid liquids and low carbohydrate vegetables.

Good combinations:
- Meat, fish, or poultry
- Low carbohydrate vegetables, no potatoes
- Soup or broth
- A vegetable salad
- Oil and vinegar, French or Russian dressing
- Cheese or low carbohydrate fruit with cream for dessert

Avoid:
- High carbohydrates and sweets
- Alcohol

A **Carbohydrate Dinner** consists primarily of carbohydrates.

Good combinations:
- Soup or broth (not cream-based)
- Vegetables, beans, potatoes
- Vegetable salad with a little Russian dressing or fruit salad
- Pasta with cheese or tomato sauce
- Bread, but no butter
- Sweet desserts, pie, low fat ice cream or ices, but no whipped cream
- A cocktail, wine or beer

Avoid:
- Protein, fats, oils, cheese and acidic liquids

Good combinations:
- Meat, fish, poultry, eggs, cheese, cream and butter
- Meat, fish, poultry, eggs, cheese, vinegar and oil,
- Meat, fish, poultry, cheese and citrus juices
- Bread and jam, honey
- Cereal, milk and sugar (if necessary)

Combinations to avoid:
- Bread and butter
- Potatoes and butter
- Meat and bread (this includes sandwiches)
- Cereal and cream
- Meat and potatoes
- Beans and protein
- Rich ice cream
- Whipped cream on a high carbohydrate dessert
- Vinegar- and oil-based dressings with carbohydrate meals

High-carbohydrate foods include:
- Potatoes, corn, beans, cereals, breads, cakes, sweets

Protein foods include:
- Beef, pork, fish, turkey, chicken, eggs, cheese

Fats include:
- Oils, butter, and cream
- Acid liquids including citrus juices, vinegar, and buttermilk

Note: See *Dr. Atkins New Carbohydrate Gram Counter* booklet for a more complete list of foods and their categories

The understanding of food combining basics allows for an increased efficiency in both the digestive and elimination systems. The ideal balance here is to eat at least two protein type meals for every carbohydrate meal consumed. For weight loss, eliminate carbohydrate meals completely for at least one or two weeks. The knowledge of whole, organic foods, as presented throughout this text, can provide additional insight into the food combining principles presented above.

Appendix B Resources for Chapter 9
Green Drink Recipe
Making a green drink is a simple matter of selecting whatever greens look good in the organic foods market, taking a handful of them and placing them in your blender. Add 6–8 oz. of purified water, strain off the blended greens, and there you have it: a homemade Green Drink. If you like, you can add a little unfiltered, unsweetened apple juice for taste. This drink will help to balance your pH and detoxify your body. Other green items that you can include in a drink are: spirulina, blue-green algae, Barley Green, and Greens Plus. You can find many of these in your local health food store.

Other sources for green drink products are listed in Appendix A under chapter 6 and 8.

Yoga Swing Exercises
The Yoga Swing is an excellent way to keep your body structure flexible and lively. Although it is not for everyone, it provides relief from the constant effects of gravity on the human body. If the slant board is not quite enough, and inversions are not a problem, the Yoga Swing may be right for you. At first, care must be taken to have a spotter close by. Use caution at all times when using the swing.

Sources for yoga swings can be found online at annecorrine.com (click on "Inversion Swings") and at http://www.yoga-swing.com

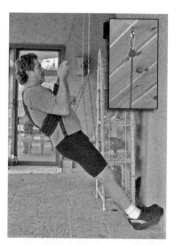
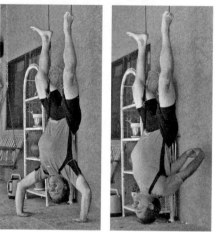

Fig. B9.1: Yoga Swing

Natural Health Practitioners
Chiropractors:
  International Chiropractic Association: www.chiropractic.org or 800-423-4690
  Applied Kinesiology: www.icak.com (click on Find an AK Dr.)
  American Chiropractic Association: www.amerchiro.org, or 703-276-8800
  National Board of Chiropractic Examiners: www.nbce.org/
  Also search online information for each chiropractic state association (for example, the Colorado Chiropractic Association).

Naturopathic doctors:
  American association of Naturopaths: naturopathic.org
  heartspring.net/naturopathic_directory.html
Osteopathic Cranial Practitioners:
  The Cranial Academy: www.cranialacademy-.com (click on "practitioners")
  Therapeutic Directory of Natural Practitioners: http://www.therapeuticdirectory.com

Candida Assessment
1. Do you have a sensitivity to one or more of the

following: perfumes, chemical smells, cigarette smoke, the smell of new carpet or furniture?

2. Do you crave sweets, bread, or alcohol?

3. Do you suffer from allergies, dry mouth, bloating, indigestion, bad breath, belching, heartburn, nausea, itching, nervous irritability, poor memory, mood swings, vision irregularities, spaciness after eating, athlete's foot, or toe fungus?

4. Have you taken antibiotics of any kind, birth control pills, or steroids?

If you answered yes to all four questions, the chances are that you have a candida yeast problem. Utilize the corrective measures outlined in chapter 9.

Goat's Milk Weaning Formula for Infants

1. 6 oz. fresh goat's milk if available, or dry goat's milk mixed according to instructions

2. Prune juice to taste

3. Infant Liquid Vitamin purchased at local health food store (use according to instructions)

4. Eugalan Topfer Forte, 1/2–1 tsp. per bottle. Order through your local health food store, call 800-877-8702, or order online at Amazon.com or Vita Net: http://vitanetonline.com/description/TO0001/vitamins/Eugalan-Forte-Lactose-Base/

Appendix B Resources for Chapter 10
Sinus Drainage Technique
Equipment

You will need a Neti Pot that can be purchased at your local health food store. Instructions come with a Neti Pot. You can also purchase a steel Neti Pot from Health and Yoga. Visit them at www.healthandyoga.com/html/product/neti.html.

Instructions:

1. Fill the Neti Pot with warm salt water (please use sea salt).

2. Insert the spout into one nostril.

3. Lower your head slightly, with one ear towards the floor and the other towards the ceiling.

4. Pour half the contents of the pot into the upper nostril and let it run out the lower one.

5. Reverse your head position and pour into the other nostril.

The procedure is much easier and less uncomfortable than it sounds, and with a little practice, it can be as simple as brushing your teeth. For more information, visit the health and yoga web site listed above.

Ideal Exercise Heart Rate

There are several heart rate formulas available today that allow you to become more aware of your ideal training heart rate. The standard heart rate formula determines your maximum heart rate by subtracting your age from 220, and a chart determines what your range of training should be. Although this formula is the most common practice used today, it often allows for too high a cardiac output, which can result in overtaxing the heart; developing symptoms of over training, such as high cortisol levels, hormonal changes, and a high resting heart rate; and even an overall weakness in your cardiovascular system.

You can also estimate your own level of fitness by determining your maximum heart rate, using the following scale: Poor shape 55, Average shape 65, Excellent shape 75, Competitor 80.

These methods of calculating your ideal training rate heart rate, and others that are much more complicated, seem to allow a person to push themselves too hard, and actually subject the body to more anaerobic training than aerobic training. Personally I espouse the method of my chiropractic associate, Dr. Philip Maffetone, whose philosophy is "Slow down to speed up."

His formula for maximum heart rate begins with 180 minus your age. Maffetone also subtracts points from this score. If you have been diagnosed with a major disease or if you are on medication, subtract 10 points. If you suffer from and injury, or have recurring injuries, cold, flu, allergies, or are new to exercising, subtract 5 points. He also adds points. If you have been exercising for two years without an injury, add 5 points. Seniors can also add up to 10 points, depending on their fitness level,

Table of Normal Blood Values and Possible Health-Related Scenarios

Test	Normal Values	Significance
RBC	Women 4.2–5.4 Men 4.7–6.1	Low: Iron, Copper, Molybdenum, B6 High: Excess Iron, Dehydration
Hemoglobin	Women 12.0–16.0 Men 14.0–18.0	Same as RBC Same as RBC
Hematocrit	Women 37%–45% Men 42%–52%	Same as RBC Same as RBC
MCV	Less than 91 Greater than 82	High: B12, Folic Acid Low: Same as RBC
Neutrophils	56%–75%	Low: B12, Folic Acid (Polys)
Lymphocytes	26%–40%	Low: Thymus, Allergies
Monocytes	1%–5%	High: Acute Injury or Inflammation Heavy Metal Toxicity, Some Infections
Eosinophils	1%–4%	High: Allergies, Parasites
Basophils	0%–4%	

CBC Blood Chart courtesy of Dr. Walter Schmitt, DC.

and kids under 16, should train at a maximum heart rate of 165. Dr Maffetone's book *Total Endurance* is recommended for any serious athlete.

No matter what your age, training with a heart rate monitor is a good idea. If you don't know your heart rate, you don't really know what your body is telling you. Heart monitors are simple to use, and are a great addition to any workout, even if you just like to walk. Heart rate monitors help to protect your deep energy stores, and help you to burn the energy of fat instead.

Check your local bike or fitness location for heart rate monitors. Some brands to look for are Freestyle, Polar, and Garmin. Be smart: Monitor your heart.

Appendix B Chapter 12
Movement Resources
Gabrielle Roth:
- *The Wave* video at Amazon.com
- The Ecstatic Dance: The Gabrielle Roth Video Collection at Amazon.com

- Also see www.gabrielleroth.com or www.shop5rhythms.com

Belly Dancing
Great resources for beginner and intermediate Belly Dance: www.bellydance.org and www.-visionarydance.com

Dance Improvisation Workshops
Ririe Woodbury Dance Company: www.ririewoodbury.com

Movement and Music
www.spiritvoyage.com

The Mozart Effect, Resource Center
Don Campbell, author of *The Mozart Effect* utilizes a variety of sounding techniques, recordings, books, and resources to educate people on the healing power of sound and music. See www.mozart-effect.com for workshop information, or call 800-427-7680 for further questions.

Bibliography

Chapter 1

Bentov, Itzhak. *Stalking the Wild Pendulum*. New York: American Elsevier Publishers, Inc., 1977.

Bohm, David and Rupert Sheldrake. *A New Science of Life: The Hypothesis of Formative Causation*. California: JP Tarcher, Inc., 1981.

Dubos, René. *Mirage of Health*. New York: Harper & Row Publishers, Inc., 1959.

McTaggert, Lynn. *The Field*. New York: HarperCollins Publishers, 2003.

Talbot, Michael. *The Holographic Universe*. New York: HarperCollins Publishers, 1991.

The World Book Encyclopedia E, Volume 6. Illinois: Field Enterprises Educational Corporation, 1977.

Chapter 2

Dubos, René. *Mirage of Health*. New York: Harper & Row Publishers, Inc., 1959.

Cannon, Walter B. MD. *The Wisdom of the Body*. New York: W.W. Norton & Company, Inc., 1939.

Palmer, Daniel David. *The Science, Art, and Philosophy of Chiropractic*. Oregon: Portland Printing House Company, 1910.

Travis, John W., MD. *Wellness Workbook for Helping Professionals*. California: Wellness Associates, 1981.

Chapter 3

Dubos, René. *Mirage of Health*. New York: Harper & Row Publishers, Inc., 1959.

Goodheart, George J. Jr., DC. *Applied Kinesiology 1981 Workshop Procedure Manual*, Volume I, 17th ed. Detroit: Privately Published, 1981.

Gray, Henry F.R.S. *Gray's Anatomy*, Twenty-ninth American edition. Philadelphia: LEA & Febiger, 1973.

Guyton, Arthur C., MD. *Organ Physiology: Structure and Function of the Nervous System*. Pennsylvania: W.B. Saunders Company, 1972.

Jacob, Stanley W., MD, FACS. *Structure and Function In Man*. Philadelphia: W.B. Saunders Company, 1965.

Jensen, Bernard. *Slanting Board*. California: Bernard Jensen Products, Publishing Division, 1976.

Lee, Dr. Royal. *Lectures of Dr. Royal Lee*. Volume I. Colorado: Selene River Press, Inc., 1998.

Maffetone, Philip. *Complementary Sports Medicine: Balancing Traditional and Non-Traditional Treatments*. Illinois: Human Kinetics, 1999.

Mortin, R.J., ed. *Dynamics of Correction of Abnormal Function,* Terrence Bennett Lectures. California: Privately Published, 1977.

Schmitt, WH Jr. (1989), *Nociceptor stimulation blocking technique,* original paper presentation, International College of Applied Kinesiology, Winter Meeting 1989, Shawnee Museum, KS.

Vigilante, Kevin, MD, MPH and Mary Flynn, PhD. *Low Fat Lies, High Fat Frauds*. Washington: LifeLine Press, An Eagle Publishing Company, 1999.

Walther, David S. *Applied Kinesiology: Basic Procedures and Muscle Testing*. Volume I. Colorado: Systems DC, 1981.

Chapter 4

Dominguez, Richard H., MD and Robert S. Gajda. *Total Body Training.* New York: Warner Books Edition, 1982.

Feldenkrais, Moshe. *Awareness Through Movement.* New York: Harper & Row Publishers, Inc., 1972, 1977.

Fuller, Buckminster. *Tensegrity.* Portfolio and Art News Annual, No.4, 1961.

Iyengar, B.K.S. *Light on Yoga.* New York: Schocken Books, 1965.

Kapandji, I.A. *The Physiology of the Joints.* Edinburgh, EH4 3TL: Churchill Livingstone, 1974. (2nd Edition, Longman Limited).

Lee, R. Paul DO. *Interface: Mechanisms of Spirit in Osteopathy.* Oregon: Stillness Press, LLC, 2005.

Magouin, Harold Ives AB, DO, FAAO. *Osteopathy in the Cranial Field.* Idaho: Northwest Printing Plus, 1966, 1976.

Palmer, Daniel David. *The Science, Art, and Philosophy of Chiropractic.* Oregon: Portland Printing House Company, 1910.

Pilates, Joseph H. and William John Miller. *Pilates' Return to Life Through Contrology.* Presentation Dynamics, 1998.

Stone, Randolph, OP, DC, DN. *Easy Stretching Postures: For Vitality and Beauty.* Illinois, Dr. Randolph Stone, 1954.

Takoma, Geo. *Complete Idiot's Guide to Power Yoga.* Indiana: Alpha Books, 1999.

The Pettibon Institute: www.pettiboninstitute.org/

Wrong Diagnosis: www.wrongdiagnosis.com/

Chapter 5

Bandy, John BN, DC. *Diet Planning & Metabolic Individuality: A Body Typing Approach.*

Casdorph, Dr. H. Richard and Dr. Morton Walker. *Toxic Metal Syndrome.* New York: Avery Publishing Group, 1995.

Cooper C, et al (1991). Journal of American Medical Association 266:513-514.

Fuller, Buckminster. *Tensegrity.* Portfolio and Art News Annual, No.4, 1961.

Goodheart, George J. Jr., DC. *You'll Be Better: The Story of Applied Kinesiology.* Ohio: AK Printing, Chp. 24.

Guyton, Arthur C., MD. *Textbook of Medical Physiology.* Pensylvania: W.B. Saunders Company, 1971.

Jensen, Dr. Bernard and Mark Anderson. *Empty Harvest.* New York: Penguin Putnam, Inc., 1990.

Leaf, David W. *Applied Kinesiology Flowchart Manual.* Third Edition. Massachusetts, 1995.

Lee, R. Paul DO. *Interface: Mechanisms of Spirit in Osteopathy.* Oregon: Stillness Press, LLC, 2005.

LIY, et al (2001). *Effect of Long-term Exposure to fluoride in Drinking water on risks of Bone Fracture.* J. Bone Miner Res. 16(5):932-9.

Maffetone, Philip. *Everyone Is an Athlete.* New York: David Barmore Productions, 1989.

_____. *Training for Endurance.* New York: David Barmore Productions, 2000.

Walther, David S. *Applied Kinesiology: Basic Procedures and Muscle Testing,* Volume I. Colorado: Systems DC, 1981.

Dr. David Williams Newsletter: www.drdavidwilliams.com

Chapter 6

Brimhall, Dr. John. *How to Clone a Successful Wellness Practice, 2001.*

Goodheart, George J. Jr., DC. *You'll Be Better: The Story of Applied Kinesiology.* Ohio: AK Printing, Chp. 24.

Gray, Henry F.R.S. *Gray's Anatomy,* Twenty-ninth American edition. Philadelphia: LEA & Febiger, 1973.

Guyton, Arthur C., MD. *Textbook of Medical Physiology.* Pennsylvania: W.B. Saunders Company, 1971.

Lee, R. Paul DO *Interface: Mechanisms of Spirit in Osteopathy.* Oregon: Stillness Press, LLC, 2005.

McCord, Kerry M., DC, DUBAK and Walter H. Schmitt, DC, DIBAK, DABCN. *Quintessential Applications (A(k) Clinical Protocol),* Florida: Healthworks!, 2005.

Oschman, James. *Energy Medicine in Therapeutics and Human Performance.* Pennsylvania: Elsevier's Health Sciences Rights Department, 2003.

Schmidt, Walter H. Jr., DC. *Common Glandular Dysfunctions in the General Practice.* North Carolina: Applied Kinesiology Study Program, 1981.

Seyle, Hans. *Stress Without Distress.* New York: Lippincott & Crowell, Publishers, 1974.

Walther, David S. *Applied Kinesiology: Basic Procedures and Muscle Testing,* Volume I. Colorado: Systems DC, 1981.

Wellness Letter. University of California, Berkeley.

Chapter 7

Abravanel, Elliott D., MD and Elizabeth King Morrison. *Dr. Abravanel's Body Type Diet and Lifetime Nutrition Plan.* New York: Bantam Books, 1999.

Bandy, John BN, DC. *Diet Planning & Metabolic Individuality: A Body Typing Approach.*

_____. Pende, N. *Human Biotypology.* Malvine, Paris, 1925.

_____. Paige, M.E. *Body Chemistry in Health and Disease.* St. Petersburg, Florida, Nutritional Development.

D'Adamo, Dr. Peter J., with Catherine Whitney. *Eat Right 4 Your Type.* New York: G.P. Putnam's Sons, 1996.

Jensen, Bernard. *You Can Master Disease.* California: American Offset Printers.

Goodheart, George J. Jr., DC. *You'll Be Better: The Story of Applied Kinesiology.* Chp 24. Ohio: AK Printing.

Leaf, David W. *Applied Kinesiology Flowchart Manual.* Massachusetts, 1995. Third Edition.

Mendosa, David. *Revised International Table of Glycemic Index(GI) and Glycemic Load(GL) Values 2002.* www.mendosa.com/glists.htm

Vigilante, Kevin, MD, MPH and Mary Flynn, PhD. *Low Fat Lies, High Fat Frauds.* Washington: LifeLine Press, An Eagle Publishing Company, 1999.

Chapter 8

Atkins, Robert C., MD. *Dr. Atkin's New Carbohydrate Gram Counter.* New York: M. Evans & Company, Inc., 1996.

Brazilian J Medical and Biological Research. 1998;31(4):467-90.

Eidner, Harry. *The Better Health Newsletter.*

Goodheart, George J. Jr., DC. *You'll Be Better: The Story of Applied Kinesiology.* Ohio: AK Printing, Chp. 24.

_____. *The Ilio Cecal Valve Syndrome.* Chiropractic Economy, Volume 9, No 6 (May/June 1967).

Gray, Henry F.R.S. *Gray's Anatomy,* Twenty-ninth American edition. Philadelphia: LEA & Febiger, 1973.

Guyton, Arthur C., MD. *Textbook of Medical Physiology.* Pennsylvania: W.B. Saunders Company, 1971.

Jensen, Dr. Bernard and Mark Anderson. *Empty Harvest.* New York: Penguin Putnam, Inc., 1990.

Lee, R. Paul DO *Interface: Mechanisms of Spirit in Osteopathy.* Oregon: Stillness Press, LLC, 2005.

Lee, Dr. Royal. *Lectures of Dr. Royal Lee.* Volume I. Colorado: Selene River Press, Inc., 1998.

Dr. Mirkin: www.drmirkin.com/morehealth/9811.html

Myth of Sunscreen, Eating Healthy website: http://smartpei.typepad.com/eating_healthy/2006/08/the_myth_of_sun.html

News Target: www.newstarget.com

1 1/2 quarts of saliva: Medical facts-www.barcharts.com/system/downloads/free/Medical%20Facts%20(QT).pdf

Price, Weston A. DDS. *Nutrition and Physical Degeneration*. Connecticut: Keats Publishing, Inc., 1989.

Satchidananda, Yogiraj Sri Swami. *Integral Yoga Hatha*. Canada: Holt, Rinehart and Winston of Canada, Limited, 1970.

Schmidt, Walter H. Jr., DC. *Common Glandular Dysfunctions in the General Practice*. North Carolina: Applied Kinesiology Study Program, 1981.

Stone, Dr. Randolph. *A Purifying Diet*. India: Radha Swami Satsang Beas, April 5, 1966.

U.S. Food and Drug Administration, Consumer Magazine (Jan-Feb 1988).

Versendahl, Dr. D.A. and Dawn Versendahl-Hoezee. *Alternative Movement Strategies*. Hoezee Marketing, 1996.

Walther, David S. *Applied Kinesiology: Basic Procedures and Muscle Testing*. Volume I. Colorado: Systems DC, 1981.

Chapter 9

Asthma and Allergy Foundation of America, www.aafa.org.

Casdorph, Richard, Dr. H. and Dr. Morton Walker. *Toxic Metal Syndrome*. New York: Avery Publishing Group, 1995.

Chaitow, Leon, DO, ND. *Candida Albicans (Could Yeast be Your Problem?)*. Vermont: Healing Arts Press, 1988.

Coca, Arthur F., MD. *The Pulse Test*. New York: Barricade Books, 1994.

Cooper C, et al. (1991) JAMA 266:513-514.

Dangers of Toxic Metals, http://www.drlwilson.com/Articles/TOXIC%20METALS.htm

Diamond, John, MD. *Life Energy: Using the Meridians to Unlock the Hidden Power of Your Emotions*. New York: Paragon House, 1985.

Epidemiology 1998;9(1):21-28;29-35, FlurorideActionNetwork.net

Guyton, Arthur C., MD. *Textbook of Medical Physiology*. Pennsylvania: W.B. Saunders Company, 1971.

Journal of American Medical Association, 1996. www.Dr-Rath-Foundation.org.

Lee, Dr. Royal. *Lectures of Dr. Royal Lee*. Volume I. Colorado: Selene River Press, Inc., 1998.

Liy, et al (2001) Effect of Long-term Exposure to Fluoride in drinking water on risks of Bone Fracture, J. Bone Miner Res 16(5): 932-9.

Toxic nature of milk: http://home1.gte.net/carriet/CowsMilk.htm

Chapter 10

Brazilian J Medical and Biological Research. 1998;31(4):467-90.

D'Adamo, Dr. Peter J., with Catherine Whitney. *Eat Right 4 Your Type*. New York: G.P. Putnam's Sons, 1996.

Gray, Henry F.R.S. *Gray's Anatomy*, Twenty-ninth American edition. Philadelphia: LEA & Febiger, 1973.

Guyton, Arthur C., MD. *Textbook of Medical Physiology*. Pennsylvania: W.B. Saunders Company, 1971.

____. *Organ Physiology: Structure and Function of the Nervous System*. Pennsylvania: W.B. Saunders Company, 1972.

Maffetone, Philip. *Complementary Sports Medicine: Balancing Traditional and Non-Traditional Treatments*. Illinois: Human Kinetics, 1999.

Takoma, Geo. *Complete Idiot's Guide to Power Yoga*. Indiana: Alpha Books, 1999.

The World Book Encyclopedia E, Volume 9. Illinois: Field Enterprises Educational Corporation, 1977.

Walther, David S. *Applied Kinesiology: Basic Procedures and Muscle Testing*. Volume I. Colorado: Systems DC, 1981.

Webster's New International Dictionary, 2nd Ed., Unabridged; G. & C. Merriam Company (established, 1831), Springfield 2, Massachusetts, U.S.A.; 1959.

100,000 miles of blood vessels: http://www.madsci.org/posts/archives/jan99/916069852.An.r.html

___. http://www.madsci.org/posts/archives/jan99/916069852.An.r.html

4000 gal every day (heart pumps): http://pddocs.purposedriven.com:8088/docs/pdym/resources/heart_to_heart_trivia.ppt.

Heart Disease Statistics: http://www.heall.com/body/healthupdates/drugs/adversedrugs.html

Chapter 11

Cousins, Norman. *The Healing Heart*. New York: W.W. Norton & Company, Inc., 1983.

Diamond, John, MD. *Life Energy (Using the Meridians to Unlock the Hidden Power of Your Emotions)*. New York: Paragon House, 1985.

Meeker, Bishop Lloyd A. *The Divine Design of Man,* Volume I. Universal Institute of Applied Anthology, 1952.

Palmer, B.J. *The Bigness of the Fellow Within*. USA: B.J. Palmer & Palmer College of Chiropractic, Reprinted 1994, 1949 by B.J. Palmer.

Talbot, Michael. *The Holographic Universe*. New York: HarperCollins Publishers, 1991.

Chapter 12

Campbell, Don. *The Mozart Effect*. New York: HarperCollins Publishers, 2001.

Gray, John. *Men are from Mars, Women are from Venus*. New York: HarperCollins Publishers, 1992.

Guyton, Arthur C., MD. *Textbook of Medical Physiology*. Pennsylvania: W.B. Saunders Company, 1971.

Halpern, Steven PhD. *Tuning the Human Instrument: An Owner's Manual*. California: Spectrum Research Institute, 1978.

Healing Currents. The Journal of the Whole Health Institute, 1987.

Total Integration Institute, www.totalintegrationinstitute.com

Stalking Truth, Tom & Flame Lutes, www.stalkingtruth.com

Chapter 13

Blair, Lawrence. *Rhythms of Vision: The Changing Patterns of Belief.* New York: Schocken Books, 1976.

Diamond, John, MD. *Life Energy (Using the Meridians to Unlock the Hidden Power of Your Emotions)*. New York: Paragon House, 1985.

Gerber, Richard, MD. *Vibrational Medicine (New Choices for Healing Ourselves)*. New Mexico: Bear & Company, 1988.

Judith, Anodea. *Wheels of Life*. Minnesota: Llewellyn Publications, 1987.

Pearsall, Paul, PhD. *The Heart's Code*. New York: Broadway Books, 1998.

Stone, Dr. Randolph. *A Purifying Diet*. India: Radha Soami Satsang Beas, April 5, 1966.

Talbot, Michael. *The Holographic Universe*. New York: HarperCollins Publishers, 1991.

The World Book Encyclopedia E, Volume 9. Illinois: Field Enterprises Educational Corporation, 1977.

Index

Italic page references indicate illustrations

About the Author

DR. JAMES VINCENT FORLEO specializes in holistic health and has over thirty years of clinical experience in chiropractic, spinal biomechanics, applied kinesiology, clinical nutrition, and cranial osteopathy. A popular workshop leader and educator, he lives in Durango, Colorado.